The
Gene
Smart
Diet

THE REVOLUTIONARY EATING PLAN THAT WILL REWRITE YOUR GENETIC DESTINY— AND MELT AWAY THE POUNDS

FLOYD H. CHILTON, PhD
with Laura Tucker

MENUS BY ANNE-MARIE SCOTT, PhD, RD

RODALE

Library of Congress Cataloging-in-Publication Data
Chilton, Floyd H.
    The gene smart diet : the revolutionary eating plan that will rewrite your genetic destiny—and melt away the pounds/ by Floyd H. Chilton with Laura Tucker.
      p.   cm.
    Includes index.
    ISBN–13 978-1-59486-840-5 hardcover
    ISBN–10 1-59486-840-9 hardcover
  1. Reducing diets. 2. Nutrition. 3. Metabolism I. Tucker, Laura. II. Title.
    RM222.2.C4795 2009
    613.2'5—dc22   2009012014

Distributed to the trade by Macmillan

2 4 6 8 10 9 7 5 3 1 hardcover

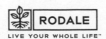

To the orphans of Africa—in particular, the
Masoyi of South Africa and the Darfur of Sudan—
for their extraordinary hope, courage, and love.
They have deeply inspired me and, in the process,
fundamentally and eternally transformed me.

CONTENTS

INTRODUCTION

THE FOUNTAIN
OF YOUTH

It Was Right in Front of Us the Whole Time

IN THE 16TH CENTURY, alchemists pored over astrological charts covered with mysterious symbols and tinkered in dark workshops over vile-smelling beakers. Their goal? To find a "universal panacea," a magical substance that could cure disease and prolong life indefinitely. They labored in the hope that some base combination of earth, wind, fire, and water would result in an elixir of life, forever unlocking the secret of human immortality.

Some of these alchemists were serious scholars, forerunners of the scientists who would one day deliver antibiotics and vaccinations that indeed extend life expectancy beyond anyone's wildest imaginings. Others were mere crackpots and charlatans. But all of these early alchemists—and indeed, the very concept of *una res*, one single thing that could transform matter, cure disease, and create life—were left behind in the dust of the scientific revolution.

Today, thanks to recent groundbreaking discoveries, modern science is closer than ever—closer, certainly, than any sensible person would ever have thought possible—to making the alchemists' quest a scientific reality.

Cutting-edge research by top-tier scientists, published over the last 5 years in distinguished peer-reviewed journals like *Nature, Science,* and *JAMA,* has delivered us to the threshold of a brand-new paradigm. I am convinced that these findings will allow us to reframe our whole approach to losing weight and fighting disease, as we move toward a more progressive, prevention-based health-care model. In the process, they will fundamentally transform our basic assumptions about wellness and longevity.

For example, would you be surprised to learn that because of what they now know, serious scientists actually consider a 120-year life span to be a credible and viable scientific challenge? I don't mean wild-eyed kooks, but leading researchers at some of the most distinguished universities and medical schools around the world. Suddenly, the unthinkable—and even the preposterous—may be within our grasp.

The craziest thing of all? It was right in front of us the whole time.

That's right: You needn't travel to the ends of the earth or buy an island to get your hands on this magical slimming, disease-defying, life-extending potion. Every single one of us has access to a highly centralized biological system, regulated by our genes, that largely controls our susceptibility to disease and how rapidly we age—a system so precisely designed that it could only have developed along with us.

Just what is this system? It's the body's genetic response to environmental stress.

No, not the sort of stress that we try our best to escape (perhaps by heading to a sandy beach to unwind). I'm talking about a more beneficial kind that triggers a stress response and forces the body to marshal its natural resources. These positive stressors—exercise, severe calorie restriction, and certain bioactive compounds in food, just to name a few—kick the body's cellular maintenance functions into high gear, so our cells take care of themselves more efficiently and thoroughly than they would ordinarily. This also happens to be how they maintained themselves when we were young and at the peak of health.

This phenomenon, known as the *adaptive stress response*, is astonishingly precise and powerful. With cellular maintenance on overdrive, our bodies can continue to protect themselves from chronic inflammation, which causes a vast assortment of serious illnesses, not to mention overall aging.

So why, with this fantastic built-in survival mechanism in place, do we get sick at all?

The answer lies in a fundamental disconnect between how the human body developed and how we actually live in 21st-century America—a disconnect that also helps to solve yet another scientific mystery: why members of affluent societies, with access to unparalleled health care, are suffering from unprecedented obesity and a host of devastating, debilitating diseases at younger ages and at higher rates than ever before. This is what I call accelerated aging, and my own work in the field of inflammatory diseases (including obesity) over the past 3 decades has examined the dietary and lifestyle triggers behind our increased vulnerability to it.

THE GENETIC CONNECTION

The adaptive stress response is a survival mechanism—a vestige of our hunter-gatherer ancestry, when 99.9 percent of the genes that make us human took shape. In other words, our bodies are designed to respond to the types of stress that our hunter-gatherer forebears would have encountered.

But marked changes in our lifestyle and our food supply—particularly the overabundance of empty, easily avoidable calories in affluent countries—have removed many of these beneficial stressors from modern existence. Twenty-first-century conditions not only deprive the body of adaptive stress, they actually drive the needle in the other direction toward overactive inflammation and the overweight and obesity, poor health, and premature aging that go along with it.

To give an example, over 70 percent of our calories come from foods that would have been unrecognizable to our ancestors. Our food supply contains far fewer polyphenols, bioactive compounds that regulate the genes that keep us healthy. Polyphenols are a casualty of modern agricultural practices—much like fiber, another bioactive that's all but stripped from processed foods. Still other bioactive compounds, like the omega-3 and saturated fat concentrations in our meat and fish, are radically different than they would have been 100,000 years ago. At the same time, we are getting way too many of the *wrong* types of calories (mostly from sugar and high-fructose corn syrup) and getting much less (and the wrong type of) exercise than our ancestors did.

Our other problem is abundance! When they had the opportunity, our ancestors ate as many calories as they could. Their bodies stored the extra calories as fat for later use—a biological process that saved them from starvation during famine. The excess fat also produced over 100 inflammatory messengers, which would have boosted their immune systems to protect them against infection and disease.

But packing on the pounds is no longer a survival mechanism. In fact, obesity-related disease is our number-one public health issue, largely because it kicks our immune systems into overdrive. You see, overactive inflammation—the result of an overaggressive and chronically activated immune system—is the central driver behind not only an array of human diseases but the aging process itself. Our eating habits and lifestyles switch on precisely those genes that trigger overactive inflammation.

On a recent trip to southern Sudan in the Darfur region, I was pondering the concept of malnutrition, and thought back to the Latin root of the word. *Mal* means "bad," so malnutrition, then, means bad nutrition. In Africa, the major problem is not so much the lack of food—there are large trucks filled with corn-based cereals, sorghum, and maize everywhere—but the inadequate nutrition in that food (90 percent carbohydrates, 8 percent protein, 2 to 3 percent fat, and very few nutrients). It is this lack of nutrition that leads to profound stunting of growth among the children there, increased susceptibility to a host of diseases, and permanent learning and behavioral problems. This has huge implications for every child and family, as well as for the community and society at large.

Sad as it might be, what does it have to do with us? More than you might think. The standard American diet is filled with empty calories. Although we eat all the time, we, too, are in a state of malnutrition. The foods we eat do not contain the ingredients our bodies require to properly regulate our brains and our immune, endocrine, and emotional responses. Make no mistake about it: In the U.S., just as in Africa, there is a severe price to be paid for this malnutrition. Ours is exacted in the form of heart disease, stroke, diabetes, arthritis, allergies, skin disease, poor cognitive function, excessive depression, and, perhaps most of all, exaggerated aging.

So the shifts in our lifestyle and food supply, in combination with our ancient genes, put *every single one of us at risk*. As you will see throughout this book, these changes have robbed the human body of the protective stress response that it so desperately needs to maintain itself in peak health and at an optimal weight. The genes that would have been so highly advantageous for our hunter-gatherer ancestors, especially during their reproductive years, are quite literally killing us today.

> The instructions that we're sending to our genes through our food and lifestyle choices may have changed, but our genes haven't.

Gene Smart is the first diet to give us the ability to control the inflammatory genes, reducing inflammatory signals—and stopping overweight, disease, and premature aging before they start.

FEEDING OUR GENES

Recently I attended an international conference on *nutrigenomics*, the study of the interaction between nutrition and the responses of our genes. I left completely convinced that this new science will revolutionize our understanding of food and medicine—and life itself. The possibilities are the stuff of fantasy. There already is a relatively inexpensive test that can give you your very own individual genetic blueprint and an itemized description of each one of the variants in some of the important genetic building blocks that make you *you*.

It's early on yet, but one thing has become clear: In the years to come, what (and how much) your blueprint can tell you will become more and more specific. You will be able to see whether you've inherited a predisposition toward obesity or breast cancer from your Aunt Millie, as well as thousands of other susceptibilities, from lambswool allergy to lactose intolerance to prematurely gray hair. But the test results will give you more than just a glimpse into your future. They will show you (and your doctor) the precise nutritional formula that will prevent your "bad" genes from expressing themselves and invoke "good" genes as protection. If you do have a disease, your blueprint will allow your doctor to pinpoint exactly which interventions and medications would most effectively neutralize it.

In short, we are entering an era of medicine that can be personalized to a degree of precision that we could not even have dreamt about a mere 3 decades ago, when I started my scientific career. It took 13 years and billions of dollars just to identify the 25,000 to 30,000 functional genes, plus the 3 billion base pairs that make up the human genome in a few dozen humans. To transform this genomic data into 21st-century gene-based medicine and nutrition, researchers must now determine which genes—and more specifically, which versions of which genes—correlate to specific medical conditions. While the best minds in science are working on establishing these associations, we're at least 10 to 20 years—

and probably billions of dollars—away from these revolutionary advances.

Everyone, both scientists and laypeople alike, can see the tremendous promise of this science. But for now, it seems, we must content ourselves with pressing our noses up against the glass.

Or do we?

I sat at that conference with hundreds of my colleagues, listening to the keynote speaker. I felt, as they did, a tremendous level of excitement at the promise dangled before us. But there was a little voice at the back of my head that I couldn't entirely silence, and it kept asking, "What can I do *now*?"

I just turned 50, and the Chilton men don't live long. Heart attacks killed my great-grandfather at 54 and my grandfather at 58, while my father died from cancer at 66. All of these diseases are driven by inflammation. I can't wait 20 years for a personalized blueprint to tell me whether or not I have inherited a devastating genetic predisposition toward heart disease or cancer. I can't wait 10 years to find out which foods I should add to my diet and which I should avoid entirely, preventing those inflammatory genes from turning on. I'll be the first in line for that genetic test when it's available. I suspect, though, that the real beneficiaries of this incredibly promising science will be the next generation—my children and the children of other baby boomers.

But what happens in the meantime? Do we have no choice but to wait?

I will sacrifice the suspense and tell you that the answer is a resounding *no*. No, we don't need maps of our individual genomes to make changes that will have profound effects on our health. Yes, there are specific things—lots of them—that every single one of us can do starting now to take advantage of the nutrigenomic advances that have been made to date. These changes—all easy to implement, with ordinary foods and lifestyle strategies—can quite literally transform our lives.

Compared to what we will know in 10 or 20 years, we comprehend very little currently. What I present in this book is not the complete picture, but it is the best that science can provide at this juncture. Further, I believe that it is enough to revolutionize our ability to turn back chronic, overactive inflammation, helping us to fight obesity, avoid disease, and extend our life spans.

HARNESSING THE STRESS RESPONSE

The adaptive stress response mentioned earlier controls many of the body's master health regulators, which in turn control the expression of an array of uniquely important genes. These master health regulators are working in one direction when you fall prey to obesity and many of the diseases of aging, and in another direction when you're enjoying the prime of your life.

I call them "master health regulators" because they are the central levers steering the genes that govern a number of essential processes. It is when we look at the effect of these regulators on the critical biomarkers of some of our most pernicious diseases that we see just how stunning the power and reach of these genetic control centers—and the adaptive stress response that drives them—can be. (Biomarkers are the specific physical and chemical traits that allow doctors to detect the presence and progression of a given disease.)

One master health regulator, for example, directs the genes that control obesity and diabetes, the cell division that leads to cancer, the formation of blood lipids that set the stage for heart disease, and the production of inflammatory messengers that result in arthritis. These are only *some* of the biomarkers under the influence of this very powerful control center—and collectively, they're responsible for an all-star lineup of our worst inflammatory diseases.

> **Groundbreaking research in the longevity field has revealed the existence of master health regulators that control inflammation.**

Many of the diseases that are under the influence of master health regulators have an inflammatory component. Inflammation is my particular area of expertise, and it's a known factor in some of our most terrible afflictions, including heart disease, asthma, arthritis, diabetes, digestive and skin disorders, as well as certain kinds of cancer.

Actually, scientists believe that even this extensive laundry list is just the tip of the iceberg. For instance, we've recently learned that chronic, low-level, full-body inflammation contributes to the aging process by eroding cells' ability to maintain themselves. The prevalence of chronic inflammation also explains why we are seeing so many "age-related" medical conditions—such as heart disease, arthritis, and diabetes—in younger and younger people: Inflammation is causing our cells—and therefore our bodies—to grow old before their time. We now know, too, that obesity is a major reason that the rate of chronic inflammation in the United States continues to climb, as it has been.

The master health regulators control how much fat we make and metabolize. They're programmed to maintain robust fat stores, so we're always prepared for famine. But when they're working properly, they also slow down the fat-storage process once the larder is full. Unfortunately, we've enjoyed such an extended period of abundance that many of these regulators have stopped functioning. Further, we've become resistant to hormones like leptin and insulin, which send instructions to these regulators. It's another sign that our bodies can't cope with the excess for which they are not designed.

With our new scientific knowledge, we can develop gene-based nutrition strategies that allow us to target the body's "control panel" and affect the genes responsible for inflammation and obesity. The emerging fields of genomics and nutrigenomics have directed us to "hinge points," crucial pathways under the influence of the master health regulators that encourage or suppress inflammation and obesity. The changes in our food supply and lifestyle over the past generation have violently aggravated these hinge points, driving us toward chronic inflammation, obesity, and premature aging.

Thanks to the discovery of the master health regulators and their role in the inflammatory process, we can finally begin to turn the tide. We can override the signals from the body's control panel that drive obesity, disease, and aging. The key is to trigger the adaptive stress response with the right number and type of calories, with certain vitally important bioactive compounds, and with specific kinds of exercise scientifically proven to alter gene expression and reduce the biomarkers of inflammation, disease, and aging.

This is precisely what Gene Smart is designed to do.

Think about it: Our genes developed so that our bodies could turn stressful environmental circumstances to their best advantage. Our modern food supply and lifestyle have taken many of these protective stressors out of play. So in order to mobilize the tremendously beneficial, health-giving machinery of the adaptive stress response, we've got to put some of the stressors back in.

> **The Gene Smart Diet can induce or mimic the primitive environmental stressors that switch on the body's life-extending adaptive stress response.**

By activating the adaptive stress response and communicating directly with the master health regulators, we can control hundreds of the very genes that turn on or turn off many of our most virulent diseases. Harnessing this response—as you will on Gene Smart—affords us the ability to strategically reprogram our genetic destiny.

If, like me, you're one of the vast majority with a family history of health concerns like heart disease and cancer, then this diet is especially good news for you. It gives you the power to influence your own fate long before the disease process is set in motion.

I believe that the landmark discoveries occurring now will propel a fundamental shift in how we approach the diagnosis and treatment of disease. At last, health care can get out of a defensive crouch and attack disease before it gains a foothold. Although relieving symptoms is a service that will continue to be essential, medicine will no longer be relegated to cleanup duty as a disease runs its course. Through the master health regulators, we can actually dictate which portions of our individual genetic blueprints get expressed, so that signals to launch the disease process are never given in the first place.

GENE SMART UNLEASHED

All of this may seem very impressive conceptually. But does it actually work in real people leading real lives and eating real food?

The answer is a resounding yes! There have been hundreds of clinical trials, conducted at prestigious research institutions and published in the best scientific journals, that support the individual aspects of the Gene Smart approach. My own laboratory just completed an 8-week clinical study involving 68 volunteers of all shapes and sizes, in which we tested the effectiveness of the strategies I put forth in this book. I'd like to share one panelist's story as an illustration of just how powerful this approach can be.

Gail Walker is a 61-year-old schoolteacher. Nothing about Gail's appearance (she was only slightly overweight), her routine blood tests (of cholesterol and other biomarkers), or other risk assessments (she never smoked, for example) would have suggested that she was in poor health. But her inflammatory profile told a different story. Indeed, it was among the most alarming I've ever seen. Gail's levels of C-reactive protein (CRP), leptin, and interleukin-6—all critically important, validated biomarkers of whole-body inflammation—were devastatingly high. Her CRP, for instance, was 36; according to at least 20 studies, anything above 5 is an accurate predictor of heart attack, stroke, diabetes, and metabolic syndrome. It's not hyperbole to say that this woman was on the verge of becoming terribly sick.

In her 8 weeks on Gene Smart, Gail not only lost 21 pounds, she restored her levels of inflammatory messengers to normal, healthy levels. Her CRP dropped from 36 to 4! This is nothing short of incredible.

I believe that we helped Gail to duck a very real and potentially deadly bullet. And there are lots of Gails out there. After all, we know that most cardiac events and strokes occur in people without elevated cholesterol, with as many as one-fifth of such incidents affecting those with no traditional risk factors at all.

The data from our study and others provide convincing evidence that the Gene Smart Diet can help you:

Lose weight. Gene Smart unquestionably promotes weight loss, a lifesaver in itself. In fact, the bioactives featured in Gene Smart have been shown to melt away pounds *even when there's no accompanying reduction in calories*. On this diet, you will modestly reduce calories as one tool for switching on the adaptive stress response. Notice that I said "reduce," not "restrict." As we'll discuss later on, calorie restriction is much more severe and not as sustainable for most people.

Those in our Hillsdale Study group lost 1½ to 2 pounds, ½-inch around their waists, and almost 0.5 percent of their body fat *per week*. These are averages, of course, but they're pretty amazing. They reflect a pace of weight loss that's healthy and safe.

What's more, sticking with Gene Smart wasn't hard. Unlike conventional weight-loss diets, the majority of our study participants reported no hunger, no confusion, and no problems with compliance. They enjoyed their meals, and they felt full and satisfied after eating.

When people in other studies followed protocols similar to those in Gene Smart, they saw their rates of weight loss improve dramatically—by as much as 28 percent.

Prevent and treat heart disease. Heart disease is the leading cause of death in the United States. Current estimates attach a price tag of $550 billion to the global pharmaceutical expenditure on cardiovascular drugs.

Gene Smart offers a nonmedical intervention at a fraction of the cost, and without any of the side effects. Numerous epidemiological and clinical trials from the best laboratories in the world confirm that the individual bioactives recommended in Gene Smart can reduce the risk of a heart attack by an average of 30 percent, of a fatal heart attack by 40 to 60 percent, and of a second heart attack by 45 percent. Such reductions are equal to those of the very best pharmaceuticals.

The bioactives and exercise recommendations in Gene Smart have also been shown in numerous clinical trials to reduce the risk of stroke; to lower triglycerides and LDL cholesterol (the "bad" kind); to raise HDL cholesterol (the "good" kind); to lower blood pressure and resting heart rate; to reduce platelet stickiness; and to lower the inflammatory messenger CRP. In our own studies, the bioactives in Gene Smart were able to correct the balance of omega fats, which a growing number of scientists believe to be an even better predictor of heart attack than any other biomarker.

In their 8 weeks on Gene Smart, our test panelists saw reductions in their triglycerides (20 mg/dl, on average), LDL cholesterol (10 mg/dl), blood pressure, and resting heart rate. The degree of change depended largely on each person's initial readings. The good news is, those with the most significant risk factors saw the greatest improvements.

Similarly, leading biomarkers of inflammation—including leptin and interleukin-6—declined over the 8 weeks of Gene Smart. Leptin, the proinflammatory protein produced by fat cells, dropped by a staggering 35 percent.

Treat and prevent diabetes. An estimated 23.6 million Americans—a mind-blowing 7.8 percent of the population—have some form of diabetes. According to several large clinical studies, the protocols that serve as the foundation of Gene Smart can help to stabilize blood sugar, a benefit that not only helps manage diabetes but protects against the disease in those who are at risk. Other studies, including our own, suggest that the dietary and lifestyle measures in Gene Smart can reduce whole-body inflammation—the primary driver behind type 2 diabetes—by more than 35 percent.

Our Hillsdale Study group showed marked reductions in their hemoglobin A1, HOMA and SCD1, among other biomarkers of insulin resistance and diabetes. Most impressively, Gene Smart reduced fasting insulin levels by more than 30 percent. A high fasting insulin level is a sign of insulin resistance and the onset of metabolic syndrome or type 2 diabetes.

Between 50 million and 75 million Americans have metabolic syndrome, defined by the American Heart Association as the presence of three or more risk factors, including abdominal obesity; high triglycerides or cholesterol; elevated blood pressure; and abnormal insulin or glucose levels. Among our Hillsdale Study participants, the number of men with metabolic syndrome dropped from 57 percent to 29 percent, and the number of women from 39 percent to 23 percent.

Gene Smart doesn't stop there. The components of this diet have been found in clinical trials to help prevent and treat cardiac arrhythmias, COPD, osteoporosis, osteoarthritis, Crohn's disease, IBS, psoriasis, and even certain cancers. (You'll read more about these studies throughout the book.) This degree of protection, and the promise of overall wellness, is not something that even we scientists believed possible without drugs. We knew that a healthy diet and lifestyle mattered, but we were convinced that what truly sealed a person's fate was indelibly written in his or her genes. However, scores of groundbreaking clinical trials involving hundreds of thousands of people—and real-life results from people like Gail Walker—have made clear that what we eat and how we live play compelling roles in determining which genes are expressed. I believe that we know enough right now to start using this information to our advantage.

YOU SAY YOU WANT A REVOLUTION . . .

The science is clear: Changes in our food supply and lifestyle have resulted in conditions diametrically opposed to the adaptive stress response so favorable to our bodies. Each one of the factors suppressing this response poses a significant threat to our health. Taken together, they confront us with a perfect storm of factors, working synergistically to make the vast majority of us overweight and seriously ill.

> Instead of benefiting from the body's natural defense against disease and aging, we have in effect short-circuited this most vital survival mechanism.

Based on what we now know, I feel confident enough to say that what we eat and how we live as Americans is sending precisely the wrong signals to our master health regulators, thus altering—for worse—the orders that these regulators send out to hundreds of genes. The Gene Smart Diet focuses on a gene-based approach to reverse the damaging effects of our overabundant society. By strategically sending health-promoting messages to our master health regulators, Gene Smart effectively restores the protective mechanisms with which our bodies were originally equipped.

And in the same way that a perfect storm of factors has fueled our current epidemic of inflammatory disease, Gene Smart unleashes a perfect storm of correctives—components that powerfully combat inflammation in their own right and are even more potent when combined. Strategies like these have never before been presented as a single, cohesive plan. They're what make Gene Smart so unique and effective.

What's more, they've never been so scientifically sound. The central underpinnings of Gene Smart draw on hundreds of epidemiological, observational, case-controlled, and/or interventional human trials that have been published in the most prestigious peer-reviewed medical and scientific journals, including *JAMA*, the *New England Journal of Medicine*, the *Archives of Internal Medicine*, *Circulation*, the *American Journal of Clinical Nutrition*, and *CHEST*. These clinical trials allow me to be prescriptive with an unprecedented degree of specificity.

You see, it isn't only that we need certain bioactives in our diets. According to overwhelming data, these bioactives must be present in the correct dosages, or we might as well not be using them. To make a difference in our health, we can't rely on guesstimates. At least four of the fundamental components of Gene Smart—calorie reduction, polyphenols, omega-3 fatty acids, and exercise—are being used by the general population in ways that offer little or no benefit.

This, of course, gives way to the frustration that characterizes so many diets: "I'm trying so hard, but I'm not seeing results!" It's not for lack of effort. You simply haven't had what you really need: specific, gene-based nutritional strategies.

Of course, having these tools at your disposal won't matter much if you can't easily and comfortably adapt them to your lifestyle. It's one reason that so many popular diets fail. In fact, yo-yo dieting—repeatedly losing and regaining weight—is one of the most destructive patterns we can fall into. It's worth noting that more than 90 percent of our Gene Smart test panelists stayed on the program until the very end. Perhaps more impressively, 74 percent of this group either maintained their weight loss or continued to lose (by following the program) a full 10 weeks after we concluded our study, which is how long we gathered data. One participant who continues to follow our program has lost more than 100 pounds so far. This suggests to us that for a majority of people, Gene Smart can be the key to long-term success.

> **The results may be radical, but the Gene Smart Diet itself is easy and enjoyable. By following its simple nutritional and lifestyle measures, you can slim down while also seeing dramatic gains in health and longevity.**

TAKING THE OFFENSIVE

What makes the adaptive stress response such a supremely powerful weapon against obesity and disease is this: It offers not just a defensive strategy but something much more proactive. Yes, it triggers the master health regulators that have the power to turn the dial away from disease, aging, and premature death. But these regulators can crank the dial all the way in the other direction, toward *optimal wellness*, by calling forth the body's amazing ability to protect itself.

The master health regulators are not just disease fighters; they're health promoters. Think of them as traffic cops, raising their hands to stop the biomarkers of disease while at the same time radioing in for reinforcements to help carry out their mission. The Gene Smart Diet, then, is more than a good defense. It's a great offense.

What's more, the Gene Smart Diet takes a strategic approach to directly affecting gene expression. This simple, scientifically sound dietary protocol—combined with equally solid lifestyle measures—is a precision instrument when compared to the blunt-force diets of the past. Because Gene Smart is the first program to account for the effects of diet and lifestyle on the adaptive stress response, it allows us to take nutrition to a whole new level. Instead of something to fear or avoid, food can truly be our medicine.

As a scientist, I would never have fathomed that the age-old quest for the philosopher's stone, the fountain of youth, the elixir of life might finally be realized within my lifetime. But as I've said, we are closer to that goal than any sensible person would have thought possible. It can take up to 10 years for discoveries in the research lab to filter down to the physicians and patients who need them most—a delay that scientists refer to as "the research gap." There are times when such a lag is necessary and beneficial; no one wants to rush the testing of a new drug's safety and efficacy, for instance. And there's no pressing need to alert the public about a breakthrough if it's going to be years before people are able to use the information to their benefit.

That isn't the case here. I am confident that our ever-growing knowledge of the adaptive stress response and gene-based nutrition has most decidedly set us on a path that will lead to countless medical breakthroughs, with plenty of blockbuster drugs—including ones that will someday grant us much longer life spans—along the way.

But the benefits of the adaptive stress response are available to all of us, through common foods—even very delicious ones! In fact, some "treat" foods like chocolate and red wine, traditionally considered off-limits to dieters, are among the best for activating the powerful master health regulators.

Our understanding of how foods interact with our genes is limited; we're just at the threshold of where we'll one day be. But we can't wait for the full picture, and we don't need to. We can take control of our weight and our health in a much fuller way than ever before, and we can do it now. That is why I have written this book—because we can, and we must.

PART ONE

The Surprising Driver Behind Obesity, Disease, and Premature Aging

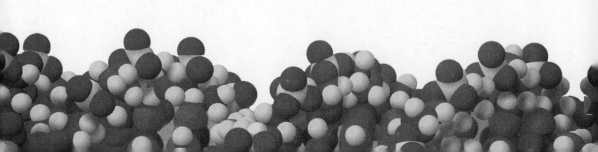

CHAPTER ONE

SHOCK AND AWE: THE INFLAMMATORY PANDEMIC

I RESEARCH INFLAMMATORY DISEASES, the kinds that come about when our own bodies viciously turn on themselves. Indeed, the question of why so many Americans are suffering from debilitating inflammatory conditions like heart disease, diabetes, arthritis, and obesity—and what steps might be taken to alleviate their distress—has been the central preoccupation of my career. More than anything, I have struggled to figure out why the incidence of these diseases has grown so astronomically during my lifetime. What could possibly explain the rapid dominance, overwhelming power, and completely devastating impact of these ailments, not just on our bodies but on a medical system powerless to affect their course?

It was only when I examined data coming from a totally unrelated field—longevity—that I began to truly understand what's driving the unprecedented surge in inflammatory illness and what the implications of this epidemic might be. I now believe that what we scientists have long considered to be "normal" signs of aging, including many of our most pernicious diseases, can be traced to specific genes. These genes developed thousands of generations ago, as a means of protecting us humans from threats to our survival. In today's world, they do anything but.

> **Understanding our massive health problems today requires insight into our genetic history.**

A BODY BUILT FOR ANOTHER AGE

Make no mistake: We owe a great deal to our genes and, more precisely, to their magnificent adaptability. We probably wouldn't have endured for so long as a species without it.

For instance, thanks to our genes, our bodies are programmed for taking in calories and storing them as fat. This ability is what allowed our hunter-gatherer ancestors to survive during times of famine, which were a fact of life for them. Back then, any number of circumstances—a change in seasons, drought, migration, or the death of a provider—could have depleted the food supply, so it made good sense for the human body to prepare to roll with the punches by replenishing its fat stores in times of plenty.

Actually, it's quite an elegant system: One of the things that extra fat does is push the immune system into overdrive—another asset for our ancestors, for whom a splinter or a cold virus might have meant death. And since their times of plenty inevitably came to an end, they weren't subjected to any of the problems caused by an overactive immune system—namely chronic, overactive inflammation.

Similarly, our bodies are hardwired to anticipate constant exposure to certain kinds of stress, because of the stressors that our hunter-gatherer forebears would have encountered on a near-daily basis. Just finding a meal would have entailed regular, often intense physical activity, which is a type of stress. And because the food supply was so uncertain, very low-calorie diets—another stressor—would have been quite common.

Over centuries, the human body adapted to these and other sources of stress by developing systems that pushed cellular maintenance into overdrive. It interpreted these stressors as cues—to stock up on calories when food was in abundance, for example, and to shift into cellular survival mode when food became scarce. We have come to depend on these systems for weight maintenance, good health, and extended life.

> **The human body is designed to accommodate environmental challenges by turning on and off the genes that help it to protect itself.**

But as you can imagine, life today is nothing like it was back then. In affluent societies as in the United States, beneficial stressors—the kind that kick our bodies into health-enhancing survival mode—are virtually nonexistent. We're nowhere near as active as our ancestors, since we no longer need to hunt for our meals, unless "hunting" means deciding which fast-food drive-thru to pull into. We are surrounded by a seemingly endless food supply, which means that we're taking in calories and storing fat in preparation for a famine that will never come. And the foods that dominate our diets are largely devoid of the bioactive compounds that directly "speak" to our genes.

In other words, in the process of enjoying the abundance and convenience of modern life, we have unwittingly turned off the genes that respond to beneficial stressors—the ones that help stave off inflammation and many of our worst medical conditions. Instead, we've turned on the genes that promote fat storage and inflammation—with awful consequences. This single, fundamental change is largely responsible for the rise in inflammatory disease that's sweeping our population.

But all is not lost. Research from my lab and others indicates that we can design rational, practical strategies to *reintroduce* the dietary and lifestyle components necessary to activate the genes that promote health and extend life. We can push back against the genes driving us to obesity and regain control over those that direct inflammation, as well as glucose and fat metabolism. By regulating these genes, we can dramatically reduce metabolic disorders and chronic, full-body inflammation. Once we do that, we won't just eliminate the scourge behind some of the worst diseases afflicting our population, we will do something that has eluded scientists for thousands of years: We will dip a cup into the fountain of youth.

This is what Gene Smart is all about: using adaptive stress, weight reduction, and bioactives in our food supply to harness our genes. But first, let's look more closely at just what chronic, overactive inflammation is—and why we so urgently need to fight it.

INFLAMMATION: THE BASICS

Based on what you've read about inflammation so far, you may think that it's a bad thing. In fact, we couldn't survive without it. Inflammation is a component of the body's immune response, a complex and elegant system with the ability to recognize and destroy invaders that have the potential to harm us.

When you catch a cold or cut yourself, an extremely sophisticated alarm system goes off inside your cells. Certain cells identify the virus or injury, report the nature of the attack, and request the necessary reinforcements to launch a counterattack. Cytokines, adipokines, and eicosanoids, the messengers produced by surveillance cells and fat tissue, dispatch ground troops—white blood cells—to combat the infection. This offensive must be carefully calibrated: sufficiently brutal to immobilize the enemy, yet controlled enough to not completely destroy the cells and tissues surrounding the battlefield.

| **Inflammation is the body's response to something gone wrong.**

Inflammation is the body's first line of defense. Without it, we're wide open to opportunistic infection, so that exposure to something as innocuous as the common cold or a paper cut could have fatal consequences.

The real question, of course, is how the normal protective process of inflammation gives way to debilitating inflammatory disease.

The Body as War Zone: Chronic, Full-Body Inflammation

Much depends on the accuracy of the early warning system that calls inflammatory cells into action. If this system is reacting to a real threat, then it's keeping the body safe. But if it overreacts—if, say, it interprets a harmless substance (like peanuts) or the body's own tissue (like cartilage) as a dangerous invader—then the normal inflammatory response becomes a disease state (severe allergies and arthritis, in the examples here).

Sometimes the threat is real, but the inflammatory response is dramatically exaggerated. When this happens, the inflammatory response never stands down, even after the threat is long gone. This, too, leads to inflammatory disease.

Another, more prevalent danger—especially in developed countries—is a relatively low-level, chronic inflammatory state, when the immune system is continuously activated by adipokines from fat tissue. This can lead to the slow but steady destruction of tissues and organs. More importantly, it places the organ systems that are most genetically predisposed to the inflammation at high and constant risk for harm. For example, chronic inflammation can cause the body to attack the islet beta cells in the pancreas. Eventually, the cells aren't able to produce insulin. The end result: diabetes.

> Inflammatory disease begins with an exaggeration of the body's normal inflammatory response.

Now a little bit of "collateral damage" is to be expected in the wake of the inflammatory response. It's a small price to pay for a successfully vanquished infection. Once the immune system has eliminated the intruder, the injured tissues should heal normally, and life goes on.

But when the body launches a full-scale inflammatory response against something inoffensive, any tissues that have the misfortune of being close by are also destroyed. As I like to say, chronic inflammation is like using a blowtorch to light a candle on a birthday cake. In a person with inflammatory disease, the body adds insult to injury by sending ever more inflammatory reinforcements to compensate for the damage from the initial inflammatory response.

Essentially, inflammatory disease occurs when the body turns its own defenses against itself in a "friendly fire" scenario. It inaccurately detects what it perceives to be a threat, or it overreacts to a real threat; it causes damage; then it overreacts again and again with subsequent inflammatory responses in an endless negative-feedback loop that scorches the battlefield. This is chronic inflammation, and it manifests itself as heart disease, diabetes, arthritis, asthma, allergies, COPD, Crohn's disease, psoriasis, and cancer, to mention only a few.

> Chronic, full-body inflammation is not just a smoke signal that something is wrong in the body; it is a forest fire that does damage in its own right.

The end result is awful. And it's location-specific, which leads us to the question that I am asked most often: How can the category of inflammatory disease encompass so many different ailments?

Same Problem, Different Location

After hearing the laundry list of medical conditions under the inflammatory umbrella, someone once asked me, half-jokingly, if there was any disease without an inflammatory component. I answered, in all seriousness, that I'm not sure there is. There are many different inflammatory diseases, yet all of them share the same underlying driver: an inappropriate inflammatory response. The difference between them is where the inflammatory response is taking place. (There are other differences, especially regarding which parts of the immune system are participating in the inflammatory response, but this explanation serves our purposes here.)

Chronic inflammation localized in the coronary arteries surrounding the heart leads to atherosclerosis and heart disease. In diabetes, as mentioned earlier, the body mistakenly identifies the islet beta cells in the pancreas as foreign invaders and destroys them so that they no longer produce insulin. When inflammatory cells such as eosinophils or neutrophils invade the small airways of the lungs, they cause asthma. Arthritis, meanwhile, occurs when the synovium—a thin, specialized tissue responsible for the production of fluid that lubricates joints—becomes inflamed.

The list goes on and on. Inflammation in the upper bowel? Crohn's disease. Lower bowel? Ulcerative colitis. The underlying process is the same; it's just the location and symptoms that change.

> **Many of our very worst diseases share one single driver: inflammation.**

In fact, scientists believe that inflammation may be behind even more diseases, including some that we weren't looking at before. In a surprising twist, some of the most interesting work in this area is focusing on the brain. Scientists have found high levels of inflammatory messengers in people with depression. In my own lab, a major research effort is under way to understand the mechanisms by which inflammation causes depression. Scientists have also identified elevated levels of certain kinds of inflammatory messengers in people with schizophrenia.

We now know, too, that normal brain molecules are disrupted as a result of chronic inflammation, which can cause amyloid beta proteins in the brain to misfold. Misfolded amyloid beta proteins are thought to play a critical role in the development of Alzheimer's disease, the leading cause of dementia. The number of people in the United States who have Alzheimer's currently stands at 4.5 million and is expected to increase to 13 million by 2050. The prevalence of the disease doubles every 5 years beyond age 65 and is approximately 14 times more common among those over 85 compared to those between 65 and 69. We now believe that inflammation contributes to—if not drives—this terrible disease.

That's not all: Scientists recently uncovered a very surprising link between inflammation and cancer.

Cancer, for a long time, was in a category of its own. As far back as the late 19th century, scientists noticed increased inflammation in the presence of certain kinds of cancer. But it was too early to connect the dots. We now have a much better understanding of how the disease process works.

First of all, researchers believe that inflammation plays a crucial role in turning premalignant cells into malignant ones. Cancer starts with a group of cells gone haywire, reproducing rapidly and then migrating into the surrounding tissue. This marks the transition from premalignancy to malignancy, and scientists suspect that the tumor essentially "borrows" the body's natural inflammatory process to aid and abet the transition.

This mechanism was discovered by a researcher at the University of London, who found that mice engineered without the ability to produce a particular inflammatory messenger (ironically called tumor necrosis factor–alpha, because it kills cancer cells under certain conditions) never developed tumors. This inflammatory messenger, when it is chronically present in low levels, essentially creates a breeding ground for premalignant cells to turn malignant.

But as one of my oncology colleagues often says, it usually isn't the primary cancer that kills: It's the metastases, when cancer cells break off, travel to other locations throughout the body, and set up camp. Here again, inflammation plays a crucial role. Researchers believe that inflammatory messengers accompany the cancerous cells on their journey, acting as bodyguards as the cells travel through the bloodstream.

This is why what we've learned about the relationship between inflammation and cancer is so chilling: As it turns out, inflammation is a key factor in two major stages of development of certain kinds of cancer. Certainly, what we now know should add fuel to the fire behind finding solutions to chronic inflammation, as these solutions will surely have their place in the cancer-fighter's toolbox.

With the addition of certain kinds of cancers under the inflammatory umbrella, we can safely say that chronic inflammation is behind the leading causes of death in the United States, including heart disease, cancer, stroke, and diabetes. But inflammation isn't the only thing these diseases have in common. They also share a strong correlation to diet, and to overweight and obesity.

As we shall see, this correlation is no coincidence.

Diseases with a Proven Inflammatory Component

Here's just a sampling of the conditions in which inflammation is known to play a part:

Allergies

Arthritis (rheumatoid and osteo-)

Asthma

Atherosclerosis

Atopic dermatitis

Cancer (certain kinds)

COPD (chronic obstruc-
tive pulmonary
disease), including
emphysema

Crohn's disease

Diabetes

Heart disease

Psoriasis

Stroke

Ulcerative colitis

Inflammation has also been implicated in a host of other health concerns, including:

Age-related cognitive decline

Alzheimer's disease

Depression

Schizophrenia

CHAPTER TWO

HELP! I CAN'T STOP EATING!

Losing weight—and keeping it off—is extremely difficult, given our ancestral biology. Obesity is another natural outcome, and a very, very dangerous one at that, when we suppress the body's innate adaptive stress response. Being overweight in itself greatly increases dangerous full-body inflammation; in fact, as we will discuss in this chapter, new science shows that many of the hormones driving obesity, like leptin, are powerful inflammatory messengers in their own right.

By using specific strategies to reintroduce sources of beneficial stress, Gene Smart activates the adaptive stress response, which prompts your genes to switch on or off in ways that quell dangerous inflammation. This genetic change-up is vital if you want to achieve and maintain a normal weight.

INFLAMMATION, OBESITY, AND DISEASE

According to the American Heart Association, more than 71 million Americans have some form of heart disease, the number-one killer in the United States. Number two on the list, responsible for about one-quarter of all deaths, is cancer. More than 50 million Americans have hypertension, which can lead to stroke, the third leading cause of death. And 23.6 million Americans—49 percent more than a decade ago—suffer from diabetes, which contributes to about 200,000 deaths each year.

Diabetes not only is a scourge in its own right—about 60 to 70 percent of people with the disease experience mild to severe nerve damage, and more than 60 percent of nontraumatic lower-limb amputations occur in this population—it also has ties to the nation's leading killers. Adults with diabetes are two to four times more likely to experience heart disease or a stroke, while more than 70 percent have high blood pressure.

When we consider all of these diseases collectively, we can readily identify a few commonalities. First, we now know that all have an inflammatory component. Second, our risk of these diseases depends to a large extent on our diet—what we eat and how much of it. And third, all are more likely to occur in tandem with overweight or obesity.

That our country has a serious weight problem is by no means news. But the impact of obesity on our collective health cannot, in my opinion, be over-estimated. As many as 70 percent of Americans are overweight or obese. In the United States, as in most Western countries, diet-related chronic diseases represent the single largest cause of mortality and morbidity. Mortality rises with obesity; a body mass index over 32 *doubles* the risk of death, mostly from inflammatory diseases like heart disease, cancer, stroke, and diabetes, to mention only a few.

> **Simply put, being fat is more likely to kill us than anything else.**

You're doubtless familiar with the connections between overweight and conditions like heart disease and diabetes. But you may not realize that, according to National Cancer Institute estimates, at least 35 percent of all cancers have a nutritional component, which includes obesity. When other lifestyle factors such as smoking and lack of exercise are accounted for, the risk associated with obesity becomes much stronger and may be as high as 85 percent.

The data on cancer and obesity are often presented in the scientific literature in a very complex—and, I might add, confusing—manner. So here are the facts as we know them: We can say with some certainty that obesity is a risk factor for cancers of the colon, breast, endometrium (the lining of the uterus), kidney, and esophagus. In fact, we can safely say that obesity increases the likelihood of developing these cancers by 25 to 33 percent. Because more studies than not show a reduced risk of cancers of the cervix, gallbladder, prostate, and thyroid in people who follow a low-fat diet and/or who engage in a higher than average level of physical activity, a link between obesity and these forms of the disease also is likely.

Though much of the research performed so far has focused on the potential for developing cancer, one of the most interesting studies that I've seen involved 752 men, ages 40 to 64, who were newly diagnosed with prostate cancer. This study, which came out of the Fred Hutchinson Cancer Research Center, suggests that men who are obese at the time they're diagnosed are much more likely to experience a recurrence and, ultimately, to die from the disease. In other words, obesity places men at an incredible disadvantage once they get prostate cancer. The marked increase in both the risk of recurrence and the risk of death among obese men was seen *regardless of the treatment protocol*, and was the same for both low-grade (less aggressive) and high-grade (more aggressive) cancers. Overall, men who had been obese one year before their cancer diagnoses were 2.6 times more likely than men with normal body mass indexes—below 25—to die from prostate cancer. Obesity also tripled the odds that regional prostate cancer, or cancer that had not spread, would eventually do so.

Similarly, a study that appeared in the journal *Clinical Cancer Research* in 2008 found lower breast cancer survival rates and a greater likelihood of breast cancer recurrence among women who were overweight or obese, compared to those who were normal weight or underweight. Women who are obese also are more likely to develop inflammatory breast cancer, which has been associated with a poor prognosis.

Insulin resistance, a critical factor in conditions like diabetes and heart disease, also appears to play a role in cancer. In insulin resistance, the body's cells no longer work properly, so insulin and glucose build up in the bloodstream. Insulin is known to stimulate cell division, so an overproduction of insulin may be partially responsible for the development of cancer.

One more potential connection between obesity and cancer: People who are obese tend to eat very few of the foods rich in the bioactives that we'll be discussing in this book. Most scientists believe that these bioactives help protect against cancer.

The observation that overweight and obesity often lead to disease and premature death is not a new one. As early as 400 BC, the Greek physician Hippocrates noted that "sudden death is more common in those who are naturally fat than in the lean." But the connection between obesity and inflammation is just now emerging, and many scientists—myself included—

are convinced that the rise in obesity and overweight is largely responsible for our current epidemic of inflammatory disease. The reason is simple: Nothing suppresses the body's adaptive stress response like eating too much.

GENETIC LINKS TO OUR ANCESTRAL PAST

So why are we so fat? Our culture of abundance certainly bears its share of the blame. That said, I don't really believe that we're gaining weight at such a desperate rate just because we are a bunch of couch potatoes with no self-control. Instead, I suspect that it's due largely to a genetic drive, one developed under living conditions very different from the ones in which we now find ourselves. Scientists refer to this drive as the "thrifty gene" hypothesis, and it helps us to understand why certain populations and certain individuals may be more prone to obesity than others.

Here it is, in a nutshell: In times when food could become scarce, the ability to take advantage of rare periods of abundance by efficiently storing energy as fat undoubtedly was a selective advantage. The better our ancestors were at storing fat, the more likely they were to survive.

> We're designed to eat as much as we can as long as food is available—and so we do.

Our ancestors' ability to hoard calories and gain weight kept them alive— and not just because the fat served as a reserve supply for lean times, although that certainly came in handy. Whatever extra fat they were able to squirrel away also afforded them extra protection against disease.

You see, fat cells aren't simply inert. Fat is an endocrine organ, like the pancreas and ovaries—one that secretes over 100 powerful inflammatory messengers. You'll be hearing more about these messengers, which have names like tumor necrosis factor-alpha and IL1-beta.

> Fat cells not only produce inflammatory signals themselves, they also provide sites for inflammatory cells like macrophages to make even more.

Normally, inflammatory messengers are our allies. We produce lots of them, for example, when we're fighting an infection; once the infection is vanquished, we stop. But fat cells manufacture relatively high amounts of inflammatory messengers *all the time*, even when nothing is going on. Persistently high levels of these messengers cause low-grade, whole-body inflammation, which dramatically raises the risk of inflammatory disease. So the heavier we are, the more inflammatory messengers we produce, and the more whole-body inflammation we have.

> **The ability of fat tissue to generate an unlimited supply of inflammatory messengers sets the stage for low-grade, whole-body inflammation, which consequently leaves us vulnerable to a host of inflammatory conditions.**

What's more, fat is the only organ with an almost unlimited ability to increase in size. For a long time, the conventional wisdom was that the number of fat cells in the body was fixed in childhood and remained constant throughout life. We now know that fat cells not only change in volume, they also change in number. In other words, they get bigger, and they multiply.

Scientists have made another, even more disturbing discovery about fat cells. Once they exceed a critical size, they turn into mature fat cells. The larger and more mature the cell becomes, the more metabolically active it is, and the more inflammatory messengers it can churn out.

For our hunter-gatherer ancestors, it was a great advantage for fat to produce inflammatory messengers. As I've said, these messengers are not, in and of themselves, bad guys. When you're under attack from a bacterial, viral, or fungal infection, inflammation helps your body fight off the invaders and heal itself. So a few extra pounds would have made a hunter-gatherer's immune system much more aggressive, helping to protect him from infection—a very useful trick in an age when even the common cold virus could have killed him.

> **For our hunter-gatherer ancestors, fat wasn't just a way to stockpile energy for the tough times. It helped to make them more disease-resistant, too.**

From a survival perspective, packing on enough fat to get through a famine far outweighed (pardon the pun) any other biological function except basic metabolism. As abundance waned, fat stores were used up, and enhanced inflammation subsided.

As unpleasant as those lean times might have been, they were powerful tools for kicking the body's self-defense mechanisms into high gear. And since our ancestors' life spans were short, they did not have to worry about the long-term effects of overproducing inflammatory messengers or whole-body inflammation—things like heart disease, diabetes, and arthritis, the very ailments that so seriously plague us today.

As we've seen, there's a fine line between an inflammatory response that acts appropriately, protecting the body, and one that acts inappropriately, putting its charge in harm's way. Gaining weight upsets this balance, tipping the scale toward very destructive inflammation, especially in those who are genetically susceptible to it. And when an entire country heads down the path to obesity—according to a paper recently published in the journal *Obesity*, Johns Hopkins researchers predict that 86.6 percent of American adults will be overweight or obese by 2030—it's no surprise that the statistics on inflammatory disease are as grave as they are.

The "thrifty gene" hypothesis helps to explain why the majority of diets don't work: They ask us to go against our own genetic programming, a system fine-tuned over hundreds of thousands of years. How could we possibly stand a chance? Gene Smart is the first diet that gives us direct access to our genes, reprogramming them instead of asking us to marshal our willpower against them.

KNOW YOUR INFLAMMATORY MESSENGERS

Our hunter-gatherer ancestors were driven to eat everything in sight during times of abundance, a genetic trait that I am afraid their modern counterparts have inherited. We are equipped with genes to ensure that we eat as much as we can when food is plentiful, as it always is in developed countries like the United States.

But that's really an oversimplified explanation of why we're so overweight. In fact, obesity manifests itself through an incredibly intricate genetic control system. There are thought to be dozens of biological pathways that promote eating, and probably several that signal satiety. However, research over the past decade has identified one signaling system—the leptin system—as particularly important.

Leptin: Friend or Foe?

Leptin is a hormone that is made by fat cells and then put into circulation. When it was first discovered, scientists thought that large amounts of leptin sent a "stop eating" signal to the brain once fat stores had been restocked. Pharmaceutical companies, as you might imagine, went crazy, producing leptin and leptin-like molecules in the hope of curbing appetite and preventing obesity.

But then another observation threw the original theory into question: It turned out that people who are obese have high levels of leptin—and high levels of the hormone, when administered artificially to people on high-fat diets, did not seem to promote weight loss. As scientists quickly realized, the human body can become resistant to the effects of leptin, just as it becomes resistant to insulin.

Under normal circumstances, leptin regulates the amount of fat that the body stores, slowing the process if fat becomes overstocked. But in people who are obese, this system breaks down; their bodies have seen so much leptin that they don't respond appropriately to large amounts of it. Exposed to enough of the stuff, their bodies simply ignore it.

In fact, leptin can work against our weight-loss efforts. When levels of the hormone fall rapidly, as they do when we lose weight, it triggers profound changes in energy and hormone balance. We end up eating more in order to restore our energy levels, as our bodies say, "Hey, I feel draggy and tired; maybe a donut would help." Again, this signaling system would have helped our hunter-gatherer ancestors to avoid starvation, since continuous abundance wasn't an issue, but the system is downright cruel to the modern-day dieter.

If all that weren't enough, a study that very recently appeared in *The Journal of Clinical Investigation* showed that low leptin levels cause behavioral changes that make resisting food very difficult. Michael Rosenbaum, MD, and his colleagues at Columbia University Medical Center found that as leptin levels declined with weight loss, brain activity indicated an increasing emotional and cognitive response to food as well as declining control over eating behavior. In other words, the more weight you lose, the harder it becomes, as you'll be less inclined to keep your hands out of the cookie jar. This helps explain why only 5 to 25 percent of people who had been obese but lost at least 10 percent of their body weight through diet and exercise are able to keep off the pounds.

Finally, we're beginning to understand why losing weight is not as easy as "eat less and exercise more." It is not a lack of willpower, but rather a genetic predisposition, one that has devastating consequences in our modern world. We're not too weak; our biology is too strong.

Here's the real kicker: Leptin itself has proven to be an incredibly powerful inflammatory signal. Structurally, it looks very similar to the highly inflammatory cytokines; it acts like them, too. Early studies showed increases in circulating leptin concentrations in people harboring infection, suggesting that the hormone is a component of the inflammatory response. We now know this to be true. Leptin causes the production of several inflammatory messengers, including cytokines and eicosanoids, and it contributes to the development of inflammatory cells. Scientists believe that the hormone plays a critical role in inflammatory diseases such as diabetes, rheumatoid arthritis and osteoarthritis, and intestinal inflammation.

The way in which Gene Smart works on leptin is one of the reasons this diet is so incredibly effective at helping people to lose weight as well as to reduce chronic, full-body inflammation. Participants in our study, the Hillsdale Study, saw their leptin levels plummet by more than 35 percent, on average. Those who started the program with especially high levels of the hormone experienced even greater reductions. In light of the connection between leptin and inflammation, this is great news.

Most interestingly, the majority of our participants did not experience the subsequent increase in appetite that's usually associated with a significant drop in leptin. In fact, they told us things like, "I rarely finished my sandwich at lunch." Honestly, we don't know for sure what additional appetite/satiety systems are being activated with Gene Smart, but I suspect that the generous amounts of soluble and insoluble fiber in the diet activate yet another genetic system, as does the exercise component.

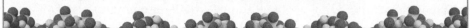
We're just beginning to unravel these mysteries, but the message is clear: There is great power in working with your genes instead of against them. It allows you to reach behind the body's control panel and reprogram the very systems that have been obstructing weight loss and feeding inflammation for so long.

Other Messengers to Watch

Gene Smart also lowers levels of other inflammatory messengers that can have especially adverse effects for people who are overweight or obese. In the Hillsdale Study, we tracked a number of these messengers, including the following:

C-reactive protein. This is the inflammatory messenger that's closest to becoming a household name. High levels of C-reactive protein, or CRP, are so closely correlated to so many virulent conditions that I sometimes think of it as a biomarker of disease and aging in general.

Data collected from more than 20 studies demonstrate that higher than ordinary levels of CRP are strongly associated with nearly all of the important cardiovascular risk factors, including high cholesterol, high blood pressure, insulin resistance, and diabetes. According to three recent studies, CRP is an important determinant of both near-term and all-cause mortality—

death, in other words. And—you guessed it—it's present like gangbusters in people who are overweight.

One study found that women who are obese are more than six times as likely as women of normal weight to have elevated CRP—levels higher than those usually associated with many infections. In the same study, men who were obese were more than twice as likely as men of normal weight to have elevated CRP.

Our own Hillsdale Study has confirmed that people who are overweight or obese have higher than normal levels of CRP. But it also showed that there is a direct relationship between a reduction in body fat and a reduction in CRP. One of our female participants entered the study with a CRP of 37, one of the highest that I have ever seen in the absence of infection. After 8 weeks on Gene Smart, her CRP dropped to just over 4—an astonishing improvement. As another participant said, "The harder you work on the program, the better you feel." This certainly holds true as we examine markers of inflammation like CRP.

Interleukin-6. An additional important inflammatory messenger is interleukin-6 (IL-6), whose role is much more complex. As we'll discuss in Chapter 12, IL-6 may have anti-inflammatory effects in people who are lean and physically active. In this group, it helps to regulate metabolism, suppress appetite, and prevent weight gain. But in people who are overweight or obese, elevated IL-6 is associated with excess whole-body inflammation and increased CRP production. IL-6 also may be a factor in cardiovascular disease and diabetes.

Data from the Hillsdale Study offer evidence that Gene Smart can lower IL-6 to healthy levels. Further, our study identified a direct relationship between reductions in body fat and reductions in IL-6.

Interleukin-8. Our fat cells also produce an inflammatory messenger known as interleukin-8 (IL-8). IL-8 plays a pivotal role in the development of atherosclerosis and other inflammatory diseases by controlling how and when white blood cells move into tissues to cause damage. One recent study showed that the amount of circulating IL-8 correlates to the obesity-related biomarkers CRP and IL-6, as well as to glucose regulation. The study further suggested that IL-8 may be the link between obesity and atherosclerosis and diabetes.

In our study, the Gene Smart Diet markedly reduced expression of the gene that produces IL-8. I feel comfortable predicting that inhibiting this gene will translate to an anti-inflammatory response.

Tumor necrosis factor-alpha. Tumor necrosis factor–alpha (TNF) is an inflammatory messenger made by macrophages, a type of white blood cell that's quite prevalent in fat tissue. In people who are lean, macrophages make up only 5 to 10 percent of fat tissue, while they account for up to 60 percent of all cells in the fat deposits of people who are overweight or obese. One study found that compared to those of normal weight, those who are obese release more than seven times as much TNF from their fat tissue.

TNF is associated with insulin resistance, diabetes, hardening of the arteries, and congestive heart failure. It also has strong ties to cancer. Although it does kill cancer cells in high enough doses, it actually promotes tumor growth when present at lower levels but over a longer period of time. When production of this messenger is turned off in laboratory mice, they don't develop tumors at all.

Other inflammatory messengers. These include prostaglandins, leukotrienes, isoprostanes (products of arachidonic acid, an omega-6) and interleukins such as IL-10, all of which are present in higher than normal levels in people who are obese. Results of the Hillsdale Study suggest that the Gene Smart Diet blocks isoprostane production.

Clearly, fat tissue has all of the weaponry to be a very powerful contributor to whole-body inflammation, and thus to disease and aging. However, as our own Hillsdale Study convincingly demonstrates, all of us have the power to turn back the clock—and the scale—when we deploy the counteroffensive that is Gene Smart.

CHAPTER THREE

OLD BEFORE OUR TIME

THE SUPPRESSION OF THE BODY'S NATURAL, protective adaptive stress response explains another statistical reality that has been driving scientists crazy for the last generation. You see, it isn't just that we're facing an epidemic of diseases characterized by full-body inflammation, including obesity. Despite unparalleled advances in science and the quality of available medical care, the epidemics are getting *worse*.

For proof, consider the following statistics, remembering that each of these diseases has an inflammatory component:

- Current figures from the Centers for Disease Control and Prevention (CDC) put the prevalence of obesity among adults at about 66 percent. A recent study from Johns Hopkins University School of Medicine concluded that if we were to continue at the present rate, "by 2048, all American adults would become overweight or obese."

- Allergies now rank sixth among chronic human diseases.

- There has been a 100 percent increase in the prevalence of hay fever in developed countries in each of the past 3 decades.

- Almost 10 percent of young children are affected by allergic dermatitis, triple the rate in 1960.

- Today, more than 25 million Americans have asthma—twice as many as in 1990. And the severity of the disease appears to be on the rise as well: More people died from asthma in 2000 than in 1970.

- Nearly 24 million Americans—8 percent of the population—have diabetes, according to statistics released by the CDC in 2008. Even more shocking have been the data from individual states. In 1991, only nine states had diabetes rates of 7 to 8 percent, with none higher. By 2001, 43 states had diabetes rates of *at least* 7 to 8 percent, with Mississippi, Alabama, and Florida exceeding 10 percent. Estimates are that by 2025, the number of Americans with the disease will be close to 50 million.

- Arthritis and joint disease affect 43 million people in the United States, almost 20 percent of the population. This number is expected to surpass 60 million by 2020.

- More than 5 million Americans have Alzheimer's disease, with the direct and indirect costs of Alzheimer's and other dementias topping $148 billion annually, according to the Alzheimer's Association.

- Depressive disorders occur in approximately 18.8 million American adults, or about 9.5 percent of the U.S. population age 18 and older.

Clearly, something we're doing is driving our genes—and the master health regulators that control them—in the wrong direction.

Now, some detractors will discount this very alarming spike in inflammatory illness by saying that we're only now living long enough to contract "diseases of aging," as they like to call them. "If we'd had longer life expectancies back then, we would have seen the same number of people falling prey to these diseases that we're seeing today," they say. A hundred years ago, they argue, humans were too vulnerable to infection and accidents to live to a ripe old age.

For years, my counterargument has been that inflammatory diseases have become more common over a time frame when life spans have *not* gotten significantly longer. While life expectancy has increased dramatically over the last century (thanks largely to the introduction of antibiotics, which led to a marked reduction in deaths from infectious diseases), it has changed little in the years between 1970 and today. Yet the rate of inflammatory disease has risen by 30 percent during the same time period. And children, not the elderly, account for a huge proportion of the new cases.

That's not to say there's no connection between inflammation and aging. In fact, I believe that there is a very strong connection, which we can interpret a couple of different ways. One is that it's coincidence: We are currently facing down an epidemic of inflammatory diseases, many of which—arthritis, heart disease, diabetes—happen to become more common with age.

The other perspective requires an entirely different view of inflammation itself—one that makes my blood run cold. Until recently, we had no idea of the widespread effects of chronic, whole-body inflammation or the number of conditions in which it is a factor. We didn't fully understand the adaptive stress response, the importance of obesity, or its impact on our genes. Ten years ago, we didn't even consider the possibility of an inflammatory component to cancer and Alzheimer's, much less investigate anti-inflammatory strategies as treatments. Are we, as a population, succumbing to the newest and most global entry in the inflammatory epidemic: aging?

Put another way, is inflammation driving us to become old long before our time?

HOW OLD *ARE* YOU REALLY?

Before we explain the connection between the adaptive stress response, obesity, inflammatory disease, and premature aging, we need to address a question for which the answer may seem obvious at first blush, but in fact is not.

What is aging?

Traditionally, aging has been defined as the deterioration of systems over time. Longevity experts have noted that not just humans but all living organisms appear to carry with them a built-in "expiration date." A downward spiral commences once we leave behind our reproductive years, as if we've outlived our usefulness once we no longer can procreate. After all, what purpose do we serve once we've stopped furthering the species? By then we're simply consuming resources that others who can still reproduce would put to better use. And so we begin to experience diminished strength and heightened vulnerability to disease, which eventually ushers in a decline in our essential systems. This deterioration can be observed through what scientists call *biomarkers of aging*, a set of readily measured functions and conditions that change as we get older.

Identifying these biomarkers of aging has been incredibly important. After all, how else could scientists find out if their newly discovered "fountain of youth" is working? Let's say that we've discovered a component of our diet that will give most of us the chance to reach the ripe old age of 120. How can a scientist test this substance in humans in order to determine that it actually works? Our life span is long enough that it makes for very unwieldy experiments; nobody is going to wait around for 30 years to see if my 50-year-old self surpasses my normal life expectancy of 80 years. Let's face it: Even if the compound works and I survive to 120, most of the scientists running the experiment will be dead.

So what the scientific community urgently needed was a set of measures that would help us determine the *rate* at which we humans are aging, in less than the full life span. These are the biomarkers of aging. By examining how this set of measures changes, we can determine if what we're doing is working—or not.

You probably don't need me to tell you what many of the biomarkers are. You've seen them in your grandparents and parents—even in your aging pets! And you, like me, are probably starting to see some of them in yourself.

The biomarkers of aging are, in short, the things that make us look and feel old. Our skin loses elasticity, so that all of the expensive potions in the world won't restore our unlined brows. Joints stiffen up, leaving us creakier, sorer, and less flexible. We're more prone to colds than we were in our prime. Our muscles atrophy, so that we eventually need a helping hand for something as routine as getting out of a chair.

Our hormone levels decline, bringing about dramatic changes throughout our entire bodies. Our bones weaken and our balance becomes less sure, leaving us vulnerable to broken bones after a fall. Our hearts are weaker, and our arteries have picked up deposits. Our glucose regulation is less efficient, increasing our risk of diseases like diabetes. The neurons in the brain change, affecting our cognitive function—those so-called "senior moments"—and contributing to the dementia that's so common in older folks. And yes, our metabolism slows, our muscle mass declines, and exercise can be more difficult, all of which can contribute to weight gain.

Some Biomarkers of Aging

Arterial deposits	Loss of balance
Cognitive decline and dementia	Loss of skin elasticity
Hormonal changes	Muscle atrophy
Joint stiffness	Slowed metabolism
Less efficient glucose and insulin regulation	Weakened bones
	Weight gain

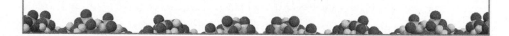

Knowing what the biomarkers of aging are does not mean that we know exactly how we should assess changes in them, or how these changes directly relate to aging. We humans are complex creatures; it's unlikely that scientists will ever find a single biological measure that accurately reflects the rate of aging in such a complicated organism. So instead, they've come up with panels of biomarkers to evaluate many of the systems within an individual, such as the brain, heart, liver, bones, hormones, and so on. Together, these give us a more complete picture of how quickly we are aging.

In fact, scientists suspect that it will most likely be the *interactions* between biomarkers for various organ systems that ultimately determine the life span of an individual. It's a complex science, since all of us inherit different sets of genes and live in different environments. But once we know how to measure and predict these variants, we'll be best able to determine how they influence our bodies' systems.

The thing I find most interesting about the concept of biomarkers of aging is the assumption that underlies it. It proves what we already, intuitively know to be true: that each of us ages at a unique rate. It also means that the standard we've been using—chronological age—is probably not the best predictor of remaining life expectancy. "50 is the new 30," the magazines proclaim, and for some people, that's true. Using biomarkers allows us a much more realistic—and personalized—picture of our individual profiles by measuring the "age" of our various tissues, organs, and organ systems. I may be 50, but how old is my heart? My lungs? My skin?

IS AGING INEVITABLE?

For a long time, the aging process—or, by our new definition, the orderly decline in the biomarkers of aging that accompanies advancing years—was considered to be completely normal, and indeed inevitable. We expected that at a certain point, weakness and increased vulnerability would kick in, giving way to an ever-steeper fall-off as we continued to grow older. And that was that.

For years, the medical community's approach reflected this view of aging as inevitable and occurring at the same rate in everyone. "You're in great shape for someone your age," your doctor would tell you as he wrote out the prescriptions: a statin for your cholesterol, an anti-inflammatory for your tricky hip, and perhaps a little something to help with your love life, since your circulation isn't what it used to be. But these were just delaying tactics—a postponement, not a real "cure" for aging.

But when scientists began looking more closely at what really happens when we get older, they noticed something interesting. In fact, the rate of decline long recognized as "normal" aging might not be inevitable after all.

Aging is not an inevitable tumble off the cliff, it turns out, but rather the result of something very specific: a decline in the body's ability to maintain itself at peak cellular condition. Although our bodies generally do work harder to sustain themselves as we get older, age and maintenance are associated, not intrinsically connected.

> The "aging process," as we know it, can happen at dramatically different rates in different people, depending on how well (or how poorly) our cells maintain themselves.

You see, when we're in the prime of our lives, we don't just look and feel good. We enjoy that youthful glow and seemingly boundless stamina because deep down at the cellular level, our bodies are working full-tilt to repair DNA, defend against free radicals, and carry out other tasks necessary to their optimal function. Robin Holliday, PhD, the author of *Understanding Aging*, describes 13 distinct maintenance mechanisms that are vital to our very existence. Repairing and maintaining our bodies is an incredibly labor-intensive process, requiring enormous energy, resources—and the precisely coordinated cooperation of thousands of individual genes.

Ensuring optimal cellular maintenance appears to be the secret to health, and the true antidote to accelerated aging. Any number of comparative studies have demonstrated unequivocally that the organisms that live longest are the ones that most efficiently and competently manage their cellular function.

This optimal maintenance also is key to the vitality that we enjoy in our twenties. We felt superhuman in our younger years because we were, in a sense. Our cells and their maintenance systems were working overtime to keep us in tip-top shape in order to give us the best shot at reproducing. That's why we could eat anything we wanted without seeing a change in our waistlines; how we could brush off a bad fall on the basketball court or effortlessly work a full day after staying up all night. Our cells were carrying out all of their maintenance activities on overdrive, so none of our bad behaviors slowed us down.

When our bodies are humming along in this fashion, we are bulletproof in many ways. We not only are impervious to lines and wrinkles and can more easily maintain the weight that's appropriate for our frames, we also can dodge a host of chronic conditions like heart disease, diabetes, arthritis, and certain kinds of cancer, which typically catch up with us later in life.

We've learned to think of these as "diseases of aging," but the fact that we're more vulnerable to them in our advancing years isn't just coincidence or bad luck. As we pass beyond our reproductive prime, our bodies' maintenance systems shift into low gear, and all the associated processes begin to decline. When our cells aren't as vigilant about housekeeping, we see changes in the biomarkers of the disease known as aging: a higher fat-to-muscle ratio, reduced cardiovascular strength and endurance, poor glucose and insulin regulation, lower energy and stamina, poor endocrine and cognitive function, less skin elasticity—in other words, all the stuff that we have come to associate with getting old.

> The systemic decline that we have traditionally regarded as normal aging is really a symptom of cellular disrepair, the result of poor cell maintenance.

Imagine that you had a maintenance crew on standby around the clock, ready to tackle any home repairs the moment they cropped up. Every board that needed replacing, every room that needed painting, every pipe that needed refitting would be taken care of before it became a major problem. Under such circumstances, your home would age at a very slow rate.

That's the kind of maintenance our cells perform when we're in our twenties. Later in life, they scale back to something a little more casual—calling the plumber in an absolute emergency, relying on the occasional Saturday project for the rest. As you well know from your own housekeeping, a couple of months of that kind of halfhearted effort, and before long you've got a real mess on your hands.

The creakiness in our joints, the lapses of memory, the extra flab around our waists—not to mention diseases like arthritis, diabetes, and heart disease—these are the body's version of scuffed baseboards and torn window screens, and closet doors that don't quite close. They're the inevitable outcome when our bodies fail to properly maintain themselves at the cellular level.

In short, we age because at a cellular and systems level, our bodies are slacking off. They're programmed for this slowdown after we leave our reproductive years and those cellular maintenance crews are no longer standing at attention, all spit and polish, as they were during our prime. Our increased vulnerability to overweight and the "diseases of aging" is a function of the fact that the body is no longer on high alert against them.

> **The key to enjoying the vitality of a 20-year-old seems to lie in the ability of our cells and systems to maintain themselves at the same rate and level that they did when we were in our twenties.**

INFLAMMATORY AGE VERSUS CHRONOLOGICAL AGE

Heart disease, arthritis, dementia—all are not just inflammatory conditions, but classic "diseases of aging." In fact, that's probably the number-one response I hear when I reel off the list of them: "Inflammatory disease sounds a lot like getting old."

Weight gain is in the mix, too. There isn't a single one of us who hasn't noticed how much more easily the pounds creep on with every passing year—and how much harder they are to take off.

The connection becomes even clearer when we consider the effects of chronic inflammation in someone who *isn't* old. If you've ever seen the hands of a young person suffering from rheumatoid arthritis, you know how her knuckles are swollen and disfigured from the inappropriate inflammatory response that's constantly being unleashed in her joints. The continuous trauma causes swelling and scarring, collateral damage from repeated assaults. The result? The hands of a 25-year-old with rheumatoid arthritis look like the hands of someone in her nineties.

The same is true of someone who suffers from chronic inflammation of the coronary artery around the heart: He has the cardiovascular system of someone who's much older than he actually is. And as we know, chronic inflammation causes certain cells to mutate more and helps certain malignant cells to move throughout the body, increasing the likelihood of developing cancer—another disease that's often associated with aging.

Why do so many diseases of aging have an inflammatory component? It's as though you keep raking your yard, only to have a gale-force wind blow through as soon as you're done. The answer is this: Those cellular maintenance crews can't keep up with the profound destruction that constantly occurs with an inappropriate inflammatory response, even if they're doing their best work. (As we'll see, our cells usually aren't doing their best work because the modern American diet doesn't give them the tools they require.)

That said, even in a best-case scenario, it simply wouldn't be possible to keep up with the chaos and disorder caused by chronic inflammation—as if two dozen partying college students converged on my immaculately clean house every single night, eating chips on the couch and spilling beer on the carpet. Eventually, no matter how good my cleaning service is, the place is going to start to look like something out of *Animal House*. And so inflammation gradually but steadily undermines the systems that it attacks, leading to something that looks very much like an acceleration of the aging process.

> **The damage inflicted by the inflammatory response undoes the good work of the cellular maintenance crews that help keep you young.**

This also explains why certain "diseases of aging"—obesity, diabetes, heart disease, arthritis, cancer—aren't limited to the aging population. At least, they aren't anymore. One of the most disturbing trends in inflammation epidemiology is watching these conditions show up earlier and earlier, in younger and younger people. Diabetes is one of the best examples of this.

> **Most of what we consider to be biomarkers of aging are really biomarkers of inflammation—or vice versa.**

By simplest definition, diabetes is the body's inability to regulate blood glucose, or blood sugar. As we've already discussed, it is astonishingly prevalent in the United States: A staggering 8 percent of the U.S. population has some form of the disease. About one-third of these people don't even realize they're diabetic. Left untreated, diabetes can give way to a host of complications—skin, eye, and foot trouble among them.

More seriously, diabetes is a primary risk factor for a host of other life-threatening conditions, including heart disease, stroke, and kidney disease. This is why doctors consider it to be the proverbial "canary in the coal mine," the first sign of more serious trouble ahead.

There are two kinds of diabetes. One, known as type 1, is comparatively rare. It's a genetic disorder, and thus unavoidable. In type 1, the body simply cannot regulate its own blood sugar. The other, type 2, also has a genetic component; some people are more disposed toward "sugar," as we call it in the South. But type 2 is largely triggered by poor eating and exercise habits, which explains its strong correlation to overweight and obesity. Not surprisingly, given our national propensity for weight problems, the lion's share of diabetes cases fall into this second category.

The percentage of the population that's living with diabetes is growing at a staggering rate. But to me, that's not the scariest part: What frightens me even more is that the people developing the disease are getting *younger and younger* every year.

Thirty years ago, if you met a young person with diabetes, it was pretty much guaranteed to be type 1. A 20-year-old simply hadn't been on the planet long enough to suffer the damage of dietary and lifestyle habits that set the stage for type 2. Back then, type 2 was known as adult-onset diabetes, because it was something that happened to older people, particularly after they became more sedentary and started packing on a few extra pounds.

The same sequence of events played out over and over. A patient would gain weight once he reached his fifties. Five or 6 years later, his physician would notice signs of insulin resistance, indicating that his body was not using insulin efficiently. Five years after that, the patient would be diagnosed with full-blown type 2 diabetes. Another 5 years would pass, and he'd be living with coronary heart disease or at high risk for stroke.

What we're seeing now is not a different sequence of events. In fact, it's the very same: Weight gain still gives way to insulin resistance, which gives way to diabetes and, eventually, to heart disease and stroke. The difference is the age of the patients. The curve has shifted so much that what was once standard for a 50-year-old is now standard for a 30-year-old. And while an 18-year-old with coronary heart disease might be an exception, he's not a complete anomaly either.

What's driving all this? Inflammation—or to be more precise, the occurrence of chronic, low-level, full-body inflammation in an increasingly younger population, most likely because so many of us are overweight.

In my opinion, the dramatic changes in physiology, disease incidence, and aging that we see with excess calories and obesity largely correlate to the degree of inflammation that we carry within our bodies. More specifically, I believe that the markers of inflammation associated with consuming too many calories are our most important signs of primary aging.

> **Eat less, lose weight, and you'll have less inflammation and fewer biomarkers of aging. Eat more, and the opposite occurs.**

Let me give you another example: In 1948, the National Heart Institute (now known as the National Heart, Lung, and Blood Institute) embarked on an ambitious research project called the Framingham Heart Study. The research team recruited 5,209 men and women between ages 30 and 62 from the town of Framingham, Massachusetts. The objective of the study was to identify common factors or characteristics that contribute to cardiovascular disease (CVD) by following its development over a long period in a large group of participants who had not yet shown overt symptoms or suffered a heart attack or stroke. Since 1948, the subjects have returned every 2 years for detailed medical histories, physical exams, and laboratory tests. As you can imagine, the study has been a gold mine of information for scientists.

Using Framingham data, Oscar H. Franco, MD, PhD, and his colleagues were able to compare 50-year-olds with and without diabetes. What they saw was a pretty dramatic demonstration of how inflammation affects aging and mortality. Dr. Franco concluded that people with diabetes have life spans approximately 8 years shorter than those without the disease. When diabetes was already present by age 50, it frequently provoked early onset of heart disease. This is a perfect example of people getting old—and indeed, dying—before their time because of a chronic inflammatory condition.

When I think about large-scale, long-term studies like Framingham, what stops me in my tracks is how the data from these studies might look 50 years from now, given the incredibly high incidence of obesity and diabetes among our young people. My fear is confirmed by recent recommendations from the American Academy of Pediatrics, which suggests that children as young as 8 could benefit from cholesterol-lowering medication, and that kids as young as 2 should be screened for high cholesterol. Horrifying, isn't it?

This isn't an anti-aging book, in any classic sense of the phrase. After all, what does "aging" really mean, if what we have always considered to be bio-markers of aging are showing up and causing disease in 30-year-olds? It isn't a diet book, either. It's about much, much more than flat abs and thin thighs. I want to give you the tools you need to revitalize your body's adaptive stress response and recruit the genes that fight inflammation.

Will you lose weight on Gene Smart? You sure will—I guarantee it. Will you look and feel dramatically younger? No question about it. We're going to do it not by following the same old approach, but rather by taking steps toward eliminating the root cause of overweight and disease. Our objective, ultimately, is to shut down the inflammatory epidemic that's making us old and overweight before our time.

The great news is that once we push the needle in the other direction—that is, when we support our bodies' built-in defense system rather than fighting it—we reclaim our good health and longevity to a degree that none of us could have fathomed.

CHAPTER FOUR

THE HUNGRY MOUSE: A SCIENTIFIC MYSTERY SOLVED

INFLAMMATION, OVERWEIGHT, and aging are what happen when the body's maintenance crews go off high alert. The switch from supervigilant to slacker is well orchestrated, and it's happening earlier and earlier in the population at large, if the inflammatory epidemic is any indication. But as scientists are discovering, the transition isn't necessarily an inevitable one.

In fact, we do our bodies a tremendous disservice when we think that the rate at which we age—and the weight we gain as we grow older—are set in stone. Our bodies have a tremendous capacity for rejuvenation. They do an amazing job of protecting and, indeed, fixing themselves—something that a normal inflammatory response is a very good example of.

Which begs a few very interesting questions, the first among them: What if we could harness this tremendous self-curative power and use it to reverse our own decline?

GENES × ENVIRONMENT = *WHO* YOU ARE; (GENES × ENVIRONMENT) × TIME = *HOW OLD* YOU ARE

It's been estimated that we humans have between 25,000 and 30,000 functional genes in our DNA. That's 25,000 to 30,000 distinct packets of the instructions necessary to correctly build and maintain a person throughout his or her life.

These packets make about 100,000 proteins that determine everything from how you develop in the womb, to what you look like as a child or an adult, to whether you have any athletic ability (and what you excel at), to how efficiently your immune system operates, to how rapidly your body's cells divide and when they die.

Perhaps most importantly for our purposes, these gene packets also control the inflammatory response, which means that they directly influence your potential for ailments like cancer, heart disease, diabetes, allergies, asthma, and arthritis. Further, scientists have confirmed without question what a quick look around the Thanksgiving table could have told most of us: that a tendency toward overweight and obesity has a strong genetic link.

But the instructions in the gene packets with which we were born are not the only factors that determine whether we become overweight or ill. It's a combination of our genes and our environment, remember? So let's say you're one of the lucky ones who got packets that predispose you to be naturally thin, with a lot of athletic potential. Well, that certainly puts you a step ahead, but it isn't the final word. What if you spend your whole life sitting on the couch watching reality shows and eating donuts? You might not gain as much weight as someone whose genes predispose them toward clumsiness and overweight, but then again, you're not going to be a picture of radiant health.

On the other hand, perhaps you haven't been blessed with the choicest genes (and again, a quick look at your family tree will probably reveal a great deal about the packets you've inherited). If you were to go on the donut-and-television diet described above, you'd find yourself packing on the pounds fast—much faster than if you were genetically gifted. Now you might be thinking, "It's not fair!" Well, as a scientist, I can tell you: It's *not* fair. But your particular gene packets are not an irrefutable sentence, either.

The central focus of my laboratory is to understand how dietary fatty acids affect the inflammatory response associated with asthma, allergies, arthritis, heart disease, and stroke. My studies, as well as those from other laboratories, have shown that different people can have different versions of genes that cause them to make beneficial or harmful fats at different rates. Further, we can manipulate the switches—the master health regulators—

that control the overproduction of harmful fats in those with the more destructive genes. So we know that it's possible to regulate large swaths of genes. But it must be done with great precision.

> **Through diet, it is possible to regulate the genes that control inflammation.**

You see, an estimated 2,000 to 3,000 genes (of the 25,000 to 30,000 in your body) control your immune and inflammatory responses. A large proportion of these gene packets are under the direction of master health regulators. These regulators, in turn, are switched on and off by bioactives, specific compounds that are present in food and that are taken in specific dosages and combinations over a set period of time.

So you can greatly improve your health outlook by changing certain environmental factors to which you expose your body—specifically, to the right types and amounts of bioactives in your diet, and to the right types of exercise. This is precisely what you'll be doing on Gene Smart.

In other words, your genes aren't a life sentence. There are quantifiable rewards for doing the best you can with what you've been given by taking advantage of our new understanding of gene-based nutrition. As long as you're careful not to trigger the genes leading to overweight and premature aging, you can keep your weight and your health on track.

In fact, I believe that a more accurate method of determining your true age is to factor together your genes (or specific variations of individual genes known as polymorphisms) and your environment, especially if that gene-based interaction gives rise to chronic inflammation. Then multiply by your time spent to date in a "Gene Smart" or "non–Gene Smart" environment.

The point is, your lifestyle choices determine whether you achieve the potential—good or bad—that's spelled out for you by your genes. Learning how to influence your genetic predispositions is what the Gene Smart Diet is all about.

I've been using weight gain as an example, but it certainly isn't the only thing that you can have a genetic predisposition for—or that you can influence through your behavior. Gene Smart is, at its heart, an anti-inflammatory program. Because when we talk about losing weight, we're really talking about controlling inflammation. And when we talk about extending longevity, we're really talking about helping our cells to maintain themselves at an optimal level, past the point when they typically might start a downward spiral. One of the best ways to do this is to avoid an environment that is likely to produce chronic whole-body inflammation.

> **Less destruction + better maintenance and repair = a normal weight, better health, and reduced aging.**

The dazzling promise of some magic dust that could help us retard the process by which all the body's systems wind down and eventually stall out has fueled research for decades. Before pursuing this path conceptually, scientists needed to come to terms with what triggers—or delays—the downward spiral in the first place. Obviously, it's not as simple as just getting up there in years; every one of us knows a 71-year-old who looks 40 and can out-hike his grandkids. Certainly, proper care—a prudent diet with the right bioactives, adequate amounts of the right types of exercise, lots of sleep, and maintaining a healthy weight—has something to do with his vitality. His lifestyle supports his cells' efforts to maintain themselves.

But doing the right stuff lifestyle-wise can't be the entire explanation, either, because each of us also knows someone who has done all the wrong stuff and still finds himself at the peak of health. "All the doctors who told me to quit smoking are dead," a 104-year-old woman recently told a *New York Times* reporter in an article about exceptional longevity, or the study of the very long lived. More tragic is the perfectly fit, clean-living 40-year-old who drops dead on his morning run without any warning at all. I'm behind that genetic eight-ball myself. Despite taking good care of themselves, my great-grandfather lived only to 54, and my grandfather to 59; my father, the most vital and energetic man I've ever met, lived to 66.

So our biological age isn't inexorably tied to our chronological age; our lifestyle plays a role, too. Still, we can't entirely control the speed at which we grow older simply by taking meticulous care of ourselves. Apparently, our cells also take their cues to maintain themselves (or not) from somewhere else. Scientists now believe that to really understand why we get old (or why certain of us get old more quickly than others), we must look at the interplay between two things: a genetic component, which we can't control, and our lifestyle choices, which we can.

Now what if I were to tell you that we've found something that overrides nature's imperative for our cells to stop maintaining themselves in their peak condition? Something that hits both the things we can control and the things we can't?

We have. And here's the real kicker: We've known about it since the 1930s.

EAT LESS, LIVE LONGER

In 1934, two scientists from Cornell University, Clive McCay and Mary Crowell, made an interesting observation. Laboratory mice given a diet that was nutritionally sound but severely reduced in calories lived twice as long as they were expected to. We know, from terrible experience, that being overweight can have serious, even life-threatening consequences. These early experiments proved that going in the opposite direction produced a very different result.

In the 70 years of research that has followed their discovery, their model—called calorie restriction, or CR—remains the only thing that has consistently and universally proven to extend longevity.

And it works. Boy, does it ever! Not surprisingly, animals on a calorie-restricted diet are as slim and trim as they come. But that's just the beginning. Over and over, across multiple species, researchers have been able to dramatically improve life span a staggering 30 to 40 percent, simply by limiting the number of calories consumed by their subjects. In human terms, that would translate to a life span of about 120 years!

A longer life is nice, certainly. But more years isn't all that CR promises. You see, CR extends life span by reversing many of the critical biomarkers of devastating medical conditions like heart disease, diabetes, arthritis, and cancer—as well as the biomarkers of aging itself.

> **Restricting calories reverses the biomarkers of aging and disease.**

Like us humans, mice tend to begin a downward spiral after reaching a certain point in their life cycle—typically after their reproductive years. But in laboratory mice on calorie-restricted diets, this decline proceeds much, much slower. The lab mice don't lose muscle when you'd expect them to, their fur doesn't thin as it usually would, their immune systems remain strong, and they don't become susceptible to diseases like cancer, as older mice—and older humans—generally do. CR mice are more physically active than they should be, they don't develop diabetes or any of the metabolic disorders associated with excess weight, and they completely duck the inflammatory ailments—everything from arthritis to heart disease. In short, they look younger, they act younger, and they don't succumb to diseases of aging.

> The lab animals in CR studies don't just live longer, they stay in their prime longer.

OK, but mice are mice. Does CR have the same effects in humans—supporting weight loss, increasing muscle tone, and promoting physical activity, even while fending off chronic disease and promoting longevity? Well, there aren't a lot of studies, for a few reasons—reasons that, incidentally, highlight why CR is not a great real-world solution for the vast majority of the population.

Measuring change in the human life span is difficult. To begin with, there are too many variables, like job layoffs, bad marriages, secondhand smoke, and a million other lifestyle factors that differ from human to human and that don't come into play in the study of laboratory animals. And because humans live so long anyway, it's hard to back up CR's biggest claim—that it extends life span. Think of it: If those researchers had started a CR experiment involving humans back in the 1930s, they'd just be seeing the results now!

But the bigger and more consistent problem with studying CR is the obvious one, the elephant in the room: Diets that severely restrict calories are difficult to conduct outside of laboratory conditions. Heck, they're difficult to conduct *within* laboratory conditions. My lab has performed studies in which we provide all the food for hundreds of humans, and I can tell you from personal experience that ensuring compliance among research subjects is hard. And that's on diets that don't leave them hungry all the time! Calorie-restrict by 30 to 40 percent, and compliance is next to impossible.

Additionally, doing CR *properly* is very difficult—but very important. Because the overall calorie count is so low, people who follow a calorie-restricted diet must take great care to ensure that they're sufficiently nourished. Otherwise, they're just starving themselves, and at the levels we're talking about, it's a pretty fine line. Generally, practitioners of CR record every bite they eat and then use a special computer program to meticulously calibrate their daily intakes of a long list of nutrients, including some that you and I never think about; we get adequate amounts just by eating as we normally do.

For all of these reasons, tracking CR in humans presents a challenge. But there have been a few studies, and the results seem to indicate that CR holds much the same promise for humans as it does for animals. For instance, in the late 1990s, scientists conducted sealed missions in Biosphere 2, an artificial closed ecology system made of steel and glass that's located in the Arizona

Calorie Restriction by the Numbers

In the very few studies that have been done of calorie restriction (CR) in humans, participants have shown various positive biological changes—just like the monkeys and mice that live longer when they're fed calorie-restricted diets. It's a relatively safe speculation, then, that humans would live longer if they practiced CR, too.

The study subjects saw a significant rollback in many of the biomarkers of aging. People lost weight, as you'd expect. But other results were more surprising. For example, the study participants:

- Lowered their systolic blood pressure (the top number in a blood pressure reading) by 25 percent and their diastolic pressure (the bottom number) by 22 percent

- Reduced their white blood cell count by 31 percent (these are the cells that participate in inflammatory responses)
- Lowered their insulin by 42 percent and their blood sugar by 21 percent
- Improved their blood lipids, with a drop in total cholesterol of 30 percent and much-improved ratios of LDL and HDL cholesterol

In addition, the thickness of their carotid arteries—an early sign of atherosclerosis—was about 40 percent less compared to the control groups.

In other words, based on a range of risk factors, it appears that long-term CR may have a powerful protective effect against heart disease and many other inflammatory disorders.

desert. For much of one 2-year study, the participants experienced marked food restrictions—that is, forced CR.

In a separate study outside of the Biosphere, a group of highly motivated individuals who had followed a calorie-restricted diet on their own for an average of 6 years were compared to a group of healthy people of the same ages, who had spent those 6 years eating the typical American diet.

The results from these studies were very impressive, suggesting that restricting calories in humans can have a highly positive effect on our old friends, the biomarkers that represent various bodily systems. The study participants showed lower blood pressure than people of the same age who had not restricted calories. Their triglycerides and LDL (bad) cholesterol were lower, while their HDL (good) cholesterol was higher. Their arteries showed fewer signs of atherosclerosis. Their fasting insulin and glucose levels were lower. In short, they had the cardiovascular systems of much younger people.

CR AND INFLAMMATION

What really caught my attention was the news about inflammation that came out of the human CR studies. What effect would CR have on this key driver for so many ailments, among them heart disease, diabetes, asthma, allergies, psoriasis, Crohn's, Alzheimer's, and even certain kinds of cancer?

We would find out through measures of a substance called C-reactive protein (CRP), an inflammatory messenger produced by the liver. CRP rises in the presence of tissue injury, which is the result of infection, trauma, malignant disease, and chronic inflammatory conditions. Elevated CRP is a major red flag that the body is either under attack or attacking itself. In fact, it is such an important sign of trouble brewing that I sometimes think of it as a biomarker for disease in general.

 | **C-reactive protein is a biomarker for disease in general.**

Indeed, the presence of CRP is known to be a specific, predictive biomarker for a number of our worst inflammatory conditions, including heart disease, arthritis, and diabetes. (Cardiologists now believe that high CRP is a much more accurate predictor of sudden death by heart attack than elevated blood cholesterol.) Further, CRP levels are much higher in the obese. It's really quite simple: Where there is CRP, there is inflammation; where there is inflammation, there is disease.

With this much at stake, you can see why I'd be so excited to find a study—published in the *Proceedings of the National Academy of Sciences* in 2004—in which CR showed a very real impact on the full-body inflammation that gives rise to elevated CRP and thus to so many insidious diseases.

In this study, the plasma CRP concentrations among the people in the CR group were extremely low—84 percent lower, on average, than among those in the control group. These people are in their mid-fifties by now, but they have the CRP levels of a very healthy 20-year-old. The implications of this finding alone are amazing, with potentially profound consequences for the health of every single American.

> **Calorie restriction dramatically reduces C-reactive protein, a biomarker of inflammation, in humans.**

But there's more. For another study, published in a recent issue of *JAMA*, a group of scientists evaluated the effects of 6 months of CR. They saw improvements in many of the biomarkers associated with aging, including insulin and thyroid hormone levels, as well as some of the other biomarkers we've already talked about. Most interestingly, this study was the first to report a significant decline in DNA damage with CR.

Now DNA damage is without question one of the most important biomarkers of aging. Think of it as wear and tear. Usually it takes one of two forms: mutation or destruction. In other words, either DNA changes in some way or it falls apart altogether.

This process is very predictable: The longer you live, the more DNA damage you have; the more damage you have, the more likely it is to give way to disease. In fact, it's so predictable that scientists think of DNA damage as the factor that sets your internal biological clock.

The connection between DNA damage and life span makes the discovery of CR's ability to slow this damage very significant indeed. Think of DNA damage as the process by which food spoils—or, to continue our aging metaphor, by

The Pros and Cons of Extreme Calorie Restriction

Calorie restriction is the only thing scientists have ever proven to extend life. Here are some of the benefits and risks:

Pros

- Lowers blood pressure
- Lowers bad (LDL) cholesterol
- Lowers triglycerides
- Raises good (HDL) cholesterol
- Lowers fasting insulin and glucose levels
- Lowers C-reactive protein
- Slows DNA damage

Cons

There's only one, but it's a biggie: "I'm *hungry*!" Severely restricting calories is unrealistic for the vast majority of us.

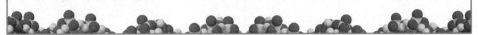

which it passes its expiration date. Slowing DNA damage is like putting a carton of milk in an ice-cold refrigerator, allowing you to preserve its freshness for a much longer time.

So two of the most significant biomarkers of disease and aging—full-body inflammation and DNA damage—are dramatically reduced by CR. That was big news in the scientific community.

Unfortunately, even results this spectacular could not overcome the one major drawback of CR: Nothing changes the fact that a severe reduction in calorie intake simply isn't a real-world solution for the masses. A doctor could never "prescribe" such a diet to her patients; compliance would be impossible to secure; and even the most agreeable and motivated patients would need to exercise constant vigilance in order to meet their basic nutritional needs.

It's not impossible, certainly, as you'll see if you check out the newsgroups or visit the blogs dedicated to the CR way of life. But for most of us average Americans, long-term severe calorie restriction is not an option—not even if it will return us to the slim physiques of our youth and no matter how many extra years it will earn us on the longevity clock.

What a frustration for us scientists! The promise of CR is spectacular, yet the fix is impossible to implement. So the key to a longer life, and more time spent in our prime, once again dangled tantalizingly out of reach.

STRESS: THE SURVIVAL SWITCH

But CR's promise was too strong to resist for long. After all, if someone could identify the critical genes—and critical gene-nutrient interactions—driven by calorie restriction, then perhaps we could figure out a way to reproduce its effects. We had to find something that mimicked CR, with all of the same health-promoting, age-defying results—but without requiring people to go hungry.

The first inkling that the CR code could be cracked came from several very different areas of biology, all converging into one central idea—and, I might add, an unlikely one.

What is it? In a word: *stress*.

Yes, I know—stress doesn't seem like an obvious link to longevity. Stress, as we generally know it, feels like it depletes us rather than restoring us. I, for one, am always startled to see how drawn and, well, old I look after a particularly difficult bank of meetings or a long day of travel.

But the stress I'm talking about isn't the normal, workaday variety—like an irritating commute or an unexpected bill. In fact, serious psychological stress may launch a cascade of internal responses that ultimately impair immune function. In one epidemiological study, for example, death from all causes increased in the months following a severe stressor—in this case, the death of a spouse, explaining the anecdotal observation that elderly folks often die soon after their spouses pass. Other consequences that have been tracked by scientists include rates of infection and HIV progression, as well as cancer incidence and progression.

But beneficial or *adaptive* stress exacts a very specific toll on the body's physiological systems. This type of stress—the kind that doesn't kill you, in other words—can actually strengthen the body's cellular maintenance.

One of the best and most obvious examples of adaptive stress at work is the physical effects of an exercise program. In a healthy person, placing a robust amount of controlled stress on the muscles on a regular basis through physical exertion—for example, aerobic activity at 65 to 85 percent of maximum heart rate or resistance training—will strengthen them and increase their endurance. It's a wonderful feeling: After a few weeks, you suddenly realize that you've effortlessly completed three sets of a resistance-training exercise with a weight that you could barely lift when you were just starting out.

| **Beneficial stress makes you stronger as your body adapts.**

To continue to improve your fitness level, you must continue inducing the adaptive stress response. You can do this by kicking up the intensity of your aerobic workout (let's say 30 minutes on an elliptical trainer at a resistance of 10 rather than 6, which is where you started) or your resistance training (e.g., increasing the amount of weight by 15 percent).

We scientists used to think that exercise damages muscle, which then repairs itself and adapts to the stressor—that is, the exercise—by becoming stronger and less fatigable. Indeed, this is part of the answer. But we now have shown exercise to be the type of stress that communicates with the master regulators of a family of genes that help you not only to get in shape but also to reduce whole-body inflammation (more on how this works in a minute).

By increasing the intensity or duration of an aerobic activity or the weight or reps in a resistance-training session, you bring about changes in your genes as well as in your muscles. And you continue to stress your muscles by challenging them to an ever-increasing degree over time. This is why exercise is such a powerfully beneficial stressor, with profound effects on inflammation in its own right.

REACHING BEHIND THE CURTAIN: A GENE-BASED SOLUTION

Your muscles are not the only place in your body where you can see this phenomenon in action. Every single one of your cells can benefit.

What we're really talking about here is an allocation of resources. Stress forces your body to put a lot of energy into the kind of high-level cellular maintenance that we've been talking about—the kind that makes your body thinner and younger.

Our bodies have a limited amount of energy and metabolic resources available to them. So we developed to respond to changes in our environment in ways that ensure our survival. For instance, an animal loses its ability to reproduce when its calories are restricted; the body shifts its metabolic resources from reproduction to basic metabolism and cell maintenance. By putting breeding on the back burner and moving survival to the front one, the body increases the likelihood that it will outlast the famine and be well enough to breed once the food supply improves.

> **We respond to changes in our environment by adapting our physiology to give us the best possible chance for survival.**

That, in a nutshell, is thought to be why calorie restriction works. If you're going to be facing down a real threat, like a famine, your cells really need to be operating at optimum levels to give you a survival advantage. There is nothing more essential to life than food, and we are genetically programmed to interpret a shortage of it—as in a calorie-restricted diet—as a real threat to our continued survival.

So when we're consuming fewer calories than we need, as we would in CR, our bodies think, "Uh-oh, we're going through some hard times." This prompts them to switch to emergency survival mode, turbo-charging all those cellular maintenance activities. Dehydration, physical exertion, certain environmental chemicals, and excess heat all have the same effect. These particular stressors require our bodies to train their focus and, more specifically, their energy on cellular maintenance to ensure survival, resulting in the kind of premium-level maintenance work that can keep us young.

> **The adaptive stress response is one of the most powerful protective weapons in our arsenal. Faced with a threat, our bodies gear up to cope.**

THE HORMESIS EFFECT:
A LITTLE BIT MAKES YOU STRONGER

Scientists such as Mark P. Mattson, PhD, of the National Institute on Aging, a division of the National Institutes of Health, have since added another, equally essential piece to the puzzle by revitalizing an older concept called hormesis. The word *hormesis* comes from the Greek meaning "to excite." Hormesis can broadly be defined as the stimulating or beneficial effect of small doses of a toxic substance, circumstance, or environmental condition that at higher concentrations would be harmful or lethal.

Let me provide you with a real-world, and somewhat embarrassing, example of this from my undergraduate years in college. My roommate back then frequented the local watering hole every night of the week and could drink until closing time. By comparison, just a few beers on a Friday night invariably sent me back to my dorm room, woozy and stupid, with a headache virtually guaranteed the next morning.

The reason for the discrepancy in our tolerance? My buddy was drinking during the week, while I was hitting the books. By having a few beers every night, he was making more of an enzyme (alcohol dehydrogenase) that effectively protected him from ethanol, the toxin in beer. I, meanwhile, had no such protection. The chemical "stress" of those small doses of poison, administered over the course of the week, built up his tolerance, allowing him to handle a higher dose of the stressor by the weekend. In other words, his body had adapted.

Another way to look at it? My roommate was effectively "training," as an athlete does, for our weekend parties. (Please note: I'm not endorsing a three-beer-a-day regimen, except as an example of the hormetic response, although it may explain some of the apparent benefits of moderate alcohol consumption.)

We can sum up hormesis this way: A little bit of something harmful, when taken in small doses over an extended period, can actually make you stronger.

The hormetic response was originally applied to plant physiology. For instance, scientists observed that the herbicide Phosfon stimulates the growth of peppermint plants at low soil concentrations and inhibits it at higher, normal concentrations. Later, in animal studies, scientists observed that challenging mice with small doses of gamma radiation shortly before exposing them to very high levels of those same gamma rays actually reduced their chances of developing cancer.

The last decade has brought a huge conceptual jump, as scientists have been able to connect the hormetic response to the adaptive stress response. Give us a little bit of something, the theory goes, and our bodies will adapt; the stress will make us stronger.

Let's consider how hormesis and the adaptive stress response work together, using calorie restriction as an example. Like gamma rays, extreme calorie restriction (also known as starvation) will kill you. But as we've already seen, just a little bit of CR can work in your favor. Thirty percent calorie restriction is stressful enough, from a dietary perspective, to trigger dramatic physiological changes, all of which fall under the adaptive stress umbrella. These changes enhance cellular maintenance, in order to allow the body to better endure the stress of making do with less food than it would like. As with most adaptive stressors, if CR is maintained long enough, it will leave the body much stronger and more resilient than before.

As we've discussed, the key to looking and feeling young, and to resisting disease like a young person, is optimum cell maintenance. Well, in the presence of physiological stressors like calorie restriction, our bodies focus their energy and resources on the areas that will enhance maintenance in order to prepare themselves for current and future challenges. From a molecular perspective, this means that environmental stressors trigger a cascade of changes in gene expression that will allow us to adapt to the stressors, priming us to take on even greater environmental challenges in the future.

> **Stressors can cause changes in gene expression that help
> the body to adapt to those stressors, strengthening it in the
> process.**

Most of these stressors also appear to have what I call crossover power. For example, exercise not only protects us by enhancing our fitness and increasing our strength, it also markedly reduces inflammation as measured by many biomarkers, including CRP. The huge tissue known as muscle is one of our most powerful anti-inflammatory organs, provided we stress it correctly.

Another example is moderate alcohol consumption. A meta-analysis of numerous clinical and case-control trials involving tens of thousands of people revealed that an alcoholic beverage a day reduces the chances of a heart attack by as much as 30 percent.

> **Certain stressors, when applied at just the right dosages and for the proper duration, dramatically alter whole-body responses such as inflammation and even aging itself.**

So scientists understood that there was a trade-off between cell maintenance and other cellular functions, and that what didn't kill us appeared to make us stronger. But they still struggled to understand the exact nature of the molecular events that laid the groundwork for the protection afforded by the adaptive stress response. Only then could they find something that had all the benefits of CR, without the risks.

As it turns out, it all comes back to controlling chronic, low-level, full-body inflammation.

CHAPTER FIVE

FLIPPING THE SWITCH TO HEALTH: THE MASTER HEALTH REGULATORS

IN 2003, A GROUP OF SCIENTISTS led by David Sinclair, PhD, at Harvard and Leonard Guarente, PhD, at MIT made several scientific observations that were nothing short of revolutionary. Indeed, in my 25 years as a research scientist, I have seen only one other discovery whose importance is on par with this one. That other discovery—of the relevance of defects in apoptosis, or programmed cell death—has delivered us to the threshold of understanding the spread of certain kinds of cancers.

Drs. Sinclair and Guarente were studying the effect of calorie restriction (CR) on the number of times a yeast cell could reproduce. Maybe not the most glamorous stuff, but that's often the way of science. What they found was the research equivalent of a gold mine: a central switchboard for controlling the genes that dictate how long yeast cells live and how many times they divide.

Actually, the switchboard is a biological pathway that the scientists called Sir2. (*Sir* stands for silent information regulator.) Simply put, Sir2 senses how many nutrients are available to an organism in its environment. If nutrients are scarce—as they are when we restrict calories—the switchboard lights up and its activity increases. This activity, in turn, has a major impact on how long an organism lives and/or how many times it can reproduce. For the yeast cells, activating the switchboard extended their life span by a whopping 30 to 40 percent, just like CR.

This discovery in yeast was exciting enough. But things really heated up when mammals, including humans, were found to have a very similar protein switchboard called SIRT1. Then came the discovery of six other SIRT forms—2 to 7—that seem to perform similar tasks to SIRT1 in mammals. The entire family of protein switchboards is collectively known as the sirtuins.

It is thought that all seven sirtuins (SIRTs 1 through 7) deploy in response to the stress of calorie restriction. They sense when the body is running low on nutrients and direct a wide range of metabolic adjustments. So if calorie restriction continues for an extended period, the body gradually reaches a new equilibrium. For instance, insulin sensitivity improves—a great thing when you consider that insulin resistance is a step on the path toward diabetes. Oxygen consumption and physical activity increase, and energy use returns to pre-CR levels. CR provides a turbo boost, too; in animals, we see a marked enhancement of their ability to endure a number of other stressors like heat and alcohol. All of these changes are hallmarks of calorie restriction in mammals.

SIRTUINS: THE MISSING LINK

The Sinclair/Guarente studies—which were published in top scientific journals—shed light on why CR is so effective. They showed that the sirtuin proteins not only dramatically extend life, they also improve health.

> By reducing inflammation, which leads to better cell maintenance, the sirtuins increase life span and overall health.

When scientists turned on the sirtuin switchboard, mammals responded with turbo-charged protection against inflammation—and therefore, against disease and the aging process. Mice with extra copies of SIRT1 did not succumb to cancer. They did not develop insulin resistance, and they showed none of the biomarkers associated with atherosclerosis. Those are diabetes, heart disease, and cancer—three of the most prevalent and most serious medical conditions among humans. Other research has shown similar beneficial changes in biomarkers of human disease when sirtuins increase.

What makes the sirtuin switchboard so remarkable is that it controls the expression of a wide swath of uniquely important genes—genes that are responsible for many of humankind's most pernicious maladies. It's like a master switch for disease. Many of the benefits associated with the sirtuins stem from their ability to control inflammation and obesity. In fact, perhaps the most important finding to date is the capacity of SIRT1 to regulate inflammatory responses by controlling another master regulator, nuclear factor–kappa B (NF-κB).

It's no exaggeration to say that NF-κB is the most important regulator of inflammatory genes that scientists have identified so far. It directs many of the most critical aspects of inflammation, including the ability of inflammatory cells to release inflammatory messengers, to generate an inflammatory response, and to remain at the sites of inflammation.

> **If you can control the master switchboard NF-κB, you
> can control inflammation and therefore most inflammatory
> diseases—including obesity, heart disease, asthma,
> arthritis, and diabetes.**

Scientists believe that the breadth of NF-κB's influence explains how powerful steroid drugs like prednisone block the inflammation associated with diseases like arthritis, allergy, and asthma. When inflammatory cells are on alert, so is NF-κB. Steroids keep the NF-κB switchboard from lighting up, which means that it can't activate the many inflammatory genes under its direction.

Unfortunately, while steroids are very effective in blocking the switchboard, they also come with a host of very toxic side effects. Every person who suffers from a serious inflammatory disease struggles to balance these serious side effects with the drugs' potential benefits. This is one reason that finding the sirtuins is so exciting: The sirtuin switchboards and their connections give us access to an incredibly potent anti-inflammatory weapon— a side-effect-free master health regulator that allows us to turn off the overactive, chronic inflammation that leads to obesity and disease.

By adding what they learned about the sirtuin master health regulator to what they already knew about the adaptive stress response, scientists finally had taken a considerable leap toward solving one of the great scientific mysteries of the last century: why severely restricting calories has such a protective effect on the body.

As we've seen, environmental stress—like the stress of CR, for instance—forces the body into a state of battle-readiness. Scientists now understood that environmental stress works by lighting up the sirtuin switchboards, thus altering which genes are expressed.

You might experience something like this if, for example, you are facing a deadline at work. Your alertness, stamina, concentration, and fluidity of thought sharpen dramatically, while your desire for the creature comforts—food and sleep, for example—decline. The environmental stress—that is, your deadline—fuels optimal performance, for a short time anyway.

So it is with the environmental stressors that activate sirtuin and other regulatory pathways, putting the body on extreme high alert. All of the cells that were sitting back with their feet propped up on the desk suddenly swing into overdrive, buckling down and giving 100 percent. They quell inflammation and fine-tune a number of crucial systems, such as glucose and energy metabolism, to the greatest degree possible.

> **Sirtuins work by shifting your body into battle-readiness, a state of optimum cellular maintenance. Not so coincidentally, this is how your body continuously maintains itself when you're young.**

All of us have heard stories of mothers who, under the influence of adrenaline, find the strength to lift cars in order to save their children. The sirtuins and other master health regulators work in the same way, at a cellular level. The power surge that they provide gives our cells the energy that they need to maintain a healthy weight, suppress inflammation, and inhibit many diseases—indeed, to influence the aging process itself.

CONTROL OVER OUR GENES

In Chapter 4, we talked about how our true biological age (as opposed to our chronological age) is the product of our gene variants and our environment, which together determine the rate at which we grow older. We've always known that we're more or less in control of our environments—which foods we eat, how much exercise we get, that sort of thing. But until recently, we thought that we were stuck with our genes. Healthy lifestyle choices could improve our odds, but inevitably, our genes sealed our fate.

As it turns out, that isn't really the case. The fact is, every one of us is walking around with "bad" genes, and lots of them. Yet not all of us get sick. Two sisters might have the infamous breast cancer gene, for instance, but only one will develop breast cancer. And even those lucky few who are born into families that seem to be genetically blessed—in which generations routinely outlive normal life expectancies and consistently sidestep diseases that befall the rest of us—have been dealt a few bad genetic cards.

As we now understand, it isn't simply the presence of bad gene variants that determines our lot. It's whether (and when) these bad genes get expressed, or turned on—and similarly, whether our protective genes are down-regulated, or turned off.

Some genes roll back processes like inflammation and help our bodies to defend themselves against aging and disease. Others unleash a host of destructive forces like obesity and inflammation, speeding our journey toward sickness and old age. It's a very complicated system that I will do my best to explain through the rest of this book. Simply put, altering gene expression is precisely what our master health regulators—in other words, the sirtuins and other genetic switchboards—are designed to do.

> Selectively controlling critical master health regulators
> allows us to dictate whether or not certain critical genes
> get expressed.

That's why what we're talking about is so powerful: The effect is multiplicative, not just additive. Given the right environmental signal, each master health regulator has the ability to send out thousands of copies of instructions to hundreds of distinct genes that provide information to make individual proteins. These proteins are responsible for all of the biological reactions, good or bad, that take place in your body.

Which master regulators we activate, of course, depends on what we eat and how much we exercise. Up to this point, I've been focusing entirely on the sirtuin pathway. But if research over the past decade is any indication, the powerful sirtuin's just the tip of the iceberg.

> There is clear evidence to suggest that several master health regulators exist.

A number of other master health regulators controlling large groups of genes have been discovered, and several Nobel Prizes have been given for studies demonstrating the importance of these crucial switchboards of gene expression. They include PGC1-alpha (peroxisome proliferator-activated receptor gamma coactivator-1); the PPARs (peroxisome proliferator-activated receptors); NF-κB (nuclear factor–kappa B, which we've already discussed as a master regulator controlling inflammation); the steroid receptors; SREBP (sterol regulatory element binding protein), and Nrf2 (nuclear factor–erythroid 2–related factor 2). Each one plays an absolutely critical role in either optimal cell maintenance or basic metabolism. And each is under the influence of environmental factors, including diet.

As I have said throughout this book, the science is very young but evolving very quickly. What we are learning is exciting indeed, especially for a scientist like me. I have devoted my career to the study of inflammation; every passing year has served to confirm my suspicion that inflammation drives many of humankind's most terrible diseases. What makes this new research so compelling to me personally is knowing, in effect, that Mother Nature agrees with me. So it's with some gratification that I can report that many of the master health regulators, not just the sirtuins, function as switchboards controlling overactive inflammation.

THE SPIDER WEB—REVEALED!

The discovery of the sirtuins and other master health regulators like them has sent a shock wave through the longevity field and a number of related fields. It provided me with a crucial piece of the inflammatory puzzle that I'd been working to put together.

One of the most valuable lessons I learned as a scientist came at the very beginning of my career from one of my mentors, Peter Henson, PhD, at the National Jewish Medical Research Center in Denver. I would often race to Dr. Henson's office after long stints in the laboratory with what I believed was convincing evidence to solve one problem or another. Never taking away the importance of each achievement, Dr. Henson encouraged me to think of medical science more in terms of a spider web, and to always examine every breakthrough within the context of the larger web.

The mastery of individual strands is certainly important in science. But for a treatment to have real and widespread benefit for a complex human disease, it must control either one central strand absolutely or many strands of the web simultaneously—and it must always take into account the web as a whole. As Dr. Henson repeatedly underscored, finding that central strand is unlikely; our chances of influencing the whole web are much better when we affect multiple strands at once.

By the same token, a treatment that targets only one strand of the web probably will be limited in its usefulness. The statin drugs are a good example of this. They excel at lowering cholesterol, yet many folks who take statins still have heart attacks. As we now know, cholesterol is just one strand of the heart disease web, and controlling this biomarker in itself is not nearly enough. We must affect numerous strands—including those that orchestrate the inflammatory response, those that direct the lipid-elevating response, and those that control insulin regulation, to name only a few.

I credit Dr. Henson with instilling in me the scientific instinct to always seek out the broader pattern of the spider web, even when focusing on an individual disease. In doing so, I've come to realize just how exquisitely complex the biological puzzle of inflammatory disease is, and how daunting an adversary.

As more of the spider web came into view, the goal of finding a single solution with sufficient centrality to impact multiple strands simultaneously appeared ever more remote. That began to change as I learned about the relationship between calorie restriction and the sirtuin pathway. It awakened me to the possibility of central switchboards, gatekeepers to health and longevity, not unlike the elixir of life that eluded the alchemists.

The bottom line is this: The 1,000 to 2,000 strands that control the inflammatory response sit squarely at the center of the spider web. And we have the means to affect tens or hundreds of these critical strands all at once, instead of plucking one at a time. How? Through a Gene Smart approach, as you'll see in the next section.

PART TWO

The Bioactive
Prescription

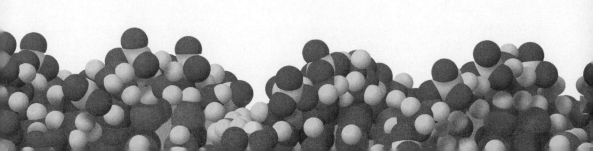

CHAPTER SIX

CR MIMETICS: RESULTS WITHOUT HUNGER

THE DISCOVERY OF SIRTUINS and other master health regulators—the switchboards that control processes as fundamental as how our genes work—is especially good news for those of us with a genetic predisposition toward devastating ailments like heart disease and cancer. It presents us with the extraordinary potential to seize control of our most important genes—in effect, to rewrite our genetic destiny. And we can do it long before the disease process is set in motion.

Looking ahead, this means a profound shift in how we as a society approach disease. At last our healthcare system can get out of a defensive crouch and attack disease before it gains a foothold.

Through the master health regulators, we can have a say in which parts of our individual genetic blueprints are expressed. More precisely, we can prevent pro-inflammatory genes from sending the signal to launch the inflammatory disease process, eliminating the threat before it can cause harm.

> Access to the master health regulators means that we're no longer limited to treating the symptoms of disease. In many cases, we can stop disease before it starts, at the most basic level of all: our genes.

What excites me most about all this is that we're not just thwarting disease, we're restoring balance to our bodies. As current statistics on disease and obesity clearly show, we've been living in a state of imbalance for quite a while. Indeed, our success at restoring balance depends at least in part on our ability to achieve and maintain a healthy weight.

As a scientist, I haven't created the Gene Smart Diet just to help people look better in their bathing suits. We simply can't allow our bodies to be sabotaged by an organ that has an almost unlimited potential to increase in size and simultaneously produce over 100 pro-inflammatory proteins. The organ that I'm talking about is body fat, and its inflammatory effects are a major reason that the obesity epidemic in the United States is such an unprecedented disaster.

Using data from the Centers for Disease Control and Prevention, I've extrapolated what our nation's obesity picture will look like by 2015. If my math is correct, obesity rates in the southeastern United States alone will exceed 35 percent, on average. We're talking about the percentage of the population that's obese, not just overweight (a number that could rise above 80 percent). Our bodies, our healthcare system, and our economy can't absorb the profound effects of this imbalance.

As I've said before, the vast majority of us weigh more than we should not because we're lazy but because we're genetically programmed to store fat, even though it's making us terribly sick. We must change the signals that we're sending to our genes. If we don't, we will be remembered not for our great accomplishments, such as unraveling the human genome, but for hosting the equivalent of a modern-day bubonic plague—ironically, even though we're blessed with the most advanced health care in the history of humanity.

Now is the time for us to act. Thankfully, with the discovery of the master health regulators—and our ability to influence them through diet and lifestyle, as you will do on Gene Smart—we have more control over our genetic destiny than we ever thought possible.

CR MIMETICS: NO STARVATION NECESSARY

The discovery of the master health regulators has been groundbreaking in itself. But even more revolutionary is the realization that there is no wizard behind the wizard. In other words, we're the ones who are manning the controls.

> What we do influences the powerful master health regulators in ways that we could never have imagined possible.

The reason that scientists were so excited about the link between calorie restriction (CR)—the only thing known to extend human longevity—and the sirtuin pathway is this: It meant that an environmental signal was regulating a large swath of our genes. So we weren't necessarily at the mercy of the genetic blueprint we'd inherited from Aunt Millie after all; we could determine whether our bodies "read" harmful genetic instructions or helpful ones simply by changing the environmental signals we were sending. This revolutionized scientific thinking about the degree to which any of us can chart the course of our own health.

Of course, the only environmental signal that scientists knew worked for sure was calorie restriction, and for all the reasons we've already covered, CR just wasn't a workable solution. (You're beginning to see how frustrating it must have been to keep running up against the "CR in the real world" problem, aren't you?)

It is here that we come to understand why the molecular events associated with CR, and their enormous impact on longevity, have been a biological Holy Grail. Knowing how the body kicks into high gear and optimal cellular maintenance when it's under duress begs the question: Can we trick it into doing so, even when it's stress-free?

> Using what we know, can we fool the body into engaging in a high level of cellular maintenance, even while it's in a relatively stable environment? I believe the answer is yes.

We're only beginning to understand this science. But it dovetails closely with dietary epidemiological evidence, interventional clinical trials, animal studies, and even laboratory experiments involving individual cells. The convergence of all of this research suggests that we already have what we need to advance the cells and systems within our bodies from what they're doing now to what they routinely did when we were young—that is, to a better quality of cellular maintenance. Indeed, I believe that activating the central pathways regulating gene expression is our best available protection against the cascade of system failures that leads to inflammation, disease, and aging.

As we now know, calorie restriction is not the only way to advance the transition to optimum cellular maintenance. Other environmental signals influence the body just as CR does; other dietary and lifestyle strategies affect the master health regulators and the genes under their control, just as CR does. But unlike CR, these are real-world solutions, available to anyone with the desire to take charge of their weight and their health.

What we do—specifically, what we eat; how much we eat, to a degree; and how we exercise—gives us a direct line to many of the most important master health regulators. These factors are known as CR mimetics because they mimic many of the effects of CR, inducing the beneficial adaptive stress response that our bodies so desperately need but without the distress that we'd experience if we were restricting calories by 35 to 45 percent. The CR mimetics are the foundation of the Gene Smart Diet. I believe that they're absolutely revolutionary.

> **CR mimetics like the ones in Gene Smart give us many of the biological benefits of calorie restriction, without the discomfort.**

By maximizing our intake of CR mimetic compounds, we can induce the beneficial adaptive stress response, which in turn allows us to directly communicate with thousands of genes. We can encourage them to make many more copies of the proteins that protect us from overweight, overactive inflammation, and premature aging while stopping production of those proteins that might be harmful. Understanding which environmental signals are best—which ones dampen expression of the most destructive genes while activating the most protective ones—is at the core of Gene Smart.

Does the promise of reaping the benefits of calorie restriction with none of the unpleasantness mean that we can disregard calories completely? Sadly, no. Burning more calories than you consume is still the only way to lose weight. But you needn't dramatically restrict calories, either. On Gene Smart, you simply reduce your calorie intake—something that's made considerably easier by other components of the plan. Strategies like eating exactly the right types and amounts of fiber, fish oil, and polyphenols, along with integrating the right types of exercise, will support your weight-loss efforts. And because these are real-world strategies, you're bound to stick with Gene Smart long enough to see results—and stay with it even after you reach your goal weight.

There is strong evidence, too, that the various components of Gene Smart work together to make weight loss a much less arduous and much more positive experience than you may have had in the past. Certainly that's what we saw in our own Hillsdale study: The vast majority of study participants were eating at least 600 calories less per day than they were accustomed to, yet none of them felt hungry. In fact, many of them reported that they couldn't finish their meals. Although we've not yet pinpointed the genes that Gene Smart is influencing, they're almost certainly among the ones that control satiety.

Of course, the "CR without CR" approach of Gene Smart offers many benefits beyond weight loss. Remember, mice with extra copies of the SIRT gene retained muscle tone and stayed in shape even without a great deal of exercise. Comparable studies have yet to be performed in humans, but there's every reason to believe that the results will hold up. Our Hillsdale study panelists, for example, reported significant increases in energy.

The best news of all is that you don't need a prescription for the CR mimetics. You can get them by making a run to the grocery store or simply lacing up your sneakers and heading out for a walk. Sure, it isn't news that "an apple a day keeps the doctor away," but for a long time we had absolutely no idea how the apple worked. Now we know a little better, to the point of being able to determine what kind of apple it should be. The time to implement what we've learned is now.

YOUNGER AND THINNER—AT ANY AGE

As we've discussed, Mother Nature has very little use for us after we reproduce, but she will go to great, almost unbelievable lengths to keep us alive when we're facing extreme environmental stress. The adaptive stress response has been shown to involve a marked increase in cellular maintenance, enhancing our ability to maintain a normal weight and dramatically extending our longevity.

The somewhat surprising observation in all this, at least for me, is that our capacity to kick into optimal maintenance mode seems to be available to

SHIRLEY SOLOMON

AGE: 73

STARTING WEIGHT: 164 pounds

LOST: 15 pounds, 5 inches from waist, 4½ inches from hips during the study; 23 pounds total

CHANGES IN KEY BIOMARKERS IN 8 WEEKS ON GENE SMART

BMI: –2.5 points

BLOOD PRESSURE: –50 mm Hg systolic, –5 mm Hg diastolic

RESTING HEART RATE: unchanged (60 beats per minute)

CIRCULATING INSULIN: Over 99 percent lower

HEMOGLOBIN A1C: 19 percent lower

FASTING LEPTIN: 60 percent lower

CIRCULATING LONG-CHAIN OMEGA-3s: 41 percent higher

" My family has a history of high blood pressure and heart problems, so I felt like I needed to do something about my weight. I want to be around for a long time!

I'd always been a very active person; I used to play tennis for hours. But then I developed macular degeneration and could no longer drive. I've always loved to cook, so it wasn't a good situation: I just stayed at home and cooked and ate! I tried Weight Watchers, but because of the macular degeneration, I couldn't count the points; it was hard enough to find something on the menu that appealed to me, let alone to do the calculations.

Getting off the sugar and starches—the cakes, the breads, the chips—was

some degree at any age. As far as we know, nature hasn't restricted it to just our reproductive years.

My neighbor, Herb, may be the best embodiment of this phenomenon that I know of. In his early sixties, Herb was what you might call a walking heart attack—overweight, with high cholesterol and insulin resistance. And he did have a heart attack, an event that he describes as the ultimate wake-up call. He adopted a very healthy diet, began a twice-a-day regimen of aerobic exercise and weight training—and, not surprisingly, lost weight. He's now in his late seventies, and when he runs around the neighborhood with his shirt off, there isn't a man on our block who wouldn't want to look like him. His only major for me. As I said, I've always loved to cook, and in my family, we discussed what we were going to have for dinner while we were still sitting down to lunch. Eating cereal for breakfast was probably the single biggest change for me. I wasn't a big breakfast eater before doing Gene Smart; when I did eat breakfast, it was a cup of coffee and a couple of Krispy Kreme donuts. Now when I have cereal for breakfast, I can eat half a sandwich for lunch and feel full. After all that fiber, I'm just not that hungry.

I don't cook as much, but I've found a whole new outlet for my energy: I'm at the gym! A friend and I try to go 4 days a week. Exercise changes the way you feel about everything. For example, my outlook on food is totally different now. I can look at a piece of cake and think, 'It's not worth it!' With exercise, it's very easy for me to say thanks, but no thanks.

It's also very motivating when you understand enough of the science to know that you are really making a difference in your health. I know that that helped me with making choices. I was doing Gene Smart for my health, and to get rid of inflammation. The weight loss was almost secondary—a nice side effect. The emphasis for me was on a healthy body.

People look at me and say, 'How much weight have you lost?' I'm down 23 pounds now; I kept losing even after the study was over. Even though I need to lose more, I'm wearing clothes that I haven't worn in years. I was a 14, and I'm back down to a 10. Also, with my doctor's blessing, I'm taking my blood pressure medication every other day; I'm going to ask about reducing the dosage again.

I consider myself very fortunate to have had the opportunity to be part of this study, and to follow Gene Smart for my health. I've never felt elderly, and I sure didn't want to look elderly, either. Guess what? I'm not one of those round ladies anymore! And if a 73-year-old can be successful on this plan, then a 40-year-old surely can.**"**

regrets are that it took him so long to "get with the program"—and that more of his friends didn't hear the wake-up call when he did, before it was too late.

It's my guess that nature never needed to worry about enhanced cellular maintenance kicking in at an older age because other factors typically killed us humans before we could achieve a maximum life span. That's probably why we've retained this capacity for so long. It's a great thing for us because it means that we can tap into the CR mimetics and the adaptive stress response at any point in life. It's never too late: Just ask Shirley Solomon, a 73-year-old Hillsdale study participant who feels as though she's not just 23 pounds lighter but 23 years younger since starting Gene Smart.

CHAPTER SEVEN

THE BIOACTIVES: NATURE'S DRUGSTORE

IN MY PREVIOUS BOOK, *Inflammation Nation,* I talked at length about the challenge facing my sister and many others with rheumatoid arthritis. She and her doctors must constantly weigh the potential benefit of alleviating her symptoms with steroids against the harm inflicted to the rest of her body by these powerful drugs. At first blush, the best solution would seem to be a steroid with fewer side effects, right? That is one option—and the scientist who comes up with it will be as rich as Croesus, which is why some of the best minds in medicine are on it.

There is another way, however. And as so often happens when we put our eyes to the microscope, we're finding that Mother Nature got to it first.

NATURE'S DRUGSTORE

We've long known that a diet rich in whole grains, fruits, vegetables, and fish is good for us. Our instinct is certainly borne out by the epidemiological evidence: People from cultures that eat more of these foods tend to be healthier. My dad used to say to me, "That white bread you're eating will kill you faster than cigarettes." I'm not sure he was right about that—but he *was* right to avoid white bread. Until recently, though, we didn't know much more than he did about why.

In the history of nutrition science, we've tended to focus on macronutrients, the big building blocks that make up foods—things like carbohydrates and proteins and fats. Further refinement led to the discovery of vitamins and minerals. More recently, as nutrition has gotten even more specific, we've become aware of certain very powerful nutritional compounds called *bioactives*.

Generally, bioactives are minor components. But just because they're small doesn't mean that we should underestimate their influence over our physiological and cellular activities. Bioactive compounds aren't nutrients in the classical sense; that is, they're usually not essential for life. But emerging research suggests that they are essential for good health—as powerful as some of our most sophisticated pharmaceuticals, but with an unerring precision that we're light-years away from duplicating in a laboratory.

Essentially, the bioactives are Mother Nature's pharmacy. They are potent and have terrific efficacy, even in very small quantities. And they are comparatively safe, because unlike pharmaceuticals, bioactives have developed along with our bodies to be used by them. More precisely, they interact directly with the master health regulators that control our genes.

> **Control the bioactives—by eating them or avoiding them— and you dictate the expression of genes or the activity of enzymes and cellular receptors that control your health.**

I believe that our new understanding of bioactives, together with advances in the field of nutrigenomics, will revolutionize how we think about food and

What's a Bioactive?

Bioactive compounds:

- Typically occur in small amounts in foods
- Are not nutrients, in the classical sense; that is, they typically are not essential for life, a fundamental criterion for a nutrient
- Influence physiological or cellular activities, usually resulting in a beneficial health effect

- Modify disease risk, rather than preventing deficiency diseases
- Act as inducers and inhibitors of enzymes, inhibitors of receptor activity, and inducers and inhibitors of gene expression
- Can mimic an adaptive stress response in animals and humans when ingested

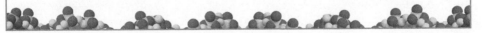

medicine. We are one step closer to understanding how the foods we eat, and those we avoid, can help to treat and prevent many of the most devastating chronic diseases affecting humankind.

Over the course of this book, we'll explore three categories of bioactives, including two that you may already be somewhat familiar with: fiber and the omega-3 fatty acids (though perhaps not in this context). But the story of the power behind the bioactives and their ability to affect gene expression begins with the category known as polyphenols.

THE FRENCH PARADOX AND THE POLYPHENOLS

Polyphenols are a large family—numbering more than 4,000, by current count—of diverse compounds widely distributed in plants and their fruits. They can be found in most legumes; in fruits such as apples, blackberries, blueberries, cantaloupe, cherries, cranberries, grapes, pears, plums, raspberries, and strawberries; and in vegetables such as broccoli, cabbage, celery, onions, and parsley. Other sources include red wine, chocolate, green tea, olive oil, bee pollen, and many grains.

Much of the initial interest in polyphenols grew from a phenomenon known as the French paradox. The French eat an astonishing amount of fat— four times as much butter as we Americans, 60 percent more cheese, and three times as much pork. Yet despite their high-fat diets—an established cardiovascular risk factor—French populations have a comparatively low incidence of cardiovascular disease. In fact, the incidence of death from coronary heart disease among French men is one-third that among American men.

The French also are considerably thinner than we Americans are. Every American woman I know who visits France comes home in complete bewilderment over how her French counterparts eat such robust meals with such obvious pleasure, yet still manage to fit into the latest Parisian fashions.

One explanation for the paradox grew out of the French habit of consuming red wine with meals. Besides eating a lot more fat, the French drink a lot more wine—an estimated 100 to 150 bottles per person per year, compared to 10 bottles for the average American.

In their attempt to understand how red wine might exert a protective effect, scientists began looking more closely at what is in the wine. We have known for a long time that grapes, blackberries, strawberries, and other purple-red fruits contain a number of polyphenols, including trans-resveratrol, anthocyanins, and ellagitannins. The health benefits of these compounds are well established.

Among scientists, the conventional wisdom was that these benefits derived from the antioxidant effects of the polyphenols. Oxidation at the cellular level is often compared to the rust that forms on metal, and is thought to contribute to both cancer and premature aging. So an entire industry sprang up around the antioxidant potential of the purple-red "superfoods."

But this may be a case where we leapt to a conclusion about a treatment modality before we were certain of its effects. According to the most recent study data, something other than their antioxidant properties is likely responsible for the polyphenols' benefits. In fact, some evidence suggests that their antioxidant properties may be harmful.

For example, a 2005 study from Johns Hopkins showed that the powerful antioxidant vitamin E actually increases mortality. This was followed by several large-scale studies, the largest of which examined data from 68 randomized clinical trials involving more than 230,000 participants. This meta-analysis, which appeared in *JAMA* in 2007, concluded that the most popular and common antioxidants may actually increase mortality.

Research from my own lab has revealed that some cancerous cells may require some amount of oxidative stress in order to produce the necessary signals that promote programmed cell death, the very thing that stops cancer from running untrammeled throughout our bodies. This may explain in part why we're seeing these disturbing connections between antioxidants and cancer: because oxidation, apparently, isn't always a bad thing.

Newer studies involving many polyphenols suggest that the health benefits of purple-red fruits have less to do with their antioxidant properties than with their impact on the master health regulators. In fact, revolutionary new research in the area of nutrigenomics has revealed that several bioactives control the master health regulators, which in turn control gene expression.

> **Polyphenolic compounds in fruits and vegetables have been shown to actively call down the protective effects of the master health regulators, just like calorie restriction.**

It was an in-depth investigation of one particular polyphenol, trans-resveratrol, that led scientists to their current understanding of the CR mimetics.

TRANS-RESVERATROL: THE CR—AND EXERCISE!—MIMETIC

Trans-resveratrol, or simply resveratrol, is produced by several plants when they're under environmental stress. Epidemiological studies confirm the role of resveratrol consumption in a wide range of health benefits, including protection against atherosclerosis, cancer, and neurodegenerative disease. We now believe these health benefits to be inextricably linked to resveratrol's effects on the master health regulators that control our genes.

Experiments from the Harvard laboratory of David Sinclair, PhD, as reported in the journal *Nature* in 2003, demonstrated that resveratrol significantly extends the life span of yeast. Subsequent studies involving worms, fish, and fruit flies found a similar effect in these organisms.

According to another paper published in *Nature* that same year, of the 18 naturally occurring polyphenol-like compounds common in our food supply, resveratrol most potently activates the master health regulator SIRT1. As you'll recall, this is precisely what calorie restriction (CR) does, too.

Even more astonishing results came from a paper that appeared in *Nature* in 2006. It revealed that mice fed resveratrol lived the same length of time and had the same motor skills whether they were placed on a "healthy" low-fat diet or on a very high-fat diet. Imagine: a compound, found in food, that has the potential to protect us from our unhealthy habits!

Duplicating CR's effects, as resveratrol appears to do, is a pretty impressive claim in itself. But scientists now suspect that resveratrol has potential not just as a CR mimetic but as an exercise mimetic as well!

That's the conclusion drawn by Johan Auwerx, PhD, and his colleagues at the Institute of Genetics and Molecular and Cellular Biology in Illkirch, France, in a paper published in the journal *Cell* in 2006. Dr. Auwerx and his team devised an animal study to test the effects of high doses of resveratrol on exercise endurance in mice. A typical laboratory mouse can run roughly 1 kilometer on a treadmill before collapsing from exhaustion. But when mice were given up to 400 milligrams of resveratrol per kilogram of body weight, they were able to run twice as far as mice not given resveratrol. Further, the treated animals were found to have energy-charged muscles (i.e., more mitochondria) and a lower heart rate, characteristics usually seen in trained athletes. "Resveratrol makes you look like a trained athlete, without the training," Dr. Auwerx says. He believes that the results of this animal study could be replicated in humans.

A more recent study, conducted by Ronald Evans, PhD, in his laboratory at the Salk Institute, reveals that activation of another master health regulator called PPAR-delta supercharged the endurance of mice by 75 percent. In a *New York Times* interview, Dr. Evans stated, "It's a little bit like a free lunch without the calories, and it's likely to apply to people."

The near-magical properties of resveratrol and other potent bioactives don't end there. They also interfere with the three stages of cancer formation and modulate the master regulator NF-κB. As you'll remember, NF-κB has an almost unlimited capacity to control inflammation, especially considering that it's closely associated with two of the most powerful master regulators, the sirtuins and the steroid receptors. It also may protect against neuronal cell dysfunction and cell death, which means that in theory, it could help in our fight against devastating diseases such as Alzheimer's and Huntington's.

By now you might be thinking "Sign me up!" And I wouldn't blame you. A lot of people would love to take advantage of a compound that could eliminate the need for exercise while preventing cancer and extending life span. Bonus: You can get it by drinking red wine!

But resveratrol is not quite ready for prime time. As its critics are happy to point out, all of the studies so far, though impressive, have been done in animals. The doses that are being given to these animals are extremely high, and impossible for us humans to obtain from ordinary foods. If you tried to get comparable amounts of resveratrol from red wine, for instance, you'd die from alcohol poisoning long before you reaped any of the health benefits. Resveratrol is available in supplement form, but right now, finding high-quality products that are safe and effective can be complicated. My laboratory is very interested in this promising bioactive, and as I learn more, I will share it with you on my Web site, www.genesmart.com.

The critics may be right regarding the amounts of resveratrol in common foods, but I think they're missing the bigger picture. For me, just realizing that science has the capacity to induce an animal to live much longer—even on an extremely high-fat diet, using only a food-based bioactive—makes this a discovery of almost unparalleled importance. The fact that we now have the ability to turn an animal of average fitness into a four-legged Lance Armstrong with no additional exercise is equally astonishing.

There's another point that the critics may be overlooking. Resveratrol isn't the only polyphenol, or the most important—even in red wine. Wine alone is reported to contain over 50 polyphenols; certainly one of them could have potent bioactivity and be present at higher concentrations. Further, one or more of them could be working synergistically to produce effects that might explain the epidemiological evidence. Right now we simply don't have all the information we need to know for sure why polyphenols work.

Certainly, polyphenols are not the only bioactives. In fact, they're the ones we know the least about. Many scientists, including myself, believe that the power of the bioactive is behind the well-known health benefits of fiber and fish oils. Unlike the polyphenols, these substances have been scrutinized in a wide range of interventional clinical trials, which collectively have shown us just how powerfully beneficial fiber and the omega-3s can be.

> **Large-scale studies have conclusively shown that when you increase your daily fiber intake as outlined in the delicious Gene Smart meal plans, you can reduce your risk of a fatal heart attack by a whopping 40 to 60 percent.**

Fiber is strongly cardioprotective, and it's a great weight-loss aid. I believe it's a major reason that our own Hillsdale study was so incredibly successful. You see, fiber is intrinsically linked to satiety—the sensation of being full. Feeling satisfied after a meal is the single most important component of weight-loss success. After all, why else would people cheat on a diet, if not because they're hungry? But the vast majority of our Hillsdale Study participants did not feel hungry at all. And we know that weight loss is a powerful anti-inflammatory strategy in its own right.

As for the omega-3s, we understand so much about the inflammatory

A Note about the Omegas

One of the definitions of the bioactives is that technically, we don't need them. That's not really true about the omega fatty acids known as long-chain omegas. We do need them, and not getting enough of them in our diets leads to a deficiency.

These omega fats do have a powerful impact on gene expression, though. So for the purpose of this book, I include them as bioactives.

diseases affected by the long-chain omegas, and the dosages necessary to make a difference, that we can be aggressively prescriptive with these beneficial fats—more so than with any other bioactive.

Harnessing the power of the bioactives is like finding a treasure map directing us to the fountain of youth. As I said before, our predisposition to disease is influenced by three factors: our genes, the time we're living in, and our environment. With our growing knowledge of the bioactive switches, we have the unprecedented opportunity to design ways to control both.

> **The bioactive prescription gives us power over both the environmental factors and the genetic factors that dictate the state of our health.**

It's a whole new world. With these discoveries, I believe that we are in position to begin directing the fundamental mechanisms that influence weight loss, health, and even aging. These powerful command centers can set in motion the biological imbalances that give rise to disease and the cascade of system failures associated with the downward spiral of aging, or they can send signals to protect us from these things. Which way the scale tips is up to us.

CHAPTER EIGHT

STRETCHED TO THE LIMIT

WHAT WE HOLD IN OUR HANDS is a double-edged sword. Before we can fully understand how the master health regulators that control our genes (and the bioactives that control them) can help us, I believe we must answer the question of what's gone wrong with these health-giving regulators. Then we may begin to solve the scientific mystery that has followed my entire career: why so many Americans currently find themselves so very sick.

AN INFLAMMATION NATION

One of the things that has baffled the scientists who are studying the epidemic of inflammatory disease (I include myself in this list) is that it comes at a time when American medicine and hygiene are unsurpassed.

Although our healthcare system is far from perfect, more Americans have access to care now than at any time in the past. And contrary to reports that try to scare you into thinking otherwise, the care to which they have access is much better than it has ever been. We have more sophisticated diagnostic tools, more advanced surgical techniques, and some of the safest, most precise and effective pharmaceuticals in the world.

And yet we find ourselves staring down an unprecedented—and everworsening—disease epidemic.

> Health care is getting better, yet the state of America's
> health is getting worse.

What is going on? Why are we so sick?

As I contemplate these questions, I wonder if we're going about answering them in the wrong way. Is it possible that the sophistication of our health care has blinded us to the real seriousness of the problem we currently face? If we're so sick, given the wisdom of our doctors and the ease with which we can tap into their knowledge, then what the Sam Hill would happen to us without them? Maybe we should stop wondering why we're so sick and instead thank God that we're not sicker.

Let me give you a very simple example. To celebrate my publisher's interest in this book, I took my family out to dinner. Now, the Chiltons are dedicated carnivores, which made a steakhouse the obvious choice for a celebration. Not surprisingly for a steakhouse, the portions were gargantuan; each of us at the table found ourselves contemplating a piece of meat five or six times larger than it should have been, containing a day's worth of fat or worse. Our plates were also piled high with classic steakhouse "vegetable" sides, including creamed spinach, potatoes whipped with butter and topped with gravy, onion rings fried crispy brown, and a wedge of iceberg lettuce topped with blue cheese.

Before digging in, I looked around at our fellow diners, all of whom were sitting in front of similarly groaning tables. It occurred to me that while our visit to this restaurant was for a special occasion, the waiter seemed pretty familiar with most everyone else—predominantly business guys eating out on their expense accounts. As I looked at their stomachs straining against button-down oxfords, I knew that if I'd been able to turn on my x-ray vision, I would have seen prescription vials in every one of their briefcases—the statins for high cholesterol, the beta blockers for high blood pressure, the insulin for diabetes, the Viagra for the side effects of the others.

I'm certainly not criticizing the guys in that restaurant; I live in that glass house, too, so I'm not about to throw stones at it. In fact, that night, I was having a party in it—to celebrate a health book, of all things! But what crossed my mind then, and what scares me now, is this: I don't think we have any idea how sick we are. Oh, we see the statistics on obesity and disease, and we know that they're on the rise. But do we truly understand how sick we are, and how sick we're going to be?

It kind of reminds me of a leaky old hose: You can keep on repairing it, but eventually no amount of duct tape will be able to seal off all of the little holes. Now think of those holes as environmental factors like poor eating habits and lack of exercise—the kinds of things that fail to trigger our protective master health regulators. The very best of modern medicine—the early interventions, the cutting-edge medical procedures, the groundbreaking pharmaceuticals—might be able to patch the hose sufficiently. But even they can do only so much.

In my previous book, *Inflammation Nation*, I noted a real surprise emerging from epidemiological studies: The more developed the country, the worse the inflammatory epidemic. In other words, the current tidal wave of disease isn't happening despite the extraordinary quality of our healthcare system and relative affluence as a country; it seems to be happening because of it. I referred to this phenomenon as *affluenza*.

It makes sense, given what we now know about how the human body kicks into high gear when it's subjected to certain stressors—like calorie restriction (CR), for example. Think about it: The only thing proven to extend life is CR, yet the United States produces 30 percent more calories for every man, woman, and child than we actually should eat. Our affluence has led to excessive calorie intake, which suppresses the adaptive stress response rather than activating it, as CR does.

Now Gene Smart isn't a calorie-restricted diet; in fact, what I'm promising is many of the benefits of CR without CR. But we need to make some correction to the amount of calories we consume, because what we as a society are doing right now is exactly the opposite of activating the adaptive stress response. And all those extra calories mean that we're also building ever-larger fat stores, which produce over 100 pro-inflammatory proteins.

> **The current conditions of American life prevent us from experiencing anything in the way of an adaptive stress response that might help protect us from disease.**

I now see our nation's health as a pitched battle between two opposing forces. On one side is the very best of modern health care, putting up a great fight. On the other—and, I fear, the winning—side are the environmental factors that continue to make us fat and sick.

WHY DRUGS CAN'T BE THE (ONLY) ANSWER

Still, why should we worry? After all, we have our world-class medications, which are getting better all the time.

Because the booming $40 billion a year "natural medicine" industry proves that many of us are willing, if not desperate, to find a solution besides pharmaceuticals to our health problems. Please don't misunderstand; I don't in any way oppose the use of pharmaceuticals. In fact, I've helped to identify the pathways for a number of medications currently on the market. I've seen how beneficial they can be—both for myself and for people like my sister, who has rheumatoid arthritis. In my opinion, they're nothing short of miraculous.

On the other hand, if you talk to people like Jeff Woosley, a Hillsdale Study participant whose story appears on page 79, you'll find that a lot of them—especially those with poor family histories like his (and mine)—would prefer to enlist the body's natural ability to protect and heal itself. Turning to drugs has consequences—costs both obvious and hidden, if you will.

For me, one of the most eye-opening and chilling statistics comes from the World Health Organization, which ranks the United States as number one in healthcare spending (by a long shot) but number 37 in healthcare performance. This is not because we charge so much more for health care (we do, but that's not the whole story), and it certainly is not because we have poor health care (it's the best in the world).

To go back to our hose metaphor, we are simply putting so many holes in the hose, thanks to our diet and lifestyle, that repairing all of them would be incredibly expensive. At a certain point, the hose would become irreparable because it's damaged so badly. That's why we're spending an enormous amount on health care, but getting poor results.

Here's an overview of some of the costs.

1. The Expense

Modern health care is expensive—for us as individuals, and for us as a society. Some of the latest data available are from 2005. That year, the United States spent over $2 trillion on health care, or about $6,700 per person. The average annual premium for an employer health plan covering a family of four was nearly $11,500.

Back then, healthcare spending was expected to hold steady at 16 percent of the gross domestic product (GDP) for 2006. By 2015, however, it could rise to 20 percent of the GDP. That's over $4 trillion.

And what are we buying with these tremendous sums? Not good health, certainly. In fact, we're barely keeping our head above water.

2. The Side Effects

Every drug, no matter how safe, has side effects. So each time we take a drug, there is a risk-to-benefit equation we must consider.

Certain side effects are truly devastating, and potentially life-threatening. I know this from sad experience. As I mentioned before, my sister Tammy has suffered from debilitating rheumatoid arthritis since we were children; watching her struggle with the disease strongly motivated my decision to devote my career to the study of inflammation. If you've ever known anyone with rheumatoid arthritis, then you understand what a monstrous disease it is. During a flare-up, even the simplest movement can cause excruciating pain.

One of the tremendous injustices associated with the disease is that we already have a category of drugs that's the next best thing to a cure. Steroids can effectively silence Tammy's flare-ups. So why doesn't she just belly up to the methylprednisolone bar and enjoy the rest of her life without debilitating pain?

Because it could kill her.

The first sentence of the side effects profile states matter-of-factly that "Side effects of methylprednisolone and other corticosteroids range from mild annoyances to serious irreversible bodily damage." It then goes on—for three more pages—to detail the profound and far-reaching damage these drugs can do.

You see, steroids work by down-regulating some genes and up-regulating others. Unfortunately, the swath of genes under the drugs' control is wide—too wide.

JEFF WOOSLEY

AGE: 42

STARTING WEIGHT: 201 pounds

LOST: 16.8 pounds, 6 inches from waist, 4.1 percent body fat

CHANGES IN KEY BIOMARKERS IN 8 WEEKS ON GENE SMART

BMI: −2.4 points

BLOOD PRESSURE: −14 mm Hg systolic, −2 mm Hg diastolic

RESTING HEART RATE: −20 beats per minute

TRIGLYCERIDES: 50 percent lower

CRP: 30 percent lower

INSULIN: 53 percent lower

FASTING LEPTIN: 61 percent lower

CIRCULATING LONG-CHAIN OMEGA-3s: 25 percent increase

❝ I went on Gene Smart because I was getting discouraged and frustrated; I wasn't happy with where I was. I've never been overweight per se, but your metabolism slows down as you get older, and I had 5 or 10 pounds that I couldn't get rid of.

For me, it was more of a health issue. Both my dad and my grandfather died of heart attacks, my dad at 58. Both had high blood pressure and high cholesterol; I'm on cholesterol medication, so I felt like this was something I really needed to address.

I didn't realize how important it was to eat enough! Before I started Gene Smart, I was having just two or three meals a day. Once I started eating more often, and the right foods, I really saw a difference. And the combination of diet and exercise is crucial. Dr. Chilton really helped us to understand that we couldn't just get on a treadmill and read a book; we had to work out.

Honestly, it was much easier than I had thought it would be. I had tried different diets, including South Beach, but they were hard to stick with. On Gene Smart, there were a lot of good foods. And it was easy: There was nothing I had to search for, nothing prepackaged I had to spend a lot of money on, no crazy preparations. I could make an albacore tuna sandwich, throw some nuts and a Fiber One bar in a bag, and that was it.

In 8 weeks, I lost 6 inches from my waist. I don't know if it was the fish oil or the exercise, but the aches and pains I was having in my shoulders and neck have gone away. ❞

Steroids are able to block critical inflammatory genes, the ones that drive the symptoms of rheumatoid arthritis. Blocking these genes, of course, is a very good thing, because it helps alleviate Tammy's symptoms. But the drugs don't stop there. They also mess indiscriminately with a host of other genes, leaving Tammy susceptible to infection and osteoporosis and suppressing the activity of her adrenal glands, which can lead to nausea, vomiting, and even shock. And then there's the potential for fluid retention, weight gain, high blood pressure, potassium loss, headache, muscle weakness, facial puffiness and hair growth, easy bruising, glaucoma, cataracts, peptic ulceration, worsening diabetes, irregular menses, growth retardation (in children), convulsions, and psychological disturbances.

Now I want to be clear on my point here, so people with life-threatening medical conditions don't refuse their doctors' orders to take steroids when necessary. I am not opposed to steroid treatment. When my oldest son, Josh, was admitted to the Johns Hopkins Hospital at age 2 with severe, life-threatening asthma, I wanted him on systemic steroids as soon as possible. Saving his life certainly outweighed any side effects that he might have experienced in the short term. I'm simply noting that the side effects are part of the package, which means that doctors like Tammy's are constantly struggling with a very cruel risk-to-benefit ratio: How well can they alleviate her symptoms without completely destroying her body in the process? It's like being surrounded by the ocean and dying of thirst.

Other pharmaceuticals, of course, are milder, and have less severe side effects. And if the trade-off is saving your life, then who's going to complain about a little depression, a little shaking of the hands, a little less vigor in the bedroom department than you used to have? Still, while the side effects might be minor—especially when compared to a heart attack—they present fairly major quality-of-life issues for the people who must cope with them.

Sure, other medications—Viagra is one example—can counteract or compensate for some of the side effects we experience when we're treating our inflammatory conditions. But aren't they just more patches applied to a leaky hose? I'd bet the farm that if there were a way to achieve the same results without any of the side effects and without additional medication, most people would take advantage of it.

Actually, I don't have to bet anything. All I need to do is look at the growing number of people who are turning to alternative therapies. As I said before, they're a $40 billion industry. Unfortunately, I'm not convinced that they're a good value either, considering that in many cases, the alternatives offer no established record of safety or evidence of effectiveness.

3. Safety

This is the big one, isn't it? We've done a good job of developing medications to help the people that they're intended for. But we have not done a perfect job, as the 2004 Vioxx disaster proves beyond a shadow of a doubt. (And just so you don't think I'm throwing stones at the pharmaceutical industry, you should know that I was an author on one of the original papers describing the novel enzyme that gave way to this category of drugs.)

Nor are the COX-2 inhibitors the only example of this phenomenon. In 2000, Bayer recalled Baycol, a popular statin drug designed to lower cholesterol, after studies linked it to a series of fatalities resulting from a rare musculoskeletal disorder. And in 2008, the diabetes drug Avandia was recalled after a report in the *New England Journal of Medicine* suggested that it might increase the risk of heart attack by as much as 43 percent.

Again, I'm not sharing this information to scare you into dumping the contents of your medicine cabinet down the drain. I simply want you to be aware that there's almost always a cost—known or unknown—to treating serious inflammatory disease, and that we (along with our doctors) must assess that cost at each level of disease management. It's called a benefit-to-risk equation for this reason.

4. Treatment of the Symptoms, Not the Underlying Driver

For me, the Vioxx story leads to the principal reason that we cannot permit our superior pharmaceutical technology to allow us to become complacent about understanding and addressing what is making us sick: While medications may be very effective, they almost always are treating only the symptoms and not the underlying driver of disease.

> When we settle for treating symptoms, it means that we are not controlling inflammation, the underlying driver of disease.

Since my book *Inflammation Nation* was published in 2005, I've spoken to hundreds of lay groups about inflammatory conditions and dietary solutions to those conditions. In many cases, these are support groups for people living with Crohn's disease, COPD, psoriasis, or severe arthritis.

Everyone is very grateful for the medications they're taking, but if I hear one thing over and over, it's a collective fear that they're treating just the most superficial manifestations of their conditions. They instinctively know that the primary underlying cause—chronic inflammation—is out of control. I don't know how they know, but they do.

Now you might be thinking, if inflammation causes arthritis, but meds allow people with arthritis to live and work without too much pain, then why bother with the underlying inflammation at all? This is where our hose analogy is really effective. You see, plugging a leak doesn't address the underlying problem with the defective hose; it's only a matter of time before the hose springs another leak, and another, and another. As systemic, whole-body, chronic inflammation persists year after year, the "hose" gets weaker and weaker.

People marvel at how different the diseases under the inflammatory umbrella are, but what amazes me is how often they occur together. For instance, rheumatoid arthritis has been associated with a 60 percent increase in risk of congestive heart failure and a 40 percent increase in risk of myocardial infarction. All of these conditions have an inflammatory component. Likewise, psoriasis has been linked to heart disease and diabetes; asthma to obesity; and so on.

Just as the only way to really make sure that no water leaks out of that old hose is to turn off the faucet, the only way to guarantee that we're free of all of these pernicious diseases is to shut down the chronic, full-body inflammation that drives them.

ARE THE REGULATORS BROKEN?

So what we have is a dramatically overweight nation in dramatically poor health, held together by a network of sophisticated if sometimes flawed pharmaceuticals and medical procedures. Hardly ideal, as I think you'd agree. And yet we just spent the previous chapters exploring a series of master health regulators, designed to keep our cells functioning optimally, especially under stress.

So what's going on? Why are we so overweight and sick when every one of us is equipped with these primitive life-saving regulators, which supposedly kick in to ensure our survival? Because our environmental circumstances, including our diet and lifestyle, have changed so dramatically.

There's nothing wrong with the master health regulators. The problem is that in some cases, we're feeding them—literally *feeding* them—the wrong signals. In other cases, we are not feeding them at all, because they don't recognize the foods we're eating or the exercises we're doing.

> It is not that our master health regulators aren't working,
> but that we're unwittingly doing something to suppress
> these genetic switches.

Either way, instead of sending the signals that call down the body's natural protectiveness, we're turning the dial toward disease and premature aging.

At this moment in time, we have access to the best drugs that science can design. These wonder drugs are keeping us around longer, with a better quality of life than we might otherwise have. But it seems very clear to me that the best health care in the history of humanity is failing to keep pace with an ever-increasing threat from our primitive genetics, which is why we find ourselves so very sick. Without our pharmaceuticals, we'd probably be much sicker.

> The harder we drive our bodies in the wrong direction, the
> more help we need.

Our life expectancy is the result of this constant tug-of-war between cutting-edge science and the primitive genetic drivers, which are tipping the scale toward aging. This is why we now find ourselves losing the battle for our health. I believe the entire problem can be summed up in a single sentence: Our medicine has become our food, instead of our food being our medicine, as Hippocrates suggested it should be.

GRASPING THE LEVERS

There is no better defense mechanism in the universe than the human body's, as long as it is fully activated and operating in top form, as it is under stress. Unfortunately, this first and best line of defense has been sorely compromised, in large part because our food and lifestyle choices are sending the wrong messages to our master health regulators. We're unwittingly instructing our bodies to deregulate destructive inflammation and shift away from optimal maintenance, putting us at increased risk for disease and the physical decline associated with aging.

> **Environmental factors, in the form of bioactives and exercise, are the levers that we use to control the master health regulators.**

While I knew that diet and lifestyle factors were not just casually linked but absolutely and directly related to the inflammation epidemic, I could not have imagined the critical strands that connected them. My eureka moment came with the emerging science from the longevity field, describing the sirtuins. It illuminated why seemingly innocuous and ostensibly unrelated environmental factors so drove the epidemic of epidemics: Each one affects the master health regulators, directly or indirectly.

With an understanding of the impact of calorie restriction and CR mimetics such as trans-resveratrol on the primitive but powerful master regulators, I began to realize something else: that we've taken beneficial stress away from our bodies, when in fact they may be genetically programmed to need it. I believe this to be a major reason that we struggle so desperately with our weight, and that we're so very sick. We must change course if we hope to regain control of our weight and our health.

CHAPTER NINE

DIET AND THE MASTER HEALTH REGULATORS

TO FULLY UNDERSTAND the feedback loop between environmental factors and the master health regulators, it might be best to consider how these regulators operated in the setting where they first developed: the primordial forest. This is the environment for which our bodies are designed.

What do I mean? Think of it this way: For more than 100,000 generations, we humans were hunter-gatherers. Then about 500 generations ago, we moved into agriculture, and we've depended on it ever since. By comparison, only three or four generations have passed since the Industrial Revolution—and only one has grown up on highly processed urbanized food.

Why is this important? Because 99.9 percent of our genes developed *before* the introduction of agriculture.

You see, over extremely long periods—say, 100,000 generations—environmental conditions determine which genes are present in a given species, as well as how and when those genes are expressed. Let's suppose you have a genetic mutation that makes it particularly easy for you to digest a certain type of food, and your tribe happens to live in an area surrounded by trees that provide the food. This is an advantageous adaptation; it means that you're more likely to flourish than your neighbor who can't tolerate the food. You then pass the gene to your offspring. This process is known as natural selection, and it represents the ongoing interaction between a species genome and its environment—including its diet—over the course of hundreds of thousands of years.

Natural selection is what happened with us humans. Our bodies developed to tolerate certain diets and environmental conditions during those

100,000 generations; these same factors determined the contents of the packets of information in the 25,000 to 30,000 functional genes of the human genome.

During our tenure as hunter-gatherers, it was not just which genes would be present that was set but also how many forms of each gene would be made, how the genes would work, and when they would be expressed. You see, our bodies also developed the ability to "translate" environmental feedback into signals that would allow us to express whichever genes were most likely to ensure survival under changing conditions.

Let's say there was an inadequacy in our food supply—calorie restriction, by any other name. Our bodies had to adapt in order to survive under those conditions, so they learned to read the information coming from the environment. If a famine was on the horizon, chemicals in our food supply—specifically, certain polyphenols like trans-resveratrol, found in particular plants—would alert our bodies to alter gene expression in preparation for the impending shortage. (Isn't it fascinating that the plant kingdom is able to "speak" to the animal kingdom in this way?) On the other hand, in times of abundance, we adapted to use any available excess by storing it as fat, in the process strengthening our immune systems to protect us from infection.

> **Our bodies developed to survive on a certain diet, with certain environmental conditions in place.**

That's what I mean by optimal gene expression: Certain environmental conditions alter gene expression to provide the best possible chance of survival under those conditions.

MODERN DIET + ANCIENT GENES = DISASTER

The question now before us is: What happens when everything changes? That is, what happens when our bodies and their patterns of gene expression, which developed over 100,000 generations, are confronted by profoundly unfamiliar environmental conditions over a relatively short period of time—say, three or four generations?

Many scientists would agree that these events would cause a dramatic destabilization of a species. Suddenly, we're not getting any of the things we need to turn on the good genes and turn off the bad genes.

Worse, the wonderfully exquisite system that's intended to protect us against famine instead is putting us at risk for disease and death by hoarding calories from our abundant food supply.

Let me tell you, the optimal diet and environment for our genes couldn't be any further from the modern American lifestyle if we tried to make it so.

> **Every one of us is walking around in a severely compromised state, a kind of modern malnutrition, simply because of the foods in the standard American diet.**

Why? It has everything to do with our master health regulators and their interaction with the food and environment typical of the primordial forest. In the primordial forest, the regulators were getting appropriate signals that they could easily recognize from our ancestral diet and environment. These signals allowed them to function the way nature intended, so they were always dialed toward survival and wellness in any given situation, at any given time. Our ancestors didn't need diet books or beta-blockers to stay healthy and trim; their lifestyle had helped to design their physiology.

For years, scientists have been trying to nail down the causal connection between our health status and our diet. With the discovery that diet (particularly certain bioactives) and environment (particularly adaptive stress) influence the master health regulators, they finally can begin to connect the dots. The problem is that we humans have wandered too far afield of the ideal grazing conditions of the primordial forest. Rather than sending proper signals to our master health regulators to ensure that they're dialed toward optimal health, we're providing instructions that they interpret as cues for weight gain, disease, and accelerated aging.

To make matters worse, we no longer recognize the signals that our master health regulators respond to. So instead of giving them what they need in order for us to truly benefit from them, we're doing the exact opposite.

MIXED SIGNALS

Because our genes developed over 100,000 generations, and because this process was driven by the environmental conditions of our ancestors, we are eating foods that are not compatible with our genes. As a result, I believe we are sending messages to our genes that are explicitly inconsistent with human health.

There's not enough room here for me to fully explore the massive changes in agriculture and food manufacturing that have precipitated the upheaval in what and how we eat. For that, I recommend reading Eric Schlosser's eye-opening (and sometimes stomach-turning) *Fast Food Nation*, or Michael Pollan's revolutionary *The Omnivore's Dilemma*. But I will touch on these changes here and in the chapters to come, because they have been nothing short of revolutionary, and they have had a truly terrible impact on our master health regulators.

Back in 1800, the vast majority of the world's population—about 97 percent—was living in rural areas. The picture changed dramatically by 2000, when almost 76 percent of the inhabitants of developed countries were living in cities. The 200 years in between gave rise to the Industrial Revolution, which, perhaps more than any other event, accelerated the shift from largely agrarian societies to urban ones. It also gave rise to the massive increase in processed foods.

Of course, all this occurred much too recently on the timeline of human existence for our genes to have any chance to adapt. A recent review in the *American Journal of Clinical Nutrition* reveals that more than 70 percent of the calories in our modern-day diet come from foods that would have been unrecognizable to our hunter-gatherer ancestors. That leaves us holding the bag. Now we must deal with the devastation that has come from eating foods that are absolutely discordant with the genes passed down from our ancestors.

The consequences of this have the potential to be even more catastrophic than the current health crisis that's plaguing our country. After all, it's basically what we believe happened to the dinosaurs, isn't it? Some catastrophic event—such as a comet colliding with the earth—dramatically affected weather patterns, which in turn altered vegetation and predator/prey ecosystems. This led to a dramatic change in the diets of most dinosaurs. Those that could not rapidly adapt to these changes became sick; eventually, morbidity and mortality led to their extinction.

> Why did the dinosaurs die out? A significant change in their
> diet made them sick.

Unlike us, the dinosaurs did not have the pharmaceutical industry to offer a counterbalance to their detrimental diets. Perhaps if they had access to the saurine equivalent of blood pressure and cholesterol-lowering medications, they would have been able to hang on a little longer. As it was, those with gene variations that allowed them to adapt to the changing conditions outlasted the rest. But eventually, they disappeared, too—most likely because they were eating food that their bodies weren't designed to handle.

Sound familiar?

A PERFECT STORM: THE FIVE FACTORS

Perhaps you're familiar with Sebastian Junger's best-selling book *The Perfect Storm*, about the "Storm of the Century"—the Halloween Nor'easter of 1991. In it, Junger describes how a series of separate, individually innocuous weather events—two low-pressure systems, cold air from one direction, warm air from another, moisture from the Gulf—came together in a terrible alchemy of their own. The confluence of these rare factors, inoffensive independently but deadly in concert, created a storm of spectacular and deadly proportion, with some of the lowest barometric pressures in recorded history.

In science, we refer to this phenomenon as synergy, when two or more discrete factors acting together create an effect much greater than the predicted combined effects of the individual elements. As an example, take the following five events, any of which might happen on a given morning: Your cat throws up on your bedroom carpet; your kid spills an entire quart of milk while pouring himself a glass at breakfast; you drop and break your iPod; you miss your 9:30 meeting because of unexpected traffic; and—when you finally get to the office—you discover that your key card doesn't work.

Now any one of these things, happening in isolation, might get under your skin. But if all of them occur on the same day, I can pretty much guarantee that your co-workers will be watching as you scream and curse at the

A Perfect Storm - The Five Low Pressure Systems

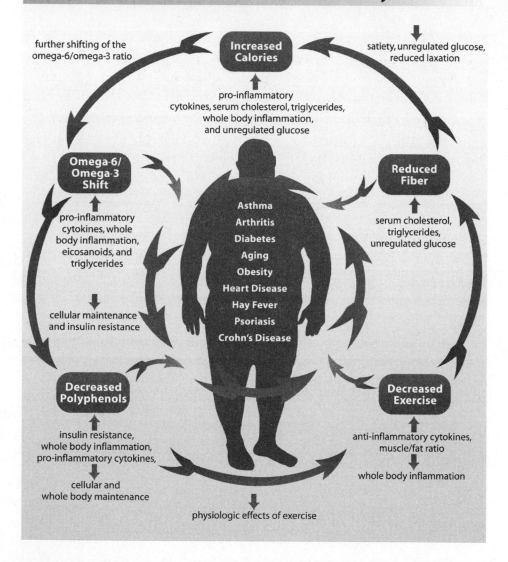

further shifting of the omega-6/omega-3 ratio

Increased Calories

satiety, unregulated glucose, reduced laxation

pro-inflammatory cytokines, serum cholesterol, triglycerides, whole body inflammation, and unregulated glucose

Omega-6/ Omega-3 Shift

Reduced Fiber

pro-inflammatory cytokines, whole body inflammation, eicosanoids, and triglycerides

serum cholesterol, triglycerides, unregulated glucose

Asthma
Arthritis
Diabetes
Aging
Obesity
Heart Disease
Hay Fever
Psoriasis
Crohn's Disease

cellular maintenance and insulin resistance

Decreased Polyphenols

Decreased Exercise

insulin resistance, whole body inflammation, pro-inflammatory cytokines,

anti-inflammatory cytokines, muscle/fat ratio

cellular and whole body maintenance

whole body inflammation

physiologic effects of exercise

key-card slot. That's synergy—a series of things working together to make the final outcome much greater than the sum of the parts.

As we consider the U.S. population today, we can see looming on the horizon an equally disastrous confluence of at least five individually significant factors, each sending the wrong signals to our bodies' cells and organ systems:

1. a massive increase in caloric intake

2. a reduction in physical activity—and, more precisely, the right kinds of physical activity

3. a reduction in total fiber intake, as well as in the right kinds of dietary fiber

4. a shift in the quantities and ratios of dietary fatty acids

5. fewer bioactive polyphenols in our diet generally, and in fruits and vegetables specifically

All of these can be traced to significant changes in our diets and lifestyles—and, perhaps most importantly, to changes in our food supply, particularly in the wake of urbanization and the Industrial Revolution. These events have caused a major disconnect between our actual diets and the foods that our bodies are designed to handle.

> **Each one of these five factors has a huge impact on our master health regulators.**

Unfortunately, the conflict between our modern diet and our genes is being decided within our bodies, turning them into battlegrounds. The result has been a dramatic rise in whole-body inflammation and a corresponding pandemic of chronic inflammatory diseases, such as arthritis, allergies, diabetes, heart disease, cancer—and, yes, what is now known as the obesity epidemic.

Why are the five aforementioned factors so devastating? Each one of them has a negative impact on the master health regulators, the switches controlling the clusters of genes that protect us from death and disease, or lead us to the same.

THE ANTI-ADAPTIVE STRESS RESPONSE

What do the five factors have in common that makes them so devastating, and so devastatingly synergistic?

In a very general sense, I believe all of them inhibit the body's maintenance systems. You'll remember that the adaptive stress response is designed to help us during tough times. Inducing this response sets into motion a complicated genetic regulatory network, leading to the optimal maintenance that helps us to survive.

The adaptive stress response revs those maintenance systems, sending the body's ability to protect itself into overdrive. These five factors *do the exact opposite.* Instead of pushing the cells to do a better job, they send critical signals to the master health regulators that instruct the cells to take a break from maintenance duty—and then to put in a DVD, order a pizza, and grab a cold one. In other words, instead of enhancing our survival, these factors push our cells hard in the opposite direction.

I'll explain exactly how we think they do this when we talk about the individual aspects of the Perfect Storm. But the short answer is that each of these factors prevents an adaptive stress response.

The objective of the Gene Smart Diet is to turn the dial in the opposite direction, giving your body the right input to trigger the adaptive stress response and all of its benefits throughout your life. Studies from the simplest animals to humans have shown it to protect health and slow aging.

That's why we must look carefully at every aspect of this Perfect Storm: because each one is an anti-adaptive response. Each one tells our bodies that all is well.

And that's why the pandemic of chronic human disease correlates so closely with affluence. The easy access to new technologies enjoyed by wealthy countries like the United States has driven many of the dramatic changes in our everyday diets. These changes, in turn, have prompted the activation of several master health regulators that control hundreds or perhaps thousands of genes. Unfortunately, this activation is having the exact opposite effect of the one associated with the adaptive stress response. Put another way, the master health regulators are making us gain weight and get sick.

Sent the wrong signals, these master regulators negatively influence everything—from energy expenditure, to glucose and insulin metabolism, to fat metabolism and storage; from how aggressive our immune systems are to how well our DNA repairs itself; from our levels of sex hormones to our cognitive development or decline. In essence, many of the cellular maintenance responses described in Chapter 3 are controlled by the master health regulators, and our diet and lifestyle are driving them in the wrong direction.

TERRIBLE SYNERGY

The fact that each of the five factors independently contributes to whole-body inflammation—a critical marker of disease and aging—is daunting enough. But it's when we examine how all of the factors work together that the view out of the porthole gets really scary.

One of the key aspects of synergy, as described earlier, is that it typically works through mechanisms that are complementary to each other. So to have a multiplicative or synergistic effect, not just an additive one, one factor must supplement another.

> The body's ability to maintain itself may be severely reduced by each aspect of the storm, but it is dramatically weakened by the collective consequences.

How does synergy work in the case of our health? As I explained earlier in the book, we can have "good" genes and "bad" genes for any given trait; these are known as polymorphisms of that gene. With a disease like diabetes, we now know that 50 or more polymorphisms—some good, others bad—may contribute to individual susceptibility to the disease. If you happen to have more bad polymorphisms than good ones, your odds of getting diabetes are much greater.

So what determines which polymorphisms are expressed? Dietary conditions, in many cases. A dietary component—or a lifestyle factor such as lack of exercise—may serve as a brake for the activity of good genes or an accelerator for the activity of bad genes that make you more prone to a disease like diabetes. It may do so by speeding up the breakdown of a so-called good protein or extending the life of a bad one. It may enhance the biological effect of a bad protein (scientists call this signal transduction) or blunt the signaling of a good one. It might facilitate the transfer of a bad protein through the cell or inhibit the transfer of a good protein. The multiple possibilities—and these are just a few—are what makes understanding the various aspects of synergy so very complicated.

What we do know is that many of the major master health regulators—those that control huge swaths of genes, such as the sirtuins, PGC1, PPAR, NF-κB, steroid receptors, SREBP1, and Nrf2—are affected by the five factors contributing to our Perfect Storm. Many of these regulators are responsible for the benefits of the adaptive stress response, while others play roles in inflammation and longevity. All control the major cellular and physiologic events that play out in our bodies.

Again, the science is in the very early stages, so we understand some gene networks better than others. But one thing is crystal clear, even now. Alone, each of the five factors—a massive increase in caloric intake, a marked reduction in the right kind of physical activity, a large reduction in dietary fiber intake, a significant shift in fatty acid quantities and ratios, and a decline in the amounts of bioactives in our food supply—chips away at our good health. Together, they transmute into something no less terrible than the wall of waves that faced the good men of the *Andrea Gail* during that other Perfect Storm.

CHAPTER TEN

HUNTER-GATHERER, MEET THE FAST-FOOD NATION

JUST BEFORE WRITING THIS, I made myself lunch. I mixed canned tuna with mayonnaise and put the combination on a slice of bread. On top of the tuna I placed a leaf of lettuce, a few slices of tomato, and another slice of bread.

Now a tuna sandwich is pretty pedestrian fare for the average American; in fact, it's one of the first things that my kids learned to make for themselves. But replicating this plebian sandwich would have been no more within my great-grandmother's reach than splitting an atom.

Tomatoes and lettuce in February? Fish caught thousands of miles away and preserved in a can? *White* bread—from a *bag?* My "ordinary" sandwich would have been completely incomprehensible to my great-grandmother. And many scientists—myself included—feel that she was quite a bit healthier for it.

Available to us today are vast categories of foods—entire supermarket aisles—that simply would have been unfathomable to our hunter-gatherer ancestors: dairy products, breakfast cereals, refined sugars and grains, and vegetable oils, just to name a few. Collectively, these products make up over 70 percent of the daily calories consumed by the U.S. population.

> **Over 70 percent of the foods in the modern American diet are vastly different from the ones that we are genetically programmed to eat.**

MIKE JONES

AGE: 52

STARTING WEIGHT: 323 pounds

LOST: 48 pounds, 17 inches from his waist, 7 inches from his hips during the study; 109 pounds total

CHANGES IN KEY BIOMARKERS AFTER 8 WEEKS ON GENE SMART

BMI: −5

BODY FAT: −10 percent

RESTING HEART RATE: −4 beats per minute

CIRCULATING WHITE BLOOD CELLS: −17 percent

TOTAL CHOLESTEROL: −9 points

LDL CHOLESTEROL: −8 points

TRIGLYCERIDES: −22 points

FASTING INSULIN: 64 percent lower

FASTING LEPTIN: 71 percent lower

EXPRESSION OF THE INFLAMMATORY GENE IL-8: 98 percent lower

❝ I've lost 109 pounds on Gene Smart. The change in me and my health has been tremendous.

It's true what they say—the longest part of the journey is the first step. But you can't be 52 years old and eat what I ate, and weigh what I weighed, and stick around for very long. I knew that. You can't live a productive life,

And that alone may be the biggest reason that we're facing an unprecedented rise in life-threatening inflammatory diseases, including obesity.

BUT ISN'T FOOD JUST FOOD?

When I mention this at lectures, someone invariably raises his or her hand in confusion. Food, after all, is food. How different can what we eat really be from what our forebears ate? It's a good question, on many levels. The short answer is not only have our eating habits changed dramatically—which doesn't seem that big of a deal because of how strongly they're reinforced by anyway. Walking was becoming hard; when you weigh 323 pounds, getting around isn't easy. Diabetes came with the extra weight, as did high blood pressure and high cholesterol. It was the right time for me to do something.

I'd just been eating too much of the wrong things. For me the biggest change was getting more fruits, vegetables, yogurt, and grains and less fast food—the pizza, the burgers, the junk. I don't eat cheese anymore. I have oatmeal or cereal and fruit for breakfast, and a fruit and yogurt mixture for lunch. I eat a lot of nuts and beans now—pintos and lentils and garbanzos. And salads, but without those high-fat salad dressings. Tomatoes have been key for me—I eat lots of stewed tomatoes, good fresh ones when I can find them.

I'm not a big wine drinker; I don't care for the taste of it. But I eat a lot of fruit. Sometimes in the evening, I'll put oatmeal, raspberries, and blackberries in a blender to get those polyphenols. The dark chocolate is a taste you get used to, and it's the only stuff we keep in the house now. It takes just a little bit to satisfy me if I start feeling like I really want some chocolate.

Since I've been on Gene Smart, I've been able to get off my diabetes medication. But the biggest change is how much better I feel. I'm back to working construction, doing ladder work and things like that, and my joints don't hurt. I've got more energy, too. Before it felt like I was drinking 10 or 15 cups of coffee just to get up and running; now I have one and I'm good to go.

We're walking again, and I joined a gym. I'm regaining my arm strength; the things I could do 20 years ago are starting to come back.

The education was critical, too. The way everything about the diet was broken down made sense to me; it felt like a commonsense approach."

our culture—the foods themselves have changed dramatically, too.

It's hard for many people to fully grasp this concept. So I'd like to suggest that we look together at one example: refined sugar.

The earliest evidence of refined sugar, in the form of crystalline sucrose, can be traced to northern India in 500 BC. Before that, honey would have been one of the very few concentrated sugars known to hunter-gatherers.

Although honey was likely a favorite food back then, our ancestors probably didn't have access to a regular supply. Honey, like most natural foods, is seasonal, and therefore unavailable a large part of the year. So even if your great-great-great-keep-going-about-500-times-grandfather found a beehive and ate himself sick, that honey would have represented a very small percentage of his diet over the course of the year.

Of course, if we get a hankering for honey, all we have to do is squeeze the little bear. And honey isn't even our biggest problem. Current population-wide intakes of refined sugars in Western countries are without precedent in human history. Refined sugar consumption in the United States was almost 70 kilograms per person in 2000, up from 55 kilograms per person in 1970. (Just to give you some perspective on what we're talking about, 70 kilograms translates to 154 pounds—the equivalent of a decent-sized human, or about 75 of those 2-pound bags you can buy at the supermarket.)

As dramatic as this annual per-capita jump is, it represents a much more significant trend that has affected all Western nations—not just the United States—since the dawn of the Industrial Revolution almost 200 years ago. In Britain at the beginning of the 18th century, the per-capita consumption of refined sugar was a mere 1.8 kilograms, or 4 pounds, a year. By 1815, that number crept up to a still-very-reasonable 7 kilograms—15 pounds, or a bag that you could carry in one arm. But it's continued to climb in the meantime, as it has in other Western nations like Norway, Denmark, Sweden, and the Netherlands.

It's worth noting that high-fructose corn syrup (HFCS)—a processed, super-sweet sugar replacement that happens to be cheaper for food manufacturers—has found its way into lots of products that once were made with sugar, like sodas, ketchup, and jams. Many people believe that HFCS, which appeared in our food supply at about the time that the obesity epidemic began gaining ground, bears its share of responsibility for our national weight problem. (Don't be fooled; a product that uses real sugar is not an improvement!) One thing is clear: Neither the dramatic increase in sucrose consumption before 1970 nor the subsequent increase in HFCS consumption over the past 30 years could have been possible on a broad-scale basis before the Industrial Revolution or "advances" in food processing technology. And sugar is just one example of the sorts of changes that have infiltrated our food supply, often without our really being aware of it.

It's next to impossible to wrap our brains around how different our modern diet is from the one our ancestors followed. Foods that would have been completely alien to them—pizza, snack foods like potato chips and baked goods, breakfast cereals, condiments like salad dressings, mayonnaise, and mustard—are standard fare for us. On the other hand, my great-great-grandmother probably would have been pretty comfortable sitting down to a meal with her hunter-gatherer ancestors, hundreds of thousands of years before. She might have been able to help them improve on the finer points, but their whole-grain porridge, small portion of meat, and selection of fresh, seasonal, local fruits and vegetables would have looked very much like her own evening meal.

The sugar story is just the tip of the iceberg. In fact, everything about our diet is different now—from the abundance of protein, to the concentrations and ratios of fatty acids, to the sources and amounts of fiber and carbohydrates, to mention only a few. Yet considering that the human genetic material has remained more or less the same for hundreds of thousands of years, the hunter-gatherer diet (and lifestyle—we can't forget about exercise) is still the one for which we are best suited, physiologically speaking.

Many scientists, myself among them, believe that if our ancestors had had antibiotics and better defenses against predators in the primordial forest, they might have enjoyed far superior health to ours, and would have lived far longer. And they may have been virtually free of asthma, diabetes, heart disease, arthritis, and other inflammatory conditions so prevalent today.

HERE'S THE (GENE SMART) SOLUTION

In the next several chapters, I will show you what is different about our modern diet and how these changes are affecting the master health regulators. I'll also tell you what you can do—right now, and without sacrifice—to reverse these changes.

There are five Gene Smart Solutions, each one of them designed to address and reverse one of the detrimental factors that we discussed in Chapter 9. These five factors, working synergistically, are a primary reason that so many of us are so very sick. But we can turn that synergistic power to our advantage.

Each Gene Smart Solution is corrective in its own right. When they work together, as they do in the Gene Smart Diet, the results are nothing short of phenomenal.

That's what we saw when we devised an 8-week study based on the Gene Smart Diet. A group of volunteers from Hillsdale United Methodist Church (thus the Hillsdale Study)—men and women of all ages and all physical conditions—came together for an initial 5-hour educational session in which we presented the same information that you now hold in your hands. These educational sessions continued once a week for the rest of the study; the group also met for twice-a-week exercise sessions. These folks had over 50 blood biomarkers tested to determine their whole-body inflammation levels, glucose/insulin status, and risk profiles.

The study was more successful in helping people than I had ever dreamed. In short, Gene Smart enabled people who didn't realize that they were on the brink of getting sick to step back from the cliff. For some with existing conditions, it meant an opportunity to once again feel in control of their health. In more than one instance, participants were able to eliminate medication (under the doctor's supervision, of course). One person with lifelong asthma stopped carrying an inhaler; a man in his forties was able to lower his dosage of statins.

Gene Smart helped people who had failed on every other diet not only to lose weight but to do it without hunger, and for good. Mike Jones, whose story is on pages 96–97, has lost over 100 pounds in just a year. That's over 2 pounds a week! Of course, it's one thing for me to speculate that you won't be hungry; it's entirely another to hear it from someone like Michelle Marcey (pages 160–161), who's back to wearing a two-piece swimsuit for the first time in 15 years.

In all cases, participants reported that they not only looked better, they felt better—more energetic, less depressed, sexier, younger. In the next section, you'll hear directly from some of them about the weight they lost and the health improvements they experienced, as well as their firsthand accounts of what it was like to follow Gene Smart, and how they feel about sticking with it.

If nothing else, I hope that what you read in the following pages will persuade you that you're in the driver's seat. You can turn the dial from disease and accelerated aging to optimal health. And it's much easier than you think.

PART THREE

The Gene Smart Solutions

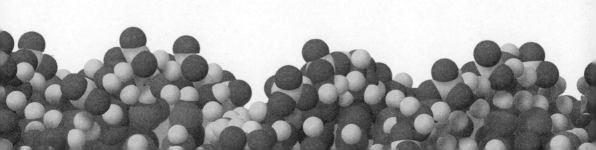

CHAPTER ELEVEN

GENE SMART SOLUTION #1: REDUCE CALORIES

THE FIRST GENE SMART SOLUTION addresses the factor that is most dramatically affecting our health: too many calories.

Oh, no! I promised "calorie restriction without calorie restriction," and then I turn around and restrict calories.

Well, not exactly. On Gene Smart, we are going to *reduce* calories. That's not the same as *restricting* calories, which means consuming far fewer calories than what you're living on right now. Plus, Gene Smart builds on one of the only real tricks in a dieter's toolbox, and it's this: Fewer calories doesn't necessarily mean less food, or going hungry.

We eat more—a lot more—than our hunter-gatherer ancestors did. But let me show you what effect that has had, and why calorie reduction is such an important signal for our genes.

MORE CALORIES, MORE PROBLEMS

Our ancestors rarely had an overabundance of food; it was simply too hard to come by. They consumed just enough calories to survive—and probably fewer much of the time. Without an excess of calories, our ancestors would never have become overweight, or suffered from the multitude of diseases associated with overweight. (As you'll remember, the only life extension method currently proven to work is an extremely low-calorie diet.)

In fact, the very genes that may have helped them to stay alive during periods of food shortage and famine may be the same ones that are making us fat. For our ancestors, the proverbial "feast or famine" would have been a way of life. At times—after a successful hunt, for instance, or during the late summer months when fruits and vegetables are in generous supply—they would have had lots to eat. But during other long periods—in the winter, for example, or during a dry hunting spell—they would have had very little. In response to these unpredictable conditions, our genes developed to ensure that our bodies store as many calories as possible as fat in times of plenty in order to sustain them through the lean times. In the process, fat cells adapted to help enhance disease resistance by revving up our immune systems to protect us from an infection or some other body challenge.

Since famine was more or less inevitable, our ancestors didn't have to worry about being fat for very long. Nor did they have to worry about the long-term downside of such a revving-up of calorie and fat storage, namely an increase in inflammatory disease. The problem, of course, is that food scarcity is no longer an issue. In Western society, abundance is the norm.

> At no time in human history has it been so cheap and easy
> to get so many calories—often with very little nutrition.

With no famine to offset it, the gene that gets greedy when presented with lots of calories stays greedy on a permanent basis. This is why we gain weight. It's also why we're at higher risk for inflammatory disease, as those extra calories end up as fat cells that keep our immune systems on overdrive.

We know that the adaptive stress response is the body's answer to an environmental challenge, such as a change in diet. In the presence of too few calories, for instance, the body's cells shift into a protective repair-and-maintain mode. In a way, the situation we now find ourselves in is the exact opposite of the health-giving adaptive stress response. It, too, is an adaptive response—an adaptive *excess* response.

Unfortunately, a generation of excess calories is not enough to change our genetics. And so our hunter-gatherer genes encourage us to have a strong appetite, and to eat as much as possible during times of abundance. We are simply heeding a primitive genetic response to excess, which allows us to stockpile as much fat as possible to prepare us for the famine that never comes.

> **Our tendency to overconsume in times of plenty is driven by a strong survival mechanism that developed over 100,000 generations.**

Combine the genetic drive to eat whatever is in sight and to store the excess as fat with the number of empty calories readily available to us, and you have a relatively predictable recipe for disaster. So it should come as no surprise that approximately 70 percent of the U.S. population is overweight or obese. If the current trend continues, a staggering 40 percent of us will be obese—not just overweight, but with a body mass index above 30—by 2015.

And so it is that the genetic adaptation that once ensured our survival now all but guarantees disaster. When we take in more calories than our bodies need, we constantly activate the adaptive *excess* response, efficiently storing fat and increasing inflammation—without ever activating the adaptive stress response necessary to push us toward optimal cellular maintenance. It's the worst of both worlds!

THE OBESITY EPIDEMIC

Make no mistake about it: We are getting fatter—at quite an astonishing rate.

I do a lot of public speaking, and without meaning to sound fat-headed, I'm generally well-received. There is one part of my PowerPoint presentation that I can safely say is a guaranteed showstopper.

It's a sequence of slides, produced by the Centers for Disease Control and Prevention, titled "Obesity Trends Among U.S. Adults." I know—it doesn't sound like a must-see. At first blush, it doesn't look like one either. Each slide depicts a map of the United States, with each state in a particular color, depending on whether more or less than 10 percent of that state's population is obese. Bear in mind, we're talking about obesity, not merely overweight. These slides illustrate the percentage of the population in which the body

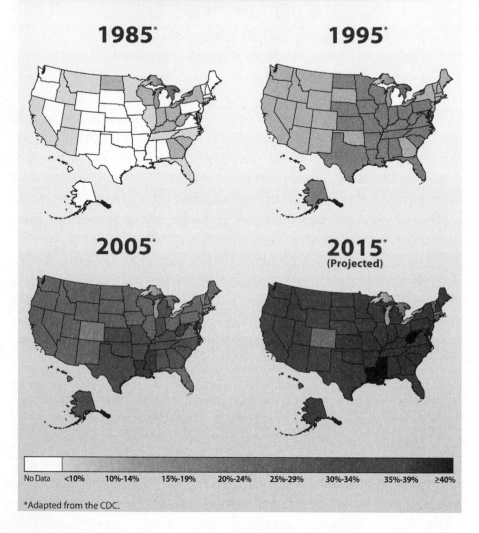

Obesity Trends Among U.S. Adults

1985*

1995*

2005*

2015*
(Projected)

| No Data | <10% | 10%-14% | 15%-19% | 20%-24% | 25%-29% | 30%-34% | 35%-39% | ≥40% |

*Adapted from the CDC.

mass index is above 30. The states in which 10 to 14 percent of the population is obese appear a darker blue.

The first slide is from 1985. It's generally light blue, with some darker blue sprinkled in. As I click through, year after year, the map grows darker and darker. By 1991, an even darker blue shows up, indicating states in which 15 to 19 percent of the population is obese. I must have given this presentation a hundred times now; I can tell you that every single time, as I click through the slides and the map progressively darkens, the room falls completely silent.

The stillness continues even through the 1997 slide, when a pale yellow is introduced to represent states in which more than 20 percent of the population is obese. I keep clicking in silence, and together we watch the map slowly turn pale yellow. But when the first red state appears—meaning that more than 25 percent of the population is obese—there's an audible gasp. By the time we have watched the South turn light red, bringing us to 2006, when we see the first blood-red states, in which more than 30 percent of the population is obese, the room is literally buzzing in shock and horror.

As of 2006, only four states in the entire United States were below 20 percent in prevalence of obesity. Twenty-two states had a prevalence at or above 25 percent; two of them—Mississippi and West Virginia—were at or above 30 percent. If we project these data to 2015, the entire Southeast will top 35 percent, with the rest of the country not far behind. Remember, we're talking about obesity, not just overweight.

I wouldn't flatter myself to think that it's my flair for presentation that holds the audience in rapt attention. And the Centers for Disease Control and Prevention certainly isn't known for its cutting-edge graphics. Even the headlines on the evening news—"Americans are getting fatter! Details at 11!"—are hardly news to anyone who owns a television set. It seems like "the obesity epidemic" is all we ever hear about, from automakers widening seats to accommodate our widening rear ends to the not-quite-good-enough political campaigns to fight fat in our children's schools. But there is something about actually seeing evidence of the steady, inexorable progression of obesity in the United States that tends to stop people in their tracks.

As my slideshow proves beyond a doubt, we're getting fatter. Men and women between ages 20 and 40 are gaining about 2 pounds per year, on average. That's an alarming trend over the long term. And it doesn't take a lot of extra calories to put on that much weight; to gain 2 pounds, you'd need to consume about 7,000 extra calories a year, or about 20 extra calories per day. That's two olives, or a single Ritz cracker!

You can imagine how just a few extra calories a day can have a catastrophic effect over time. In fact, it may account for the so-called weight creep that seems to accelerate once we reach middle age. If we're gaining about 2 pounds a year starting in our twenties, we can easily be toting an

The Cost of All Those Calories

We're much fatter than our friends in Europe, and it costs us! A study conducted at Emory University and published in the journal *Health Affairs* found that American adults are twice as likely to be obese—and that treatment of obesity-related chronic conditions like heart disease, cancer, and diabetes comes with a price tag of between $100 and $150 billion per year.

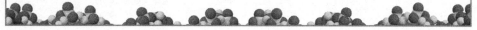

extra 40 pounds by the time we reach middle age—even if we think we've been careful about watching what we eat. For most of us, 40 pounds makes a big difference in our self-image, not to mention our health.

THE CALORIE CULPRITS

"Why are we getting so fat?" I'm invariably asked. My answer? "Because we can."

We find ourselves in a period of endless abundance that would have been unthinkable to our ancestors. According to data from the Food and Agriculture Organization of the United Nations, the United States produced almost 3,800 calories per day for every man, woman, and child in 2002. That's up 300 calories per day from 1991, and 600 calories per day from 1981. Now that's not intake; it's how much food is available for every U.S. citizen. And it's two times what the average adult male needs on a daily basis.

It's a dramatic change, even from a generation or two ago. My parents grew up in the Deep South during the Depression, a time of scarcity not so dissimilar to the ones our hunter-gatherer ancestors might have endured. They didn't have a lot of money when I was growing up, so their constant reminders to clean my plate were necessary to make sure that I got the 2,500 calories a day that my active and growing body required. But I welcomed my first grandchild, Grace, in 2008, and I can tell you that my message to her will be very different. It has to be. If she eats as many calories as are available to her, she'll be consuming more than twice as many as she needs.

Apple or Pear?

It's the question that has struck fear in the heart of many a woman: "Does this make my butt look big?"

Would it surprise you to learn that the answer—for women and for men—is an indicator of the potential health effects of whole-body inflammation? It's true: If you're overweight or obese, the location of your extra padding makes a big difference in how much damage inflammation can cause.

If you carry most of your excess weight around your middle (the so-called "apple" shape), you're releasing significantly more inflammatory messengers in critical locations than if you carry most of it in your buttocks and thighs (the so-called "pear" shape). And it doesn't take a whole lot of fat in the wrong place to contribute to harmful whole-body inflammation. Recent studies have demonstrated that even people who are mildly obese but who are prone to abdominal or visceral fat are much more likely to develop inflammation that leads to coronary artery disease.

How do you know if you're at risk? Get out the tape measure and wrap it around your waist, at the level of your navel. Is the measurement more than 40 inches if you're a man, or 35 inches if you're a woman? If so, you have what's known as abdominal obesity, a defining characteristic of the metabolic syndrome, which also encompasses high blood pressure, elevated cholesterol, and increased insulin resistance.

An estimated 20 to 25 percent of American adults already have metabolic syndrome, which is recognized as a major risk factor for heart disease and diabetes. Some research suggests that by the year 2020, metabolic syndrome may affect 40 percent of the U.S. population. And yes, scientists have determined that a second defining characteristic of the syndrome is increased whole-body inflammation.

Why is abdominal fat so dangerous? One reason is that it's located right next to the internal organs, most importantly the liver. The inflammatory messengers produced by abdominal fat are released directly into the portal vein that feeds the liver, prompting the liver to produce more of its own inflammatory signals, creating a vicious cycle.

But don't think you're off the hook if you carry your extra pounds in your butt and thighs. True, your risk of heart disease and diabetes is probably lower than for someone whose fat sits across the abdomen. But it's still considerably higher than for someone who's a normal weight. Overweight and obesity contribute to low-level whole-body inflammation, regardless of whether you're an apple or a pear.

So no matter which produce basket you belong in, it's essential for you to lose the extra pounds. Don't worry! Gene Smart will help.

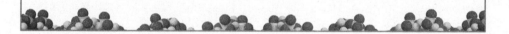

There are a number of reasons that we're in such caloric trouble. These include:

Portion sizes. Portion sizes have gone through the roof, correlating exactly with the rise in overweight and obesity among the general population. Marion Nestle, PhD, MPH, and Lisa R. Young, PhD, RD, both nutritionists at New York University, have published evidence that portion sizes offered by fast-food chains are two to five times larger than they were when the same foods were first introduced. Today's "small" soda is yesterday's large; a "child-size" meal now would easily have fed an adult back then. Thanks to our primordial genes—genes that developed in response to an uncertain food supply—we're programmed to eat what's in front of us. And so we do, and do, and do.

Fewer vegetables, more domesticated meat. One of the results of the population shift from a rural environment to an urban one has been unprecedented growth in the livestock industry. Cities have the infrastructure to support the distribution of perishable livestock products like meat, poultry, milk, and eggs before they spoil.

According to the USDA's Economic Research Service, total meat consumption (including red meat, poultry, and fish) in the United States amounted to 200 pounds per person in 2005, 22 pounds more than in 1970. And it's not just us; both industrialized and developing countries have seen sharp rises in their domesticated meat consumption. The world's livestock consumption has gone up a staggering 50 percent over the last 30 years.

It goes without saying that meat packs more calories per serving than vegetables. You'd have to eat a garbage bag full of baby spinach to get the number of calories in a hamburger.

More heavily processed foods. There's another reason that we're eating so many more calories than our ancestors, and it has to do with processing. In the beginning of his book *Eat This, Not That,* David Zinczenko ranks the 20 unhealthiest foods in America. The top 7 deliver over 2,000 calories each. That's a day's worth of calories for an adult male in a single sitting, not to mention a whole week's worth of saturated fat. It would be quite hard to match those amounts by eating nothing but whole foods.

Recently I was sitting next to someone on a plane who was reading a biography of legendary gourmand and glutton Diamond Jim Brady. Although Diamond Jim was known worldwide for his legendary appetite—and for a girth to match—both of us found ourselves marveling at the same thing: He actually wasn't all that fat. Don't get me wrong; he was obese, as someone famous for starting the day with a couple of roasted chickens would be. But he wasn't what I think of as 21st century fat, simply because the food he was eating—even in the vast quantities he was eating—wasn't engineered to deliver the ultra-caloric punch that our highly processed, fiber-poor, sugar-laden fast foods do.

HOW GENE SMART GETS IT RIGHT

At a genetic, physiologic, and emotional level, our genes are telling us to eat everything we see to prepare ourselves for the famine ahead. But there's no famine coming. We can eat as much as we want to, whenever we want to. And that's doing a real number on our genes.

> **We should be sending the master health regulators the sort of signals that can spark a protective anti-inflammatory cascade. Consuming too many calories does exactly the opposite.**

Don't get me wrong: Even if genetics had kept pace since the Industrial Revolution, our current eating habits still would increase our risk of becoming overweight or obese and developing life-threatening inflammatory illness. But our genes haven't kept up. It has been only three or four generations since the Industrial Revolution, and just one since it was

The Magic of Fiber

Every single person who participated in our study of the Gene Smart Diet will tell you that the single most important key to losing weight without hunger is dietary fiber. There's something almost magical about dietary fiber and weight loss—although the results are no illusion. Studies confirm a direct relationship between the amount of fiber you eat and the number of pounds you lose. Although we don't yet have evidence of it, I suspect that fiber somehow activates a gene cascade that controls satiety. More on this later; for now, suffice it to say that the key to reducing calories on Gene Smart without hunger or discomfort is to get plenty of fiber.

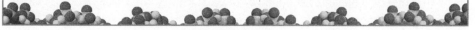

JAMES TERRELL

AGE: 44

STARTING WEIGHT: 234 pounds

LOST: 19 pounds, 4 percent of body fat, 5½ inches from waist, 4 inches from hips

CHANGES IN KEY BIOMARKERS AFTER 8 WEEKS ON GENE SMART

BMI: –2.7 points

BLOOD PRESSURE: –18 mm/Hg diastolic

RESTING HEART RATE: –14 beats per minute

FASTING INSULIN: 72 percent lower

FASTING LEPTIN: 52 percent lower

CIRCULATING LONG-CHAIN OMEGA-3s: 99 percent increase

❝I deal with numbers in my job, so I wanted to be scientific in the way I approached this diet. I meticulously accounted for every single thing that went into my mouth over the 8 weeks of the study. I even counted my omega capsules, which supplied 15 calories each.

Just doing that was a tremendous education for me. I had no idea that a hot dog bun has half the calories of a candy bar! And I was surprised to find that a lot of the foods I thought were really fiber-rich and healthy—like granola bars—had just 1 gram of fiber in them.

Until you condition yourself to keep a food journal, you're going to have a hard time seeing any change in the number on the scale. You have to pay attention to food labels, and to what you're actually putting in your mouth. Because most of the time, we don't really think about what we eat. Maybe someone brings donuts into the office, so you grab one on your way to a meeting. That's 280 calories right there. Those things add up quickly. You can't fool your body; if you don't burn more calories than you're taking in, you're going to gain weight.

vitally important for me as a child in rural North Carolina to eat everything on my plate. So it's no wonder that two of every three of us have become overweight or obese.

The adaptive response currently in play is the adaptive *excess* response—the body's reaction to too many calories. This response activates a whole host of relevant genes, triggering a propensity toward not just overweight but other diseases as well. It is why the obesity epidemic is the first low-pressure system

People say, 'I can't write down everything I eat!' But I had the drive to do it. I had all these clothes I couldn't fit into, and I'd say, 'Maybe I'll lose some weight next year.' Well, next year came. I didn't like what I was seeing in the mirror, or how I felt. I'd get out of breath just putting my socks on in the morning because there wasn't enough room for my diaphragm to move when I was bending over! I'd have to take a break halfway through tying my shoes to catch my breath.

I'm a large-framed guy. I love food, and I can put it away. On this diet, though, I was eating only 1,800 calories a day. That's not a lot for a man my size, but I wasn't hungry, and I'm sure it's because I was getting the recommended amount of fiber. In fact, I think I went a little overboard with it sometimes, but it really helped me so that I wasn't hungry. Every morning, I have 9 grams of fiber with my morning cereal and a cup of green tea. I have another cup before I go to bed.

I love sweet things. Now I use Splenda in my green tea, and that's my sweet fix. Those fiber bars are great, too. I used to love ice cream, but if I stick a low-fat yogurt in the freezer for a little more than an hour, I have something creamy and cold that's just like ice cream. I ate a lot of carrots. I'd buy a 10-pound bag from Costco and keep them in the fridge at work. They're low in calories and high in fiber. And they're cheap!

I'm thrilled with the results. There's a picture on my desk from a year ago, and my face looks totally different now. I lost a large amount of belly fat, too. Unfortunately, I wasn't able to do the exercise the way it was prescribed. I had knee surgery 20-odd years ago, and my knee still flares up really badly if I do vigorous exercise. But I followed the rest of the program, and I still saw really impressive results. Sometimes I wonder what would have happened if I'd been able to participate in the exercise sessions.

Even without them, I feel like my reflexes have improved. I work outside 60 percent of the time, and whether I'm on the job or doing stuff around the house, I feel as though I'm catching things before they hit the ground.

Gene Smart is a lifestyle change, but it's not hard. That's what my wife kept saying—'It's so easy!' I'm very happy; the benefits of this new lifestyle are tremendous.**"**

affecting our master health regulators—and, I might argue, the real eye of the Perfect Storm. What Gene Smart does is send the needle in the other direction.

We know that in times of calorie restriction—as would have been common for our hunter-gatherer ancestors—the adaptive *stress* response shifts cells into optimal maintenance mode, greatly increasing our chances of survival. Those times of scarcity can't have been pleasant for our forebears, but they nevertheless were very beneficial. Restricting daily calorie intake by 15 to 40 percent has been shown to improve glucose tolerance and insulin action, lower blood pressure and heart rate, reduce oxidative damage to DNA, help nervous system neurons resist degeneration, block inflammation, and reduce the incidence of spontaneous and induced cancers. Perhaps most impressively, in all animals in which it has been examined, calorie restriction has consistently been proven to dramatically increase average and maximal life span.

We have talked about how the adaptive stress response is influenced by a number of complex gene networks under the control of the master health regulators. We also know that calorie restriction isn't a real-world solution for the majority of people.

So how can we turn this information to our advantage? We have to utilize what we know about both adaptive responses, which is precisely what Gene Smart does.

Markedly reducing our fat stores prevents them from pumping out an overload of inflammatory signals. So our first order of business is to stop feeding the adaptive excess response. We can accomplish this by reducing our calories and losing weight, which is precisely where Gene Smart comes into play.

As you'll learn, one of your most important strategies is to write down what you eat and how much. This in itself is an education for many people. It certainly was for James Terrell, who lost almost 20 pounds in 8 weeks. Together, we'll redefine portion sizes, so you can get back in line with what your body and your genes really need, as opposed to what your neighborhood restaurant says is a serving.

On Gene Smart, you'll also be getting the omega fats in the proper ratios, which has been proven to enhance weight loss. (We'll discuss the omega fats in much greater detail in Chapter 14.) Perhaps most importantly, we'll make sure that you have lots and lots of delicious, easily available food choices, and in satisfying portions, so you're never hungry or at a loss for what to eat. You don't need to restrict calories, but you do need to increase your servings of fiber- and nutrient-dense foods, while eliminating most "empty-calorie" foods. Once you do that, you'll find that you can easily reduce (not restrict) your caloric intake without hunger or discomfort.

Along the way, you'll be reaping all of the rewards that come from following a high-fiber, protein-rich diet—you know, little things like lots more energy and lower disease risk. In fact, losing weight the Gene Smart way is sure to have a profound effect on your health because it will have a profound effect on your inflammatory profile. Remember, the more body fat you have, the more inflammation you have. Numerous studies have identified a direct relationship between body mass index, waist girth, and visceral fat tissue and levels of the inflammatory messenger C-reactive protein (CRP), interleukin-6, and leptin. Drop the excess pounds, and you can dramatically reduce whole-body inflammation, one of the most significant risk factors we know of.

> **When you lose excess weight—as you will on Gene Smart— you dramatically reduce whole-body inflammation.**

In our study, we saw dramatic reductions in leptin, a pro-inflammatory marker, and in fasting insulin levels, a strong predictor of insulin resistance and diabetes. Both of these changes are a direct result of fat loss. The news is even better for CRP: Many participants saw greater reductions than have been reported in the scientific literature. One woman, Gail Walker, whose story you'll find on pages 180–181, entered our study with one of the highest levels of CRP I've ever witnessed, a shocking 36 mg/L. After 8 weeks on Gene Smart—weeks that Gail describes as totally painless, even enjoyable—her CRP dropped dramatically to 4 mg/L. For Gail, Gene Smart was quite literally a life-saving intervention.

CRP levels above 3 mg/L are generally accepted to be associated with a high risk of inflammatory disease, especially heart disease. More than 20 major studies suggest that high CRP is correlated to high cholesterol, high blood pressure, insulin resistance, and diabetes, not to mention all-cause mortality. CRP levels above 10 mg/L are commonly observed in cases of acute or chronic inflammation. That fact should help to put the following in perspective: A recent study in the *Archives of Internal Medicine* analyzed the mean change in CRP levels and the mean change in weight, comparing "before" and "after" values from 33 separate studies. The overall data showed that every 2.2 pounds of weight loss prompted a mean change of -0.13 mg/L in CRP level.

Wow! I know of very few drug interventions that could get similar results. Lose 20 pounds, and you lower your CRP by 1.8 mg/L; lose 50 pounds, and CRP drops by almost 5 mg/L. Depending on your starting

CRP, this reduction alone can take you from a relatively high risk of a cardiac event to a low risk.

Honestly, science has not been able to dissect whether the improvements that we see with weight loss occur because all that excess fat is no longer pumping pro-inflammatory messengers into the body, or because calorie restriction—working through sirtuins or other master health regulators—shifts the body to optimal maintenance mode. Getting rid of any excess fat certainly helps. And since people don't need to restrict their calories in order to lose weight (reducing by 10 to 20 percent, as you'll do on Gene Smart, is enough), it's probably a combination of the two that's producing the effect.

In some ways, it really doesn't matter. What does matter is that we lower whole-body inflammation, and that we do it now. This is what Gene Smart is all about.

HOW GENE SMART CAN HELP

The Gene Smart Diet will kick-start your body's adaptive stress response by reducing your calorie intake by 20 to 30 percent for the first 3 weeks. Depending how much weight you need to lose, you may stay in this first phase for a bit longer. Many of our study participants were in this phase for the full 8 weeks.

When you're ready, you'll increase your daily calorie intake so that it's just 10 to 20 percent below where you started. You'll stay at this level for another 2 weeks—or longer, again depending on your starting weight.

Unlike other diets that you may have tried, many of the components of Gene Smart—like the omega fats and the fiber—will help you to lose weight, instead of taxing your willpower and leaving you feeling hungry and deprived. In this way, we will override and eliminate the adaptive *excess* response, the body's natural reaction to too much. As you'll see, we can add other healthy stressors to create benefits similar to those provided by calorie restriction—only without the discomfort.

CHAPTER TWELVE

GENE SMART SOLUTION #2: EXERCISE TO FIGHT INFLAMMATION

ON GENE SMART, you're going to move more. But—and here's the key difference from other diets that you may have tried—you're going to do it the right way and for the right reasons.

Our activity level is certainly one area where we've ventured very far from our hunter-gatherer roots. Having to hunt and gather their food meant that our ancestors routinely got lots and lots of exercise. (I've never hunted a woolly mammoth, but I'll bet it's a workout.) Imagine how trim you'd be if you had to forage for the lettuce and tomatoes in the side salad you ate with your lunch!

From drive-thru ATMs to television remote controls, modern conveniences have dramatically reduced the amount of physical exertion necessary for us to go about our daily business. When it's time for our next meal, we'll forage no further than the refrigerator—or, worse, the takeout menu drawer. In other words, we get a lot less exercise than our genes would like. And it's had a devastating impact on our inflammatory profiles.

WORK OUT FOR WEIGHT LOSS? MAYBE NOT

You might have been expecting me to say the devastating effect was on our waistlines. In fact, I think that the constant commingling of exercise and weight loss has been one of the most damaging health myths out there. It's frustrating to do something with the expectation of a result that never comes. That, for me, is what happens when you exercise with the objective of losing weight.

Of course, you can lose weight by exercising; the weight-loss equation boils down to burning more calories than you take in, and exercise is a way to burn calories. But it's a pretty inefficient system, and in my opinion, it sets up a lot of people for failure.

Think of it this way: To burn 100 calories, you'd have to bike at 5 miles per hour for 32 minutes, walk at 3 miles per hour for 23 minutes, swim slowly for 20 minutes, or engage in vigorous aerobic activity for 10 minutes. That's a lot of work! By comparison, it's easy to consume 100 calories; you can do it in the blink of an eye. Just eat one medium-size banana, one medium-to-large apple, or 1 ounce of American cheese. One cup of sweet tea or a cookie, and—calorically speaking—you might as well have skipped your bike ride altogether.

Not to mention that when you exercise a lot, your body compensates with mechanisms to maintain your current weight. For example, it naturally decreases your non-exercise-induced energy expenditure—that is, the number of calories your body burns just performing its usual functions.

One study, involving overweight college students, is especially insightful. For 16 months, one group of students exercised for 45 minutes a day, 5 days a week. The other group (the control) didn't exercise at all. The students continued their usual diets for the duration of the study.

The gender differences in the results were startling. The male students who exercised lost only 4 to 6 pounds, on average, while those who didn't exercise maintained their body weight. The female students who exercised broke even, while those who didn't exercise *gained* 5 to 6 pounds. These numbers suggest that losing weight through exercise alone may be quite difficult, especially for women.

Now, I certainly don't oppose exercise; I actually love it. When I want to shed a few pounds, the first things I do are increase my fiber intake and step up my workouts at the gym. If you want to lose weight through exercise, I recommend that you gradually work up to 60 minutes per day of moderate to vigorous physical activity.

In my opinion, though, the real reason to exercise is to reduce whole-body inflammation. That's right: The data are far more positive and conclusive on the association between exercise and inflammation than between exercise and weight loss.

> **Numerous studies show that increasing your level of physical activity is critically important to reducing inflammation.**

Observational studies reveal that you're 47 percent less likely to have elevated levels of the inflammatory messenger C-reactive protein (CRP) if you exercise regularly, compared to being sedentary. Fitness is a separate and independent factor in regulating chronic low-grade inflammation. An interventional study conducted by researchers at Louisiana State University demonstrated that aerobic and resistance training very similar to the workout recommended in Gene Smart reduced CRP levels in both old and young participants by 50 to 60 percent. These are *huge* effects.

> **Studies show that the sort of exercise protocol in Gene Smart can help reduce CRP by at least 50 percent.**

Synergy is on your side here, too, as exercise is an adaptive stress inducer that provides independent anti-inflammatory benefits. In fact, a recent study by Patricia Aronson, PhD, and colleagues reveals that metabolic factors—like body mass index, fasting glucose, HDL cholesterol, and triglycerides—and exercise are *independent factors* regarding chronic whole-body inflammation. In other words, reducing one of these—your weight, for instance—will lower CRP a certain amount; then exercise will further lower that amount.

Considering that an improvement in all of these metabolic factors is a reasonable expectation when you follow Gene Smart, that's very compelling. But it's just more evidence for what we already know: Exercise is unbelievably powerful. In fact, it's so powerful that many researchers now believe it to be just as effective as many medications for reducing overall inflammation.

BRAWN—AND BRAINS, TOO!

Many scientists, including myself, believe that exercise works to curb inflammation through the master health regulators, similar to the pathways activated by calorie restriction.

We already know that exercise is a great example of the adaptive stress response. When we put a certain amount of controlled stress on our muscles by working them, they undergo a series of changes that eventually make them stronger. This is the adaptive stress response, in a nutshell: rapid damage, repair, adaptation, increased strength. This process is known as the exercise-induced stress response—or, as I like to call it, getting in shape.

Another adaptive stress response also occurs when you exercise. You see, a bout of physical activity actually increases concentrations of pro-inflammatory cytokines and CRP. That's right: Your step class actually elevates blood levels of inflammatory messengers. However, a regular, rigorous, long-term physical training program reduces basal concentrations of inflammatory markers. Why?

As I explained earlier in this book, our understanding of fat tissue has changed radically in recent years. Instead of being a mere storage unit for energy, fat is more like an organ, capable of controlling biological processes in its own right—including the production and release of a number of dangerous, highly inflammatory messengers.

We used to think that the muscle tissue in our bodies was there simply to help us to move. But more recent research has turned that understanding on its ear. There's more brain in our brawn than we thought, meaning that the muscle tissue in our bodies has a very important function, beyond moving our bones.

Every time we exercise in a moderate to vigorous fashion, gene expression in the active muscles is altered. The muscles then release signaling molecules that communicate with the rest of the body. In this way, like fat tissue, muscle tissue acts as a very large and powerful endocrine organ.

When they're voluntarily contracted, muscles release compounds called myokines, which provide instructions to the body about how it should function. Myokines also play a role in controlling chronic whole-body inflammation. The most important myokine identified to date is the chemical messenger (also known as a cytokine) IL-6. When muscle contracts, IL-6 is released.

What was so confusing for so long was that IL-6 was considered to be inflammatory. A bout of exercise will increase plasma levels of IL-6 exponentially—up to 100 times—with a total decline in the chemical messenger during the post-exercise period. The IL-6 response is followed by elevations in circulating levels of inflammatory markers, including CRP. Basically, these are the levels we'd associate with a pretty serious infection. Disaster, right? And the magnitude of the response depends on the intensity, duration, and mode of exercise. On the face of it, then, it seemed that the more intense an activity was, the more harm it could do.

But as researchers kept looking, they discovered something highly counterintuitive: If IL-6 is released from muscle in high concentrations without the presence of several other inflammatory messengers, it is actually *anti-inflammatory.*

While physical activity was associated with an increase in IL-6 comparable to the levels observed during severe infections, researchers found little or no increase in the really nasty pro-inflammatory messengers, such as TNF-alpha and IL1-beta. The reason? IL-6 actually reduces the amount of several other inflammatory messengers in circulation. At the same time, it triggers the release of a very important anti-inflammatory messenger known as IL-10.

> **IL-6, an inflammatory messenger, actually has an opposite, anti-inflammatory effect when it's released by the muscles during exercise.**

As your muscles contract, the genes controlling IL-6 production are turned on. The more your muscles contract, the more IL-6 they produce; the more muscles used, the greater the response. When muscle energy stores begin to decline, even more IL-6 is released. So increasing exercise intensity and depleting energy stores proportionally enhance the release of IL-6 from the muscles. In other words, the more you do and the harder you do it (within reason), the more it helps.

Of course, this makes sense from a genetic standpoint. Exercising initially produces a strong inflammatory response, as the body tries to repair itself by releasing pro-inflammatory messengers. But new studies suggest that as you keep exercising, resting levels of these messengers fall very low, and levels of inflammatory markers such as CRP are cut in half. This is an exercise-induced stress response—an adaptive response—for inflammation.

Actually, adaptive stress induces muscle to protect us against inflammation, and therefore against inflammatory disease and aging. So yes, your muscles would become stronger. Even more importantly, though, the exercise-induced stress response leads to lower pro-inflammatory messengers and increased anti-inflammatory messengers, leaving you much less vulnerable to inflammatory disease.

> **The more frequent and more intense the activity level, the lower the risk of elevated, chronic whole-body inflammation.**

The IL-6 effect is emerging as a first line of defense against inflammation. Indeed, understanding the important role of muscles in the production of inflammatory and anti-inflammatory messengers is revolutionary. After all, skeletal muscle is the largest organ inside the body. And our new understanding of how this system works explains why exercise has such profound health benefits.

In particular, it sheds light on the positive relationship between exercise and chronic disorders associated with systemic low-level inflammation. For a long time, we scientists were puzzled by the beneficial effects of exercise on a number of highly inflammatory diseases, such as rheumatoid arthritis. RA was a particular mystery; the notion that anything that worked sore, inflamed joints could help and not hurt was completely counterintuitive. But RA patients and their doctors often swear by exercise. The actress Kathleen Turner, for instance, has often talked in interviews about how important exercise has been in managing her RA symptoms.

Now it appears that Turner and others with RA knew something that scientists didn't: Exercise has profoundly anti-inflammatory effects. This certainly helps explain why exercise can be so beneficial for RA and other inflammatory diseases.

So you can see why I'm promoting exercise as an inflammation-buster and moving away from the long-held party line about exercise as a weight-loss tool. That's not to say that it won't help your efforts there, too; it definitely can. I just would like for us to abandon the notion that exercise is *the* solution to our collective weight woes.

Further, I strongly believe that the tremendous anti-inflammatory powers of exercise have everything to do with the other health benefits that it can take credit for. After all, doctors have been "prescribing" exercise for what seems like forever, calling it the wonder drug. And indeed, when we look at studies of exercise—especially at the levels in Gene Smart—the benefits are amazing indeed.

Exercise helps you live longer! Ah, yes. We can talk all we want about inflammation and biomarkers of aging, but it is nice to actually measure life span. It's easier done in animals than in humans, but the science we have to support the claim that exercise extends life span is solid.

In 2005, Oscar H. Franco, MD, PhD, published in the *Archives of Internal Medicine* an analysis of data from the Framingham Heart Study. According to this analysis, people whose exercise habits were similar to the Gene Smart activity recommendations added almost 4 years to their life spans.

> **Exercising in the manner described in Gene Smart has been proven to extend life span by almost 4 years.**

In 2008, another very important study—also published in the *Archives of Internal Medicine*—identified a mechanism that could be responsible for the effect of exercise on longevity.

Telomeres are extra DNA sequences that sit at both ends of each chromosome. Every time a chromosome replicates, a small amount of the DNA at either end is lost. We don't know why this happens, but it does. As a result, telomeres naturally get shorter and shorter over an individual's lifetime. This is one of the signals that tells our cells that we are getting older. The length of the telomeres is, in a sense, a biological clock.

The study mentioned above involved 2,400 adult British twins, who provided blood samples and completed surveys about their health histories, smoking habits, and physical activity. The twins who engaged in moderate to vigorous exercise—similar to what is prescribed in Gene Smart—had longer telomeres, suggesting to the researchers that "inactive subjects may be biologically older by 10 years compared with more active subjects."

Exercise fights depression. Extensive research has shown that exercise is an effective if underused treatment for mild to moderate depression. It likely takes the amount and intensity of activity that's recommended in Gene Smart to see any effect. But even smaller bursts—as little as 10 to 15 minutes at a time—can improve mood in the short term.

We don't know exactly how exercise alleviates symptoms of depression and anxiety. There is evidence to suggest that it raises levels of certain neurotransmitters in the brain, such as endorphins, while reducing the stress hormone cortisol. It also increases body temperature, which may offer a calming effect. We'll have more answers once we better understand the role of inflammation in depression.

Exercise can help improve your cholesterol profile. Specifically, exercise increases the amount of HDL cholesterol (the good kind) in your blood, while reducing the amount of LDL cholesterol (the bad, artery-clogging kind). A relatively high volume and intensity of exercise is necessary to bring about these changes; clinical trials show that in 12 to 16 weeks, it can reduce total cholesterol by 10 to 20 percent.

> The exercise protocols recommended in Gene Smart can help lower your total cholesterol by 10 to 20 percent.

It's important to work out at the recommended volume and intensity. In 1990, researchers reported significant increases in HDL levels in men who exercised at or above 75 percent of their maximum heart rate (HRmax) three times a week for 12 weeks. Those who exercised at 65 percent HRmax did not see similar changes. The authors concluded that an intensity of at least 75 percent HRmax is necessary to increase HDL levels in men. That's why I believe it's so important to pay close attention to the Gene Smart targets set for you in Part 4.

Exercise can improve your sex life! Numerous studies support the contention that exercise may increase sexual drive, sexual activity, and sexual satisfaction.

For example, one study reported that women were more sexually responsive following 20 minutes of vigorous exercise. Among males, short bouts of intense exercise have been linked with increased testosterone levels, which may stimulate sexual interest and behavior.

Exercise also can enhance your sexual performance. Erectile dysfunction (ED) shares several modifiable risk factors with cardiovascular disease, including atherosclerosis, hypertension, hyperlipidemia (elevated blood lipids), diabetes mellitus, smoking, obesity, and sedentary lifestyle. One cardiologist I know calls ED "the canary in the coal mine" because up to 75 percent of patients with chronic heart failure (an increasingly common cardiovascular disorder) report erectile dysfunction.

> **Improving a man's physical fitness level with an exercise program like the one in Gene Smart significantly lowers his chances of ED.**

A 2005 study, published in the *American Journal of Cardiology*, demonstrated that short-term, moderate aerobic activity—similar to what's recommended in Gene Smart—improves sexual activity in men with stable chronic heart failure. This effect was correlated with improvements in functional capacity and quality of life, and was not influenced by medication.

Exercise can help manage your diabetes. Clinical trials involving people with type 2 diabetes proved that an exercise regimen like the one in Gene Smart improved insulin control by 23 percent, on average, and reduced CRP by a whopping 40 percent, on average.

Exercise will also improve your bone density, your resting heart rate, your lung function, your glucose tolerance, your sleep habits—the list goes on and on! And in all of these cases, the best results are seen when exercise is done for the intensity and duration adopted for Gene Smart.

HOW GENE SMART CAN HELP

Both the American College of Sports Medicine and the American Heart Association recommend that adults between ages 18 and 65 engage in 30 minutes of moderate-intensity aerobic exercise for a minimum of 5 days a week or 20 minutes of vigorous-intensity aerobic exercise for at least 3 days per week. In addition, adults should engage in some type of strength-training activity that targets the core muscles (those in the belly, pelvis, and lower back) at least twice a week.

Unfortunately, I believe that most of us seldom exercise in the proper dose and duration for optimal benefit, especially as it relates to whole-body inflammation. When I go to my local YMCA, I always check out the folks around me. On one side of the gym, people are barely breaking a sweat on the elliptical, even though they've been on the machine for an hour. On the other side, the bulky weightlifters are heaving huge amounts of weight for two or three reps, then talking to their buddies for 5 minutes before the next set.

Sadly, neither of these approaches is going to get you where you need to be to reduce whole-body inflammation. (It's not going to help you to lose weight, either.) They are not physically rigorous enough to force your body to adapt. In other words, they're not providing enough stress.

The American Heart Association recommends aiming for 50 to 85 percent of your maximum heart rate during your workouts. This is what's known as your target heart rate range, which I'll show you how to find. If you're not exercising in this range, then you may be just wasting your time.

On Gene Smart, you will be aiming for the low end of your target heart range (50 percent) for the first few weeks of aerobic and strength training. This is to ease you into physical activity, especially if you've not been exercising regularly. Gradually you will build up to the high end of your range (85 percent). This may seem quite intense right now, but there is a very important trade-off: You will never do an aerobic activity for more than 30 minutes. This is what makes Gene Smart so efficient; you'll never spend 2 hours at the gym again. You'll see better results than you've ever gotten before, only in a fraction of the time.

Every day of the Gene Smart Diet includes an exercise recommendation. Later in the book, you'll find a chart of moderate and vigorous aerobic activities, as well as a series of resistance and circuit-training moves that you can practice at the gym or in the privacy of your home, using nothing more complicated than a pair of inexpensive hand weights.

CHAPTER THIRTEEN

GENE SMART SOLUTION #3: ADD FIBER

HOW ARE YOU SUPPOSED TO LOSE WEIGHT when you're hungry all the time?

As anyone who's been on a conventional diet knows, hunger is a powerful driver—more powerful than anything else. And it's no wonder: According to a recently published article in the *Journal of Nutrition*, many of the most popular diets are shockingly—the American Heart Association would say dangerously—low in fiber. Yet fiber is the *only* thing proven to keep hunger pangs at bay, which is how it helps you lose weight. And as you'll soon see, it comes with a wealth of cardioprotective, cancer-preventing, blood-sugar-stabilizing benefits, including some that rival the best pharmaceuticals. That's something none of those other diets can claim.

When you follow Gene Smart, you'll be getting 15 grams of fiber for every 1,000 calories you consume—approximately 15 times what you'd get during the first 2 weeks on a diet like Atkins. That's why you won't find yourself "cheating" on Gene Smart: You're reaping all of fiber's health benefits, and you won't be hungry!

Just ask Claude Horn, one of our Hillsdale Study participants (see Claude's story on page 128). I believe our program "suited" Claude, as he says, because he was finally getting enough fiber to reduce his daily calorie intake. This allowed him to lose weight without effort because he wasn't hungry. I believe that's why Gene Smart will suit you, too.

NOT JUST TOO MANY CALORIES, BUT EMPTY CALORIES

More food, less exercise, more inflammation: We've already seen how these synergistic forces gain strength, depressing the adaptive stress response that's meant to help our bodies help themselves. But they're only the beginning.

Yes, we have what seems to be an endless food supply, and we eat far more than our genes would like us to. And yes, we aren't nearly as active as we ought to be. But these factors alone can't explain our dual epidemics of obesity and inflammatory disease. There's one more factor to add to the mix,

---

CLAUDE HORN

AGE: 74

STARTING WEIGHT: 210 pounds

LOST: 20.4 pounds, 2.6 percent body fat, 3.7 inches from waist, 4 inches from hips

CHANGES IN KEY BIOMARKERS AFTER 8 WEEKS ON GENE SMART

BODY MASS INDEX: –2.8 points

BLOOD PRESSURE: –12 mm/Hg diastolic

RESTING HEART RATE: –4 beats per minute

TOTAL CHOLESTEROL: –21 points

TRIGLYCERIDES: –89 points

FASTING INSULIN: 51 percent lower

FASTING LEPTIN: 66 percent lower

❝ I've been on other diets before; after they're all over, you just give them up. You buy stuff, and you don't follow through. Gene Smart is more of a way of life.

It's all about education—not just learning what to do and what not to do; you learn about the foods and how they affect your body. I cut out the sweets and pies and stuff like that, but somehow, the system overall seemed to suit me, without any major effort. There's no pain; you're just not hungry. That means it's something you can continue. I think that's one of the most important things for a weight-loss program.❞

---

and it's the quality of the food itself. As we've discussed throughout this book, it bears virtually no resemblance to what our hunter-gatherer ancestors were dining on.

> **Industrialization has brought changes in technology, leading to fundamental changes in the food itself.**

The refined grains so prevalent in our diet are one of the best examples of this. Hunter-gatherers wouldn't have known any kind of processed grain—no bread, no breakfast cereals, nothing. Before the Industrial Revolution, cereals would have been made using stone milling tools. And it's unlikely that the flour would have been sieved, which means that it would have contained the whole grain, including the germ, the bran, and the endosperm. Talk about a high-fiber diet!

By contrast, more than 85 percent of the cereals currently consumed in the United States are made from highly processed, refined grains. With "advancements" such as steamroller mills and automated sifting devices, the germ and the bran are removed in the manufacturing process, leaving us with flour that's made up mostly of endosperm with a uniform particle size— the building block for all those crunchy, sugary cereals and all that squishy white bread.

The difference between a diet of mostly whole grains and one that's almost entirely devoid of them has a truly profound impact on our health. Again, this change in technology—and the accompanying change in our food supply—is something that could have been possible only after the Industrial Revolution.

A recent study by Gladys Block, PhD, professor of epidemiology and public health nutrition at the University of California, Berkeley, reveals that three food groups—sweets and desserts, soft drinks, and alcoholic beverages— account for almost 25 percent of all calories consumed by Americans. Salty snacks and fruit-flavored drinks make up another 5 percent, bringing the total energy derived from nutrient-poor foods to at least 30 percent of total calorie intake.

"What is really alarming is the major contribution of 'empty calories' in the American diet," Dr. Block says. "We know people are eating a lot of junk food, but to have almost one-third of Americans' calories coming from those categories is a shocker. It's no wonder there's an obesity epidemic in this country."

It pretty much goes without saying that all the saturated fat and sugar in those desserts and all the high-fructose corn syrup in those sodas isn't good for us. But we're suffering as much from what's *not* in there as from what *is*. And one thing that is drastically, sorely missing from our diets also happens to be something that offers phenomenal health benefits: fiber.

FIBER: THE MIRACLE DRUG IN YOUR CEREAL BOWL

I'm a scientist, so I don't often give recommendations without qualification. But I will say this: The argument for increasing the amount of fiber in your diet is absolutely, positively unassailable.

Usually we think of fiber as something recommended to improve digestion, and it does. For instance, one study found that children with chronic constipation were consuming only one-quarter as much fiber as children who were not constipated.

There has also been much discussion about whether fiber prevents colon cancer. The largest study examining this topic—the European Prospective Investigation into Cancer and Nutrition study, involving over 521,000 people in 23 European countries—did find a correlation between low fiber intake and colon cancer risk. What's more, in populations with low fiber intakes, doubling dietary fiber could reduce the colon cancer risk by 40 percent.

But digestive health is really just the tip of the iceberg when we're talking about fiber's health benefits.

| Fiber's health benefits go far beyond digestive health.

It's absolutely astonishing to me that a recommendation as simple and easy as increasing fiber intake can reduce chronic full-body inflammation, as well as lower heart disease and diabetes risk. Honestly, what drug can promise all that? Fiber can—and does when taken at the dosages you'll be consuming on Gene Smart. Yet its virtues remain, in my opinion, largely unsung.

The fiber portion of the diet was unquestionably one of the big surprises for our Hillsdale Study participants. Many of them thought that increasing fiber intake was just something they did when they wanted to become more regular. Almost none of them had any idea how much fiber they were eating over the course of a normal day (or, perhaps I should say, how little)—or how many more fiber-rich foods they'd have to incorporate into their diets in order to make the minimum requirement. Their surprise was even greater when they realized how much fiber filled them up; in fact, every single one of the people we spoke to directly credited fiber with the fact that they hadn't been hungry.

Fiber 101

I am classifying fiber as a bioactive because it meets the definition of something that influences cellular activities to modify disease risk, rather than preventing deficiency diseases. Please note that it is *not* a nutrient in a classical sense, which is to say that it isn't essential for life—a fundamental criterion for a nutrient.

So what is it? Dietary fiber is plant material that humans can't digest; it's not absorbed into the bloodstream to be used as energy, so nearly 100 percent of it reaches the colon. That's why so many high-fiber foods are so low in calories.

Fiber comes in two forms: *soluble* and *insoluble*. Insoluble fiber passes through our intestines largely intact. It's the insoluble type of fiber that takes the credit for fiber's positive effects on constipation and digestive health, as it facilitates the movement of toxic substances through the colon in less time. Foods that are high in insoluble fiber include whole wheat breads, wheat cereals, wheat bran, cab-

bage, beets, carrots, brussels sprouts, turnips, cauliflower, and apple peels.

Soluble fiber forms a gel when it's mixed with liquid, while insoluble fiber does not. The soluble form is thought to be primarily responsible for lowering total cholesterol and LDL cholesterol (the so-called "bad" kind), therefore reducing the risk of heart disease. It is also credited with regulating blood sugar for people with diabetes.

Foods that are high in soluble fiber include oat bran, oatmeal, beans, peas, rice bran, barley, citrus fruits, strawberries, and apple pulp.

On Gene Smart, you'll get plenty of both kinds of fiber. In fact, I've designed the diet so that you get not only the correct amount of fiber, but what is considered an optimal ratio of insoluble to soluble (approximately 70/30). Fiber supplements are also available, although I encourage you to get your fiber from whole foods whenever possible.

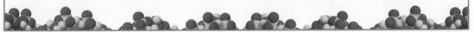

There is a tremendous amount of research on the benefits of fiber, which allows us to be very prescriptive with this powerful bioactive. As you will see, the fiber recommendations in Gene Smart are drawn from a large number of massive, long-term studies. Here's what they tell us:

Fiber in the dosages recommended in Gene Smart is strongly cardioprotective. The data are absolutely clear that a high-fiber diet can dramatically reduce your risk of heart disease.

To be honest, there are so many great studies demonstrating this that I can pick and choose. For instance, in one study of over 31,000 Seventh-Day Adventists, those who ate whole-wheat bread instead of white bread lowered their risk of nonfatal cardiovascular heart disease by 50 percent. That's right: Whole-wheat bread cut their risk in half.

The Iowa Women's Health Study showed that eating just one serving of a whole-grain product each day can reduce the risk of cardiovascular heart disease by one-third. The Health Professional Follow-Up Study, involving 43,757 male health professionals, showed that those with the highest fiber intake—about 29 grams per day—had a 55 percent reduced risk of cardiovascular disease. And in the Nurses' Health Study, which tracked 68,782 female nurses, those who ate 22.9 grams of fiber per day had a 66 percent reduced risk of heart disease. These are gigantic studies, and their results are conclusive.

Fiber's cardioprotective benefits come from, among other things, attacking the biomarkers of heart disease. Cholesterol is, of course, the cardiovascular biomarker that everyone knows about; it's the first thing your doctor tests for. The fiber dosages recommended in Gene Smart have been shown to reduce LDL cholesterol by an average of 10 to 15 percent.

And if you already have high cholesterol and are taking a medication for it, fiber will give your meds a turbo boost. In one study, total and LDL cholesterol concentrations were 4.7 percent and 6.7 percent lower in people on cholesterol medication who increased their fiber intakes compared with people taking meds alone.

A high-fiber diet like Gene Smart improves blood sugar levels. By delaying the absorption of nutrients, fiber increases insulin sensitivity, which lowers the risk of diabetes. In 33 out of 50 studies, fiber was shown to significantly reduce glycemic response, or the rise in blood sugar that occurs after a meal.

When you eat refined carbohydrates like those found in white bread and candy, your blood sugar levels go up, up, up and then crash precipitously, leaving you feeling sick and starving, as your body scrambles desperately for more energy and something to sop up the extra insulin you released to deal with all that sugar. High-fiber foods provide a much more measured response—another one of the reasons you'll be much less hungry on Gene Smart than on other diets you may have tried in the past.

Blood sugar is, of course, intrinsically linked to diabetes—another way in which our diets are making us sick. In one study of people eating low-, medium-, and high-glycemic-load diets, medium or large daily doses of cereal fiber dramatically reduced diabetes risk—by 50 percent, on average, in the case of large quantities of fiber. In our Hillsdale Study, we saw significant reductions in fasting insulin, a critical indicator of insulin resistance. Taken as a whole, studies to date reveal that by following the dietary recommendations for fiber and whole grains outlined in the Gene Smart meal plans, it's possible to reduce your risk of becoming diabetic by 30 to 40 percent.

That's something, given that diabetes is one of our fastest growing health problems—affecting over 20 million Americans, according to the Centers for Disease Control and Prevention (CDC)—and a leading cause of death for both men and women.

What explains fiber's cardioprotective, blood-sugar-stabilizing effect? Inflammation likely plays a big role, of course.

FIBER AND INFLAMMATION: LOOKING AT THE MESSENGERS

Fiber's terrific impact on diabetes and heart disease—both inflammatory conditions, as you'll remember—cannot be separated from its strong anti-inflammatory properties.

We can really see fiber's tremendous power over inflammation when we look at the impact of increased fiber intake on some of the most notorious inflammatory messengers, such as C-reactive protein (CRP). For example, results from huge epidemiological studies such as 1999–2000's National Health and Nutrition Examination Survey (NHANES) found that the more fiber people eat, the less likely they are to have high circulating concentrations of CRP.

> CRP concentrations were 63 percent lower in study partici-
> pants who reported consuming the most fiber—levels
> comparable to the ones you'll be eating when you follow
> Gene Smart.

In a very recent observational study involving 524 people, the likelihood of elevated CRP concentrations was 63 percent lower in participants who ate the most fiber compared to those who ate smaller amounts. These results reveal that dietary fiber is protective against high CRP—the molecule I think of as a general biomarker for disease—and certainly support current recommendations for a fiber-rich diet.

Another recent study in women with diabetes indicated that whole grains and bran were associated with significantly reduced amounts of CRP and TNF-alpha receptor, another inflammatory messenger strongly associated with insulin resistance, diabetes, congestive heart failure, and cancer. Finally, a study in people with hypertension, diabetes, or obesity revealed that dietary fiber intake results in a reduction of circulating CRP, concluding again that higher dietary fiber is strongly linked to a reduction in inflammatory markers in individuals with traditionally high levels of CRP—like people with diabetes, hypertension, or obesity. The relationship was even stronger when the study subjects had two or more of these conditions. In other words, the sicker you are, the more fiber can help.

Fiber, then, is really a stealth weapon. It gives us an inexpensive, non-pharmaceutical, risk- and side-effect-free (and I might even add delicious) solution to our most pervasive health problems, and to the chronic inflammation that drives them.

> There is overwhelming evidence that dietary fiber can play
> a pivotal role in lowering whole-body inflammation, in those
> who are sick as well as those who are healthy.

How does fiber work this magic? It probably signals which genes should be expressed and which should stay silent, although I will confess that we are not advanced in our understanding of the gene networks and master health regulators by which dietary fiber influences whole-body inflammation. Certainly part of its ability to affect whole-body inflammation may be a result of its capacity to cause weight loss in people; as you're already aware, there is a clear and direct relationship between weight loss and decreases in CRP and other inflammatory messengers in people who are obese. And fiber really does support weight loss.

There likely are many other ways in which fiber blocks whole-body inflammation. For example, some studies suggest that butyrate—a fatty acid found especially in fermentable fibers—may act as an anti-inflammatory. This claim is backed by clinical trials showing that butyrate has anti-inflammatory properties when used in chronic inflammatory diseases such as inflammatory bowel disease.

FIBER AND THE ADAPTIVE STRESS RESPONSE

I believe that one of the reasons fiber is so amazingly effective at stabilizing blood sugar, preventing heart disease, and fighting inflammation is that it works through the adaptive stress response. Admittedly, this is just a hypothesis, and one that needs to be rigorously tested. In truth, we don't know precisely why fiber engenders the adaptive stress response, but one explanation does seem plausible to me.

As you might imagine, a hunter-gatherer did not have a steady supply of food. How much and what he ate depended on a variety of factors—the season, the weather, drought, animal or plant diseases, his hunting ability, and his luck. For big chunks of time, he would have been on a regimen that looked very much like calorie restriction. And in those times, he would have turned to what was available to him.

In other words, when woolly mammoths were scarce and other delicacies were in short supply or buried under a layer of ice and snow, our hunter-gatherer forebear probably munched on things like tree bark. This would have kept his belly feeling full, even if tree bark wasn't a good energy source.

This adaptive strategy may have led to a number of very important health attributes, consistent with the regulator-triggered cellular "optimal maintenance" mode that we have talked about throughout this book. We may not know exactly how fiber does this, but observational and clinical evidence clearly indicates that fiber shifts several body and cellular systems into high gear.

RICK WHITESELL

AGE: 45

STARTING WEIGHT: 203 pounds

LOST: 13.2 pounds, 3.2 percent body fat, 3 inches from waist

CHANGES IN KEY BIOMARKERS AFTER 8 WEEKS ON GENE SMART

BMI: –1.9 points

CRP: 27 percent lower

FASTING INSULIN: 63 percent lower

FASTING LEPTIN: 55 percent lower

CIRCULATING LONG-CHAIN OMEGA-3s: 55 percent higher

❝ I knew I had to start taking care of myself. I'm not getting any younger, and my family history isn't very good. Both of my parents were diagnosed with type 2 diabetes in their mid-fifties; my dad had heart disease; and I have a family history of cancer. After the holidays last year, I weighed close to 210 pounds, which is too much for my frame. My cholesterol was high, too. I suffered through a bout of plantar fasciitis a few years back, which makes it very painful to walk; I don't know if that was related to my weight, but I think it was.

Now I've exercised on and off my whole life—I'm a runner—but I've never eaten very well. My weakness was fast food. I travel a lot for my job, and I'm always in a hurry, so I got into the habit of going to the drive-thru when I

> Our hunter-gatherer ancestors turned to fiber to fill them up, especially when a depleted food supply meant significant calorie restriction. That's likely why it activates so many protective genes.

Much of the evidence around fiber calls out its effects on hunger and satiety, based on its indigestible bulky properties and its influence over hormonal responses. Dietary fiber has clearly been shown to have a higher satiety value when compared with digestible complex carbohydrates and simple sugars. Eating fiber means that you eat less and stay more comfortable between meals, due to its bulk and relatively low energy density. So, you can feel full on far fewer calories.

Further, the chemicals and genetic machinery unleashed within the hunter-gatherer's body as a result of his fiber intake would have reduced his needed something to eat. Of course, I'd exercise to try to take some of that off, but it wasn't working that well. Between work and taking care of the kids, I started to put on the extra pounds. I was feeling it, too. I just didn't feel good; I didn't have the energy I should have had.

This program helped me put good eating and exercise together. The key to it was learning what to eat, and how it affected my body.

For instance, I had no idea there were so many benefits to eating as much fiber as we were on Gene Smart. I had been eating a little, but nothing even remotely close to the recommendations; in fact, I bet I was getting less than 10 grams of fiber a day before going on this program. I substantially increased that by eating more fruits and vegetables. I started eating high-fiber cereal with polyphenol-rich fruits like blackberries and blueberries, and I started drinking pomegranate juice. I hadn't known anything about polyphenols before. We're also eating a whole lot more fish in our family. I knew about omega-3s, but I didn't know about the importance of the ratios between omega-3s and omega-6s.

I'm very pleased with the results. The fiber helped keep me from getting hungry; that had always been my biggest challenge in the past. I'd try to cut back sometimes, but I'd get hungry, and then I'd cheat and end up eating more than I would have in the first place! I could always eat less during the day, but by dinner, I'd be so hungry that I'd eat everything in sight. I enjoyed the food that I learned to eat on this diet, and I wasn't hungry, so I was able to maintain my calorie intake.**"**

appetite, improved his health, and allowed him and his family to be more comfortable surviving during times of scarcity. In fact, estimates are that hunter-gatherers consumed about 40 grams of fiber per day—about three times more than the average American eats.

If hunter-gatherers turned to these high-fiber foods during times of calorie restriction, it makes sense that eating high-fiber foods would be one of the things that would put our bodies on high alert—the high alert that quells inflammation, prevents disease, and staves off premature aging.

This also gives us a hint as to why fiber is so great for weight loss. And fiber is *great* for weight loss. In fact, I think fiber is the single biggest key to losing weight and successfully reducing calories. Further, it's one of the reasons that Gene Smart is so effective at reducing not only your inflammatory profile, but your waistline as well.

BEST OF ALL: FIBER HELPS
YOU LOSE WEIGHT!

One thing has been proven beyond all doubt: The less fiber we eat, the fatter we become.

There is a strong and proven inverse correlation between high fiber consumption and obesity. In 1994, Jennie Brand-Miller, PhD, and her colleagues at the University of Sydney in Australia published a small study in which they found that dietary fiber was typically lower for obese men and women than for lean men and women. The researchers concluded that obesity is driven in part by a fiber-poor diet.

Much larger observational studies have confirmed this link between fiber intake and obesity. For example, a study involving more than 5,000 Swedes associated obesity with decreased consumption of fiber-rich foods like fruits and vegetables. And several population studies report that higher fiber consumption is related to lower obesity rates.

High-fiber foods are low in calories and add bulk to your diet. That's great news if you're dieting; it means that when you consume lots of fiber, you feel fuller for longer periods of time, and you eat less. All of this helps you to lose weight.

You might wonder how people following a calorie-restricted diet can stick with it without starving. Simple: They eliminate calories by eating nutrient-dense foods that contain fiber.

This strategy works. The proof is in the pudding—or the oatmeal, in this case. Studies have shown that in 12 weeks, dieters can lose 7 to 10 pounds *even without reducing calories*, just by adding fiber and exercise to their diets in the concentrations prescribed in Gene Smart. That, to me, is incredibly compelling.

Other studies show that you can get synergy on your side by adding fiber to calorie-reduced diets. When the people in these studies increased their fiber while watching what they ate, they were able to lose 28 percent more weight than with calorie reduction alone. That's an amazing turbo boost, considering how easy it is to implement.

If you're already overweight, the fiber recommendations in Gene Smart can really help. Many interventional studies have confirmed the potent effects of dietary fiber in treating obesity. In 2000, Grethe S. Birketvedt,

MD, PhD, and her colleagues found that the addition of dietary fiber to a low-calorie diet improved weight loss by 37 percent. In another study published in the *Journal of the American Dietetic Association*, both higher fiber diets and very low-fat diets without calorie restriction were associated with significant weight loss (8 percent of initial body weight over 8 months). And in a 12-week, randomized, controlled study that did involve calorie restriction, a high-carbohydrate, fiber-enriched diet caused significant reductions in body weight (approximately 7 pounds) and body fat (about 2 percent) in older men and women. This is doubly significant because older people tend to have a harder time losing weight.

I know from personal experience—and the Hillsdale Study data support this—that the main reason fiber helps you to lose weight is that it makes you feel *full*. In this way, high-fiber foods can displace high-calorie foods in your diet.

GENE SMART MAKES IT EASY TO INCREASE YOUR FIBER LEVELS

Despite all these health benefits, and the fact that increasing fiber is a surefire (and painless!) way to lose weight, the average adult intake in the United States is only about 15 grams, according to the American Heart Association. That's seriously shy of the recommended 25 to 35 grams of fiber per day for adults, which is why too little dietary fiber is another critical low-pressure system contributing to our Perfect Storm.

> **Increasing fiber intake, in the right types and dosages, will be one of your first priorities when you follow Gene Smart.**

Given what we now know about fiber's effects, not only on health but on weight loss, you would think that all modern diets would utilize increased fiber as a strategy to get people to eat less, wouldn't you?

To address this important question, James W. Anderson, MD, and his colleagues at the University of Kentucky examined the fiber levels of popular diets. In a survey using a 1,600-calorie weight-loss diet as a benchmark, dietary fiber intakes ranged from 4 grams per day for the Atkins diet to 49 grams per day for the Ornish diet. A more recent analysis found that several high-protein, low-carbohydrate diets—including Atkins and South Beach—were very, even dangerously, low in dietary fiber.

Joanne L. Slavin, PhD, RD, of the University of Minnesota recently published the dietary fiber content of these currently popular diets, based on representative menus shown on their websites, in the *Journal of Nutrition*. These data are shown below.

CALORIC AND DIETARY FIBER CONTENT OF POPULAR WEIGHT-LOSS DIETS

DIET	KCAL/DAY	DIETARY FIBER (GRAMS/DAY)
SOUTH BEACH DIET		
Phase 1	1,043	4.4
Phase 2	1,088	7.6
Phase 3	1,026	3.0
ATKINS DIET		
Induction	1,015	1.6
Ongoing weight loss	1,297	7.2
Premaintenance	1,027	9.3
Lifetime maintenance	1,681	5.0

The dietary fiber content in the Atkins diet is extremely low throughout the diet, but especially in the early phases (only 1.6 grams per day in the induction phase). The South Beach diet was also extremely low in dietary fiber, always less than 10 grams per day.

Doing these diets "properly" cheats you out of most of the fiber that the American Heart Association recommends you get—and all the cardioprotective, anti-inflammatory benefits we've discussed in this chapter. And I personally feel that the very design of these diets makes them tough to stay on—unless you like the feeling of being hungry.

On Gene Smart, you will be eating lots of high-fiber cereals, breads, whole grains, beans, vegetables, and fruits. In the adaptive phase, you'll be getting 16 grams of fiber for every 1,000 calories you consume; then you'll adjust to 15 and eventually 14 grams for every 1,000 calories as you progress through preconditioning to optimal maintenance. (Current fiber recommendations are tied to calorie intake, which explains why the standard recommendation for men, up to 38 grams per day, is higher than the recommendation for women, at 25 grams per day. With the Gene Smart recommendations, you can be more precise, so you get exactly what you need.)

These recommendations allow you to reap all the benefits of increased fiber—to your heart, your overall health, and your waistline. It is indeed very disappointing that many popular diets have missed out on this opportunity.

Unlike with the polyphenols, which we'll discuss in Chapter 15, we have a very good idea of how much and what types of fiber are in the foods we eat and how much fiber we ought to eat. With that information in hand, Gene Smart utilizes this bioactive to its fullest potential, to help you to melt away those unwanted pounds *without feeling hungry*—not to mention all the other health benefits you'll enjoy.

CHAPTER FOURTEEN

GENE SMART SOLUTION #4: CORRECT THE OMEGA FATS

THE LONG-CHAIN OMEGA-3 and omega-6 fats are some of the most powerful bioactives available in our food. That is precisely what makes them so dangerous when they are deployed at the wrong concentrations and in the wrong ratios, as they are in the standard American diet. And it is precisely what makes them such a boon to our health when those ratios are corrected—as they will be on Gene Smart.

When the concentrations and ratios are correct, there is simply nothing like it for human health. The long-chain omega-3 fatty acids in particular have a profound effect on inflammation, and the correct ratio of these bioactives have been found to prevent and reverse cardiovascular diseases (heart disease and stroke) in a large proportion of the populations of developed countries. The also have been shown to produce positive effects in diabetes, allergies, asthma, arthritis, psoriasis, and cancer, to name just a few—as well as other diseases with an inflammatory driver, including cognitive decline with age and depression. And they can help you to lose weight.

We know a great deal about the omega fats. We know, for instance, how rich various food sources are in these fats. We have some information on how they affect the master health regulators that control our genes, and in particular how some of these fats are converted to the messengers that control inflammation, for good and for bad. The fact that we know so much about the omegas—and their potential to harm or help us—makes the dramatic change in the type of fats we routinely consume a very alarming one.

> **Changes in our food supply have led to radical—and very dangerous—changes in the type of fats we consume.**

I can tell you, it is a change that has *not* gone unnoticed by our genes.

But knowing so much also makes it possible to be very precise in our Gene Smart solution. I personally love this area of science; the omega fats (and their effect on inflammation) have been my primary area of interest for over 30 years. In this chapter, we'll look at the scientific research on those fats— the good, the bad, and the ugly—and I'll help you to distinguish the facts from the fiction about them. Trust me, there are a lot of both. The conversation about fats in this country has become very confusing over the last 30 years. The good news is that we now have enough data to offer you proven strategies to get enough of what you need without too much of what causes overactive inflammation.

FATS 101

Since fat is such a troubled topic for Americans, let's start at the beginning. Fat can be divided into two categories: saturated and unsaturated. Although I don't believe in labeling fats as "good" or "bad"—they all perform very important functions—the proper balance is essential, and it is that balance that has been upset. Suffice it to say that we now eat many more saturated and monounsaturated fats than we used to, and get far fewer polyunsaturated fats—a development that has not been good for our health.

The long-chain polyunsaturated fats (PUFAs) can be further divided into two categories: the omega-3 fatty acids and the omega-6 fatty acids. Again, while we do need omega-6s for various reasons, you will see in this chapter that the omega-3s tend to be anti-inflammatory and cardioprotective, while consuming too many omega-6 fats (especially long-chain omega-6s) can lead to an overproduction of inflammatory messengers.

It's useful for us to remember that not all of these bioactives are beneficial. For instance, I wrote extensively in *Inflammation Nation* about one long-chain omega-6 fatty acid called arachidonic acid, or AA. AA is directly responsible for the production of inflammatory messengers. If we eat food that contains too much AA, we're likely to produce too many inflammatory messengers, and too many inflammatory messengers means inflammatory disease.

> **High levels of AA in our diets cause us to produce abnormally high numbers of inflammatory messengers.**

AA has been linked to heart disease in humans. It's a good example of how something in your food can have whopping consequences for your health. And yet, this is news to most people—including most doctors.

AA is present in large quantities in our food because of the series of changes in our food supply that we'll be discussing in this chapter.

OMEGA FATS AND THE INDUSTRIAL REVOLUTION

The shift in the ratios of which type of fats we eat that has taken place in the last hundred years is truly radical and very scary.

For hundreds of thousands of years, hunter-gatherer humans consumed an estimated ratio of omega-6 to omega-3 fatty acids of 2:1. These ratios were maintained for over 100,000 generations, until the Industrial Revolution. Then—unbelievably—in just three short generations, everything changed.

My laboratory examines this ratio in study patients every day, and we tend to find that even in young, healthy volunteers, that ratio is now greater than 15:1. It is often much, much worse in those with poor eating habits. Three generations is .003 percent of how long humans have existed on this earth—the equivalent of less than a single second in a 24-hour day. But in that period of time, less than the blink of an eye, we completely changed the fat bioactives in our food supply.

To make matters worse, the majority of the omega-3 PUFAs that we consume in our modern diet are not the beneficial long-chain omega-3s, but the short-chain omega-3s, alpha-LNA. In fact, alpha-LNA—which is derived from oils such as flaxseed oil—is the short-chain omega-3 that makes up more than 90 percent of our omega-3 PUFA intake. Not only would a hunter-gatherer's ratios have been better, but the majority of his omega-3s would have been long-chain, from fish or other marine products.

Once again, we appear to have gotten incredibly far away from the nutrients our bodies are designed to eat.

How did this dramatic shift take place?

More vegetable oils: With the Industrial Revolution came mechanical still expellers that could crush oil-bearing seeds, and solvent extraction procedures that could efficiently extract the fats in the form of oil. In the past century, there has been a dramatic increase in the occurrence of vegetable oils in the food supply of Western nations such as the United States. For example, margarine consumption has increased by 410 percent, shortening consumption by 136 percent, and salad and cooking oil consumption by 130 percent. That means that we get a much larger proportion of our fatty acids as saturated and monounsaturated fatty acids.

More meat: We're also eating a great deal more meat than we have at any other point in history. The short-term economics of the massive animal feedlots where the majority of the meat in this country is produced are very favorable, which means that the producers can pass along those savings to the consumer. The fact that meat is so much less expensive than it has ever been is one of the reasons we're eating so much more of it—but it also means that almost all of it comes from grain-fed animals, raised on factory farms.

Why does that matter? Because expeller presses and the availability of inexpensive meat aren't the only way that technology has affected the fats we consume. In fact, technological advances in wide-scale food production have changed the food we eat at its most fundamental level. It's not just what we eat that has changed, but *what our food eats*.

Before the Neolithic period, all animals consumed by humans would have been wild. The absolute quantity and type of fat in these animals would have been dependent upon several factors, including the species, body mass, age, season, location, and food supply.

As you've probably noticed, mammals store energy as fat. The dominant fatty acids in these fat deposits are saturated fat, the kind that drives up cholesterol, which is why your doctor tells you to stay away from the ribeye when you're trying to decrease your LDL. (Those deposits are visible as white streaks throughout the meat—the "marbling" so coveted by steak connoisseurs.) The dominant fatty acids in other parts of the animal—in muscles and organ tissue, for instance—are polyunsaturated and monounsaturated fatty acids, the so-called "good" fats.

Now wild animals in prehistoric times were dealing with the same seasonal food shortages that their human counterparts were. So they too were lean for much of the year, with monounsaturated and polyunsaturated fats making up the greatest percentage (much greater than 50 percent of the animal's energy stores) of the edible fatty acids in the animal. And the omega-6 to omega-3 ratios were much closer to 1:1, which meant that the humans who were killing and eating them were getting mostly poly- and monounsaturated fats—the "good" ones—from their steak dinners.

As agriculture and animal husbandry developed and advanced, the animals were no longer left to their own devices. And the constitution of the animals the humans were eating changed drastically as a result. Instead of catching a skinny pig who was snuffling through the snow for something edible, you went out and killed the pig in your backyard, all fattened up on the corn you'd grown, harvested, and stored for precisely this purpose. Unlike their wild counterparts, domestic animals maintained a steady body-fat content—and the humans eating them were consuming a corresponding increase in saturated fatty acids as a result. Because the farmer was in control of the situation, it also became possible to slaughter animals at their peak body-fat composition, as opposed to when that pig and your arrow happened to be in the same place at the same time.

The shift was widely embraced. In the United States before 1850, virtually all cattle were free-range or grass-fed, and were typically slaughtered between the ages of 4 and 5. By the late 1800s, fattening systems and feedlots had advanced so much that it was possible to produce a very large steer (more than 500 kilograms) for slaughter in just 2 years. The meat from that cow would have been "marbled"—something you don't find as often in wild, free-range, or grass-fed cattle. As a result, this meat contains much higher concentrations of saturated fat and omega-6 PUFAs—which markedly affect blood lipids like cholesterol and worsen whole-body inflammation.

So not only has the amount of meat we're eating increased dramatically, but the nutritional content of the meat we're eating in such great quantities has also changed—again, dramatically.

> Today's meat has more saturated fat and fewer polyunsaturated fats, and most of the polyunsaturated fatty acids that *are* present are omega-6s.

It's pretty simple: We are what we eat—and what the animals we're eating ate. If we feed cows corn, we are feeding them short-chain omega-6s, as opposed to the short-chain omega-3s they'd be eating if they grazed on grass. That means the ribeye on your plate is delivering a whole lot more omega-6s than it would have in your ancestors' day. One study put the omega-6 to omega-3 ratio in conventional beef at 4:1, as compared to 2:1 in grass-fed beef; moving to grass enhanced beneficial omega-3 content by 60 percent. Grass-fed beef is also leaner and lower in calories than conventional beef because of what these cows eat, with total fat and saturated fat levels often more than 40 percent less than comparable cuts.

During the same period of time, other technologies advanced on a parallel track. These were food processing procedures that allowed us to store various forms of saturated fatty acids—in the guise of delicious cheese, butter, and tallow—for consumption throughout the year.

So once again, we see that some of the most primary foods in our diets either didn't exist in hunter-gatherer times—cheese and lard, for instance—or have a fundamentally different nutritional profile than they did when our ancestors walked the earth—like feedlot beef. But while the food has changed, your genes haven't. And that's pretty important, when the bioactive ingredients in those foods—or the lack thereof—are determining how your genes function.

OUT WITH THE BAD, IN WITH THE GOOD

As I have said, I believe that a major reason that we are so ill is that we consume too many long-chain omega-6s. But there's another side to that coin, one that's also contributing to the inflammation epidemic, and that's the lack of omega-3s in our diets.

As I have said many times, when the omegas are good, they're very, very good. That's never truer than when we're talking about the long-chain omega-3s found in fatty fish and fish oil.

THERESA STANLEY

AGE: 47

STARTING WEIGHT: 121 pounds

LOST: 12 pounds, 8 percent body fat, 5 inches from waist, 4 inches from hips

CHANGES IN KEY BIOMARKERS IN 8 WEEKS ON GENE SMART

RESTING HEART RATE: –8 beats per minute

CIRCULATING WHITE BLOOD CELLS: 13 percent lower

TOTAL CHOLESTEROL: –17 points

LDL CHOLESTEROL: –31 points

CIRCULATING INSULIN: 99 percent lower

C-REACTIVE PROTEIN: 51 percent lower

FASTING LEPTIN: 73 percent lower

CIRCULATING LONG-CHAIN OMEGA-3s: 189 percent higher

66 I was small when I went on Gene Smart; I just had lots of body fat. I never got out of a size 2, but my body fat was 30 percent. I was shocked to find out that it was that high, but I knew I had a lot of fat on me, especially in my midsection. And I lost 8 percent of my body fat in 8 weeks.

The change in my energy level has been absolutely amazing. I think a lot of it has to do with the exercise, honestly. Before I did Gene Smart, I felt awful, probably because I ate sugar all the time. I was really depressed, and my energy level was very low. I'd just drag all day and want to take a nap as soon as I got home. My sleep was terrible; I'd wake up four or five times a night. After a couple of weeks on the diet, I was waking up in the morning, thinking: 'I can't believe I slept through the night!' That helps your energy level, too.

I really feel like the world needs this knowledge. I had tried other diets, but the difference with this one is that you're never really hungry, because the fiber makes you feel so full. I love ice cream and all that stuff, but I'd eat berries frozen with low-fat milk and Splenda, and it was better than ice cream.

The weight came off really fast. My goal was just to lose 10 or 12 pounds; I lost just what I wanted to! It just kind of fell off of me. I look totally different now. I don't know if it's the confidence, or my new muscles, or the fact that my waist is so much smaller, but everybody is telling me that my posture is better, and I'm not standing any differently. 99

> **No other food has been so proven to promote health as the omega-3 polyunsaturated fatty acids, which are found predominantly in fatty fish and fish oil supplements.**

Unfortunately, in too many cases, they have been forced out of our diet by the pro-inflammatory omega-6s.

The bounty of the ocean is not to be underestimated. Many fish are astonishingly high in omega-3 polyunsaturated fatty acids, and there is incontrovertible evidence demonstrating the health benefits of these.

> **Fish is our primary source of very beneficial long-chain omega-3 fatty acids.**

As recently as 50 years ago, our last real bastion of wilderness—and our last source of truly "wild" food—was the ocean. But this has also changed, and the concomitant change in the fatty acid ratios of the fish we eat has had an equal impact on our inflammatory profiles.

You see, these fatty acids, whether from wild fish or fish oil supplements, have been extensively studied. About this there can be absolutely no debate: They unquestionably reduce the risk of heart attack and other problems related to heart and blood-vessel disease, as well as the risk of a variety of other inflammatory diseases.

> **The data at every level (epidemiological, clinical, interventional, animal, and isolated cell) show that long-chain omega-3s dramatically improve cardiovascular health, with a direct impact on killers like atherosclerosis, heart disease, and stroke.**

The recommendations for omega intake and ratio have been shown to be powerfully effective at reducing independent risk factors for cardiovascular disease and heart attack. If blood work and other assessments have shown you to be at high risk for heart disease, convincing clinical studies indicate that you can expect to see significant favorable improvement in your test numbers in as little as 12 weeks. Specifically, fish oils at the dosage recommended in Gene Smart have been shown to:

Reduce the likelihood of a first heart attack. Several very large population studies report significantly fewer heart attacks and deaths from heart disease among people who regularly eat fish. These data suggest that by following the dietary guidelines of Gene Smart, including the fish entrees and fish oil supplements prescribed, individuals can reduce the risk of nonfatal heart attack by greater than 25 percent on average.

Lower high triglycerides. Here the evidence is overwhelming. A recent analysis of 17 large, population-based trials revealed that high circulating triglyceride levels are a critical independent risk factor for cardiovascular disease. Numerous clinical interventional trials have demonstrated that in people with high triglycerides, taking fish oils at the concentrations and duration prescribed in Gene Smart can reduce triglyceride levels by an average of 20 to 30 percent.

Lower elevated resting heart rate. In people with elevated resting heart rates—a significant predictor of sudden death—the fish oil concentrations and duration prescribed in Gene Smart have been shown to reduce heart rate by 2.5 beats per minute, or over 10 million fewer heartbeats in an 80-year lifetime.

Lower risk of death by a heart attack and prevent a second heart attack in those with a history of heart disease. Nobody likes to think about it, but a million Americans will die of a heart attack this year. The concentration and duration of fish oil supplements prescribed in Gene Smart have been shown to reduce chances of death from a heart attack in folks with a history of heart disease *by as much as 50 percent*, on average.

According to the American Heart Association, one out of four men and one out of three women who survive a heart attack will die within the following year. There's evidence that the concentration of omega-3s prescribed in Gene Smart can cut that risk by 45 percent.

In many of the studies to date, patients were using standard heart medication. This suggests that fish oil adds to the beneficial effects of other therapies.

> The long-chain omega-3 fatty acids are more effective at reducing mortality from heart disease than practically any pharmaceutical currently on the market.

The science so far suggests that the astonishing efficacy of the long-chain omega-3s, particularly in quelling overactive inflammation and the diseases connected to it, has a great deal to do with their ability to communicate with the master health regulators—the survival switches—we've been discussing in this book, and consequently with our genes. In fact, it appears that the omegas may be one of the most powerful bioactives we have in this regard.

OMEGAS AND YOUR HEART: THE WHOLE STORY

Over 40 years ago, two scientists, Hans Olaf Bang, MD, and Jörn Dyerberg, MD, began the first studies to link low mortality from cardiovascular disease among Greenland Eskimos (when compared to age- and sex-matched Danish controls). They believed that the low levels of heart disease they found were due to the consumption of high concentrations of long-chain omega-3 PUFAs in the Greenland Eskimo diet—and they were right.

Since then, study after study has shown that long-chain omega-3s reduce heart disease risk. I personally began to take fish oil religiously after reading two pivotal studies, together involving over 90,000 individuals. In 2001, results of the GISSI-Prevenzione study (11,323 patients with a recent heart attack) were published, convincingly demonstrating that long-chain omega-3 PUFA supplements significantly lowered all-cause mortality, resulting largely from a 45 percent reduction in sudden cardiac death during 3.5 years of follow-up. What was so interesting to me was that there were statistically significant differences (in other words, mathematics tells us that what we are seeing has a 95 percent chance of being real) between the omega-3 and placebo groups after *only* 3 months. This difference only grew larger every month as the study continued for 3.5 years. I know nothing else that can do this, especially in this patient population.

Then, in the Nurses' Health Study of 84,688 women, those without prior cardiovascular disease showed a much lower risk of heart attacks, fatal and nonfatal, with increased intake of fish or omega-3 PUFAs. More recently, a meta-analysis that examined fish consumption and coronary heart disease (CHD) in 13 cohort studies confirmed that the more fish a person eats, the lower his or her chances are of having coronary heart disease, as well as sudden cardiac death. The additional news from this study was truly groundbreaking because it allowed us, for the first time, to quantify the benefits. The study's authors found that for each 20 grams a day (a little more than half an ounce) increase in fish consumption, there is an associated 7 percent reduction in fatal coronary heart disease.

Here's what that means in English: We typically eat about 3.5 ounces of fish in a single sitting; if we ate that every day, it would translate into a *35 percent reduction in fatal coronary heart disease.*

> One serving of fish a day results in a **35 percent reduction**
> **in fatal heart disease.** You'll be consuming the equivalent of
> *two to three times* that when you follow Gene Smart.

Given the benefits outlined above, the big question is: What would it mean for heart disease mortality if people utilized this anti-inflammatory strategy? Given an approximate 36 percent reduction in heart-related deaths, intake of fish or fish oil would reduce all mortality by an average of approximately 14 percent in all populations. Isn't that staggering? According to another study that analyzed all placebo-controlled, double-blind, randomized trials since 2003, long-chain omega-3s would reduce all mortality by 17 percent.

Just for fun, let's compare that to the best-selling pharmaceuticals in the world, the statin drugs. The combined sales of the two leaders in this category, Lipitor and Zocor, add up to more than $13 billion a year. Meta-analysis of statins suggests that they reduce all mortality by 15 percent. The omega-3 bioactives, taken by enough people, have the potential to save more lives than the most used and profitable pharmaceuticals we can produce.

THE OMEGAS AND INFANT BRAIN DEVELOPMENT

Evidence reveals that infants have improved problem-solving skills if their mothers consume foods containing docosahexaenoic acid (DHA) during preg-

A New Biomarker of Cardiovascular Disease?

In a recent article in the *American Journal of Clinical Nutrition*, Clemens von Schacky, MD, and William Harris, PhD, proposed that an "omega-3 index" (EPA + DHA as a percent of total red blood cell fatty acids) be considered a new risk factor for death from heart disease. (Red blood cells are easily obtained cells that give an indication of the level of dietary long-chain omega-3s.)

The preponderance of studies that have looked at long-chain omega-3s have shown that levels of 6 percent or above are cardioprotective, and levels below 4 percent are associated with an increased risk for CHD. Using data from the Physicians' Health Study and another study examining primary heart attacks, the omega-3 index was clearly related to risk of having a heart attack. For example, there was a greater than 90 percent risk reduction for the one-quarter of individuals with the highest levels of long-chain omega-3s in their red blood cells.

This predictive value was far greater than that associated with C-reactive protein (a 65 percent reduction in risk with the lowest CRP) or total cholesterol levels (a 35 percent reduction in risk with the lowest cholesterol).

These studies are remarkable. I believe they suggest that the levels of long-chain omega-3 fatty acids should be routinely measured in all individuals, but especially in those at risk of an inflammatory disease like heart disease. Your cholesterol is measured at every check-up, and yet there may not be a great association between this biomarker and a heart attack. In fact, according to a study published in the *New England Journal of Medicine* in 2002 and another one published in *JAMA* in 2003, *most* cardiac and stroke events occur in individuals without elevated cholesterol, and one-fifth of all events take place in individuals without any traditional risk factors. The omega-3 index study would seem to indicate that we'd do better to check our omegas.

Unfortunately, it is difficult to find reputable laboratories that measure long-chain omega-3 levels in human blood. For more information on this test and where it can be done, go to www.genesmart.com.

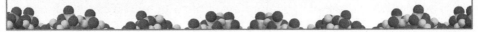

nancy. Although it's possible that children born to women who eat large amounts of mercury-containing fish could see their IQ scores fall slightly (up to 1.5 points), the Harvard Center for Risk Analysis proposes that the risk would be far outweighed by the benefits of eating small amounts of fish. I'm concerned about mercury, too, but I think the public hysteria on this topic has done more harm than good. Based on clinical studies, children born to pregnant women who eat enough fish to get the equivalent of 1 gram of DHA per day would be likely to see an increase in IQ scores ranging from 0.8 to 1.8 points.

On a national level, this small amount (8 ounces) of the right type of fish would translate into some tremendous annual benefits, according to the researchers.

> If everyone in the United States consumed 8 ounces of salmon (a low-mercury fish) per week, it would mean 20,000 fewer deaths from cardiovascular disease, 4,000 fewer nonfatal strokes, and an aggregate increase of more than 2 million IQ points in newborn children.

THE OMEGAS AND OTHER INFLAMMATORY CONDITIONS

But heart disease is just one of the inflammatory conditions that the omega-3s can affect. In addition to heart disease and cognitive function, long-chain omega-3s have been shown to be beneficial in treating a host of other inflammatory conditions, including arthritis, allergies, asthma, depression and bipolar disorder, inflammatory bowel disease, and psoriasis—to mention only a few.

Here are some highlights from a selection of other studies that have looked closely at the power of these fats.

Critical-care patients in intensive care: I know—this would seem to lack relevance in a consumer book. But I'm including these studies because there are few scientific areas where the power of the bioactives in long-chain omega-3 fats and in combinations of long-chain omega-3 fats with gamma-linolenic acid (GLA, a fatty acid found in borage oil) is more evident than in critical-care patients. And while the results may not be as applicable to the population at large as, say, knowing that fish oils are cardioprotective, I think there's something to be learned from them. These patients are the sickest of the sick. They are often overwhelmed with whole-body inflammation in ways that would never be seen in healthy people. So if fish oils can make an appreciable and beneficial difference in them, doesn't it make you wonder exactly what they can do for those of us who aren't—thank God—so sick?

The fish oil effect first reached the public's attention when Randall

McCloy, Jr., was pulled from a West Virginia coal mine in January 2007 with brain, heart, kidney, and liver failure caused by exposure to carbon monoxide. His neurologist, Julian Bailes, MD, administered high doses of fish oil concentrate as a regular part of McCloy's treatment regimen. It is claimed that the fish oil helped to reduce the inflammation in his organs—rebuilding his brain and reversing the damage to his heart, kidneys, and liver.

To be quite honest, I typically dismiss such stories because they involve only one person, but in this case, the science was there. You see, there was already a relatively large database of clinical and animal trials supporting the use of long-chain omega-3s, or the combination of long-chain omega-3s and GLA found in borage oil, in critical-care patients—with sometimes almost miraculous results.

Axel Heller, MD, PhD, and colleagues have recently presented outcome data from a multiple-center trial (82 centers, 661 patients) investigating the addition of omega-3 fatty acids to a standard soybean lipid emulsion in critical-care settings. Overall, the administration of omega-3 fatty acids significantly improved survival and diminished mortality, infection rates, and length of hospital stay.

Similarly, long-chain omega-3s in combination with GLA have provided dramatic benefits in at least three clinical studies. The fact that we see such amazing efficacy in the sickest of the sick only reinforces what we know about the role these bioactives play in the health of those of us who are not yet at the very brink of survival.

Mental health (depression, schizophrenia, bipolar syndrome, aggression, dementia, and Alzheimer's disease): There's quite a bit of evidence that the omegas play an important role in the mental health area as well. Joseph Hibbeln, MD, a researcher for the National Institutes of Health, has been a pioneer in this field. He has shown convincing epidemiological evidence for a correlation between depression and fish consumption.

In a study by my own laboratory, in collaboration with Carol Shively, PhD, of Wake Forest, 41 percent of monkeys fed a high-fat diet with few omega-3s showed signs of depression. That's an astonishing number, considering that we see little depression in monkeys that are fed low-fat monkey chow.

Dr. Hibbeln also pointed out a significant correlation between omega-3 deficiencies and aggression. Other studies have shown that long-chain omega-3s help with the treatment of depression, bipolar disorder, and schizophrenia.

Interestingly, the long-chain omega-3 EPA (eicosapentaenoic acid) has already been used to treat several psychiatric and neurodegenerative diseases due to its anti-inflammatory and neuroprotective effects. In fact, six out of seven clinical trials have shown that EPA significantly improved depressive symptoms when compared with the placebo-treated populations.

In animal models of Alzheimer's disease, dietary depletion of DHA (docosahexaenoic acid) dramatically worsens the disease, while DHA supplementation markedly improves cognitive function.

This is a rapidly growing and very promising area of research; if you'd like more information, I would suggest you read *The Omega-3 Connection* by Andrew Stoll.

Cognitive function: Decreased cognitive function is one of the worst parts of getting older. Not only do these "senior moments" reduce our productivity, but they erode our self-confidence and perceived ability to function in the world. "It's humiliating," an elderly colleague of mine told me, after forgetting the name of a molecule he'd spent the last 30 years researching during a lecture to a hundred scientists. "I feel like a doddering old fool."

Here, too, it looks like correcting our omega ratios—as we will do in Gene Smart—can help. In 1997, a study involving almost 1,000 men found that those who consumed the largest amounts of omega-6 fats showed a 76 percent greater decline in general cognitive function than those who ate the lowest amounts.

Much more recently, in 2007, a study published in the *American Journal of Clinical Nutrition* examined data on fish consumption among 210 participants who were between 70 and 89 years of age in 1990. Data on cognitive functioning collected in 1990 and 1995 were used in the study. The intake of EPA and DHA (EPA + DHA) was calculated for each participant. Participants who consumed fish had significantly less cognitive decline over the intervening 5 years than those who didn't eat fish. Further, the more fish the participants ate, the slower their decline was. The study concluded that "moderate intake of EPA + DHA may postpone cognitive decline in elderly men." While this is not a large study, it certainly provides me with enough data to recommend this simple strategy to my elderly loved ones.

Help! I Don't Like Fish!

At every talk that I give, someone raises their hand to ask me what they should do if they (a) are vegetarian, or (b) can't tolerate fish.

There is no answer for my strict vegetarian friends, unfortunately, although I believe there will be shortly. But if you're one of the people who can't eat fish due to an aversion to its smell and taste, you probably can tolerate fish oil supplements, especially the encapsulated type. And many vegetarians, like Michelle Marcey (pages 160–161), make an exception for fish oil.

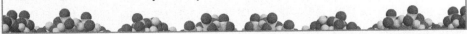

Allergies: Animal experiments strongly suggest that Mom ingesting long-chain omega-3 fats while she is pregnant may prevent allergies in her offspring. However, there have been only a few human trials in this area. In the studies that have been done, perinatal supplementation had some positive impact on allergy susceptibility. More studies are needed.

There have been few studies examining omega-3s for allergies in children. One, in Australian children, found that those who were fed oily fish were 75 percent less likely to develop allergic asthma. Researchers at Jikei University School of Medicine in Tokyo found that long-chain omega-3 supplementation produced an improvement in asthmatic symptoms and a decrease in airway responsiveness.

In adults, we know that long-chain omega-3 fats reduce inflammatory messengers (eicosanoids and cytokines). In fact, my own laboratory has demonstrated that shifting circulating ratios of omega-6s to omega-3s from greater than 15:1 to less than 5:1 in humans turns down the genes that cause inflammation and allergy.

Asthma: A few clinical trials have shown that long-chain omega-3s improve signs and symptoms of asthma. In particular, Timothy Mickleborough, PhD, and his colleagues at Indiana University have shown that fish oils are especially effective in blocking exercise-induced asthma, improving lung function by 69 percent, and reducing inflammatory messenger levels in respiratory fluids by greater than 70 percent.

While we know that long-chain omega-3 fats do many of the things that we would predict to prevent asthma, there have not been enough human clinical data to say that they are a treatment, or that they can be used to prevent asthma. That said, it has recently been shown that fish oil supplementation reduces airway narrowing, medication use, and pro-inflammatory messenger generation in nonallergic elite athletes with exercise-induced asthma. These findings are very exciting and raise the possibility that long-chain omega-3s can be used to treat exercise-induced asthma.

Pulmonary disease (COPD): COPD, the fifth leading cause of death worldwide, is characterized by chronic inflammation. There are few studies that have addressed the effect of long-chain omega-3s on COPD. One study, published in *CHEST* in 2005, examined 64 COPD patients who received either a long-chain omega-3 supplement or an omega-6 diet for 2 years. In a 6-minute walk test, the rate at which these patients got oxygen significantly improved in the omega-3 group. Inflammatory messengers— leukotriene B4, our old friend TNF-alpha, and interleukin-8—also decreased significantly in the omega-3 group. There was no significant change in the omega-6 group.

Crohn's disease and ulcerative colitis: Research is very preliminary in the area of inflammatory bowel disease, which includes Crohn's disease and ulcerative colitis. Again, however, there is every reason to believe that researchers will find a connection; these are inflammatory diseases, and we know that the right omega combinations can powerfully address inflammation.

Rheumatoid and osteoarthritis: Rheumatoid arthritis (RA) is one of the few areas (other than heart disease) where there have been enough studies to say with confidence that omega-3s demonstrate clinical benefits.

Numerous randomized, controlled trials since the 1980s have shown that long-chain omega-3 fats (either with supplementation or an increase in fish consumption) improve clinical symptoms. This has been proven by factors including decreases in nonsteroidal anti-inflammatory drug (NSAID) requirements, decreases in morning stiffness, and decreases in the number of painful joints. As any RA patient will tell you, that's a big deal.

More recent research has focused on the master health regulators and the analysis of inflammatory messengers. Interestingly, the medium-chain omega-6 GLA found in borage oil has had clinical benefit similar to that with long-chain omega-3s.

While not as extensive, a few studies have shown promise with osteoarthritis, the type of arthritis we most often associate with aging.

Psoriasis: There have also been some indications for the use of long-chain omega-3 acids in dermatology. This is an area where the clinical trial results are mixed. One of the best studies to date took 20 patients hospitalized for acute psoriasis, with a minimum of 10 percent body surface area involvement, and randomly assigned them to receive daily infusions of either an omega-3 fatty acid–based lipid emulsion (EPA + DHA 4.2 g daily) or a conventional omega-6 lipid emulsion (EPA + DHA < 0.1 g daily). The severity of disease decreased markedly in all patients of the omega-3 group, with significant improvements in all score systems ranging between 45 percent and 76 percent within 10 days.

Some cancers (breast, colon, and prostate): This is an area of science that is in a state of flux at the moment. In 2006, Catherine H. MacLean, MD, PhD, and her colleagues published a large meta-analysis in *JAMA*, in which they concluded that "dietary supplementation with omega-3 fatty acids is unlikely to prevent cancer." It is clear that several epidemiologic studies examining the effects of fish consumption demonstrate a protective effect against malignancy, while others do not support this premise; I believe that statements such as those by Dr. MacLean are premature at this time. The food frequency questionnaire and dietary records used in this study often correlate poorly with direct measurements of fatty acids in patient samples and are prone to measurement error. This is especially the case for some fish (such as farm-raised fish) that are poor sources of long-chain omega-3 PUFAs. I talk about this more in just a bit. I therefore think that a more accurate conclusion of this study is that a preventive effect of omega-3 fatty acids on all cancers is still uncertain.

FREE SPEED: HOW THE OMEGAS CAN HELP YOU LOSE WEIGHT

OK, now we're getting to the good stuff. It appears that supplementing with the right omegas, in the right combinations—as you will do on Gene Smart— can help you to lose weight.

That's what we've seen in animals, anyway. Several animal studies have shown a reduction in fat mass after supplementation with omega-3 fats. Few studies have specifically investigated the effect of omega-3 fats in humans, but those studies are under way, and the early news is promising. For instance, very recently, a study showed that omega-3 fats reduce body fat by improving bloodflow to muscles during exercise.

Other preliminary studies have shown that overweight people who supplemented with omega-3 fatty acids at the levels recommended in Gene Smart burned up to 26 percent more calories from fat than a placebo group, and had *half* the insulin levels, markedly reducing their chance of insulin resistance and diabetes. In another study, the fish oil concentrations prescribed in the Gene Smart Diet enhanced weight loss by an average of 24 percent in obese women on a diet.

MICHELLE MARCEY

AGE: 46

LOST: 17 pounds, 4 percent body fat, 6½ inches from waist, 3½ inches from hips during the study; more than 40 pounds to date

CHANGES IN KEY BIOMARKERS AFTER 8 WEEKS ON GENE SMART

BMI: −3 points

BLOOD PRESSURE: −6 mm/Hg

RESTING HEART RATE: −4 beats per minute

TOTAL CHOLESTEROL: −26 points

LDL CHOLESTEROL: −33 points

FASTING INSULIN: 99 percent lower

FASTING LEPTIN: 80 percent lower

CIRCULATING WHITE BLOOD CELLS: 7 percent lower

CIRCULATING LONG-CHAIN OMEGA-3s: 120 percent higher

66 On Gene Smart, I went from a size 12—almost a 14—to a size 6. I'm wearing my teenage daughter's shorts right now!

Weight wasn't an issue for me when I was younger, but it has been for the last 10 or 15 years. After the birth of my second child, I just couldn't take the pounds off for good; I would diet and gain back, diet and gain back.

FEWER FISH, FEWER FISH OILS, FEWER BENEFITS

Unfortunately, even with all this evidence, fish consumption in America is low compared to many other countries, and it hasn't increased significantly in recent years. In 1999, per capita fish consumption in the United States was only 15.4 pounds. It decreased to 15.2 pounds in 2000 and to 14.8 pounds in 2001, before increasing to 15.6 pounds in 2002 and to 16.3 pounds in 2003. When you compare that to per capita consumption of chicken (80 pounds), beef (65 pounds), and pork (50 pounds), you can see that fish accounts for only a small fraction of the animal protein consumed every year. More importantly, it accounts for a very, *very* small portion of the fat that Americans consume every year.

I wasn't seeing any health issues yet, but I definitely wasn't as energetic as I had been. I got tired easily, and I found myself getting out of breath when I was going up the stairs—that kind of thing. I'd avoid putting on a bathing suit to go to the pool. If my husband and my kids wanted to go on a hike while we were on vacation, I'd stay behind so that I wouldn't hold them up. It scared me; 46 isn't old, but time passes quickly. I wanted to be around for my kids.

So for me, it was not just about weight loss but about wellness; it was about getting better and feeling better, and about changing the inside, too. And the change feels permanent. I enjoy working out now in a way I never did before. The big thing was that I wasn't hungry; all the fiber helped me to feel full. I'm a vegetarian, and I've learned that it's easy to get protein in non-fattening foods. I cut out a lot of fast foods; I just realized that they don't have anything for me. And I drank a lot of water and liquids.

Seventeen pounds doesn't sound like a lot, but my body composition is completely different. My face looks thin. I have a waist; I have curves again. My family and friends can't stop talking about how much better I look; it's very noticeable. And it's been really fun shopping for the clothes. I actually bought a two-piece bathing suit for this cruise we went on.

I feel so much better about myself, too. On our cruise, I went kayaking, snorkeling, and swimming—all these things I wouldn't have done before Gene Smart.**"**

In some populations, fish consumption may actually be declining. After the FDA released a mercury advisory in 2001, one study showed a 17 percent decrease in fish consumption among pregnant women in the United States. Concerned that this trend could spread to the general population, the researchers from the Harvard Center for Risk Analysis calculated what might happen if everyone reduced their consumption of fish. They found that even if the decrease were as little as 3 to 4 percent, it would translate into significantly higher rates of cardiovascular disease, as well as more heart attacks and strokes. Talk about throwing the baby out with the bathwater!

What about Flax?

Flax seeds and flax-seed oil are often put forth as sources of health-giving omega-3s. So every time I talk, someone raises their hand to ask me about flax.

I welcome the opportunity to try to straighten this out. Let me be clear: Flax seed and flax-seed oil are not and cannot be considered substitutes for the omega-3s found in fish.

Don't get me wrong: Alpha-linolenic acid in flax-seed oil is a very good thing to be eating—much better than long-chain omega-6s. However, we do not efficiently convert this botanical fatty acid to the potent bioactives, long-chain omega-3s. Humans, cows, and pigs are limited in an enzyme called delta-6 desaturase, which aids in that conversion. Without the enzyme, we just don't do it very well.

If we're going to get the benefits of these bioactives, we have to take them *correctly*. And given our genetics, we humans are unlikely to get the same benefits from flax that we do from the fish oil. So if you're feeding your kid flax in the hopes of increasing long-chain omega-3s in her brain in order to improve her cognitive function or vision, stop. According to the current scientific evidence, her body can't efficiently make those fatty acids from flax. If you're taking flax to combat arthritis or heart disease, the science says that you won't get the same benefit, either.

But don't throw out your flax seeds just yet. In fact, there's a really good reason to eat flax seeds, and it has to do with a critical bioactive. It's just not an omega-3. Rather, it's *fiber*. Flax seeds are very rich in both soluble and insoluble fiber, and so they fit beautifully into the Gene Smart program. Nutritionists generally suggest that you buy them whole and crush or grind them yourself in order to get the maximal benefits. Sprinkle

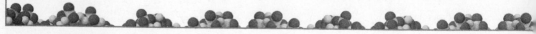

WHAT IF THE OMEGAS AREN'T IN THE FISH?

There's another threat to our omega-3 consumption, and that's the presumption that those beneficial long-chain omega-3s are actually *in* the fish. Changes in the food supply, however, make that a more dubious claim.

In the 1970s, the demand for fish began to outstrip what we could reasonably catch. Public awareness of the health benefits exacerbated the shortage, and (forgive the pun!) spawned a tremendous expansion in aquaculture and fish farming. It is now the fastest-growing form of producing food *on the planet*, expanding at a rate of 10 percent per year since 1990.

My laboratory has spent the last few years monitoring what the explosion

them on cereal, oatmeal, or yogurt, or bake them into whole-grain quick breads or muffins, and enjoy!

The growing popularity of flax seed (even if it's ineffective for the purposes for which it's being used) exposes something important: For a lot of reasons (taste, smell, compliance, and acceptability to vegetarians), there is a very strong demand for a botanical source of omega-3s that can be converted by the human body to the bioactives we so desperately need.

Finding a plant-based solution to the problem of enriching the American diet in a meaningful way with long-chain omega-3 PUFAs would have enormous public health impact, and would presumably reduce the incidence and severity of several complex human diseases, including coronary heart disease, stroke, hypertension, diabetes, and obesity.

In fact, this is one of the major focuses of my own laboratory. A novel idea that we have explored is to use a botanical oil that is enriched in a fatty acid known as stearidonic acid. Stearidonic acid bypasses the limiting metabolic step in the formation of long-chain omega-3 fatty acids from alpha-LNA. My laboratory has demonstrated that this fatty acid is converted to the potent long-chain omega-3s. It reduces triglycerides and affects gene expression in a way that is comparable to fish oil.

Botanical fatty acids that can be converted to long-chain bioactives—and then added both to our food supply and to the feed of the animals we eat—will have a huge impact on our future. It is worth noting that a UK company, Croda, has just received permission to sell echium oil, which is enriched with stearidonic acid. So it is likely it will be hitting the marketplace soon—stay tuned!

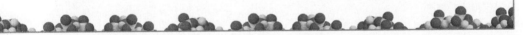

in aquaculture—as it is currently practiced—has done to our fat ratios, and it is nothing short of a disaster. The focus of the concern so far has been on mercury and PCBs in our fish supply; these make the editorial pages on a regular basis. But without sounding like an extremist, I believe that the threat doesn't even approach the gravity of the problem we're looking at, with the altered concentrations and ratios of omega-6s to omega-3s in our most popular fish. Fat is never far off the media radar, and I am convinced that the realization of the terrible damage that our consumption of long-chain omega-6 fats is doing to us will be the next big "bad fat" story.

Tilapia is one of the most widely farmed fish on the planet. It's inexpensive, and it doesn't smell or taste strongly "fishy," which is why the market for it is one of the fastest growing. Consumption of tilapia is projected to increase from 1.5 million tons in 2003 to 2.5 million tons by 2010; experts expect that it will surpass farm-raised Atlantic salmon as the most eaten farmed fish in the United States within a few years. Similarly, consumption of farmed catfish has dramatically increased, from 0.3 million metric tons in 1994 to 0.7 million metric tons in 2003.

But my laboratory has recently shown that tilapia and farmed catfish have several fatty acid characteristics that would generally be considered by the scientific community and doctors as detrimental. This paper was published in the *Journal of the American Dietetic Association* in 2008.

First, they have much higher saturated and monounsaturated fat to PUFA ratios than other farmed or wild fish. Ratios this high in diets have been shown to be directly associated with increases in cholesterol and atherogenesis (the development of arterial plaques) in both humans and non-human primates.

Perhaps more importantly, the concentrations of long-chain omega-6 PUFAs—and more specifically, the long-chain omega-6 PUFA, AA—are high. In fact, these fish contain some of the highest levels of AA found in the human food chain. Long-chain omega-6 fatty acids alter gene expression in such a way that it upends blood lipids (cholesterol, LDL and HDL, and triglycerides) and induces whole-body inflammation by producing several families of messengers that markedly exacerbate inflammation and inflammatory disease.

In isolation, this would be problem enough. But the inflammatory danger we face from the long-chain omega-6s is largely exacerbated by the fact that there are so many long-chain omega-6s in the Western diet when there are so *few* long-chain omega-3s. When the ratios of the two primary long-chain omega-6 and omega-3 PUFAs (AA and EPA, respectively) were examined, both farmed tilapia and catfish contained high AA/EPA. While there was a great deal of variability in the AA/EPA ratio in farm-raised tilapia, the average ratio was approximately 11:1. Two fish samples harvested in Central America had over 20 times more AA than EPA.

> **The most commonly eaten fish have omega ratios that are harmful to our health.**

This is very far away from what is optimal for our cells; the science to support the connection between an imbalance in our fatty acid concentrations and ratios and our ill health is convincing. Hundreds of clinical trials, including six from my own lab, support the connection between an imbalance in certain types of fatty acids and inflammatory disease.

By replacing beneficial long-chain omega-3s with long-chain omega-6s in these fish, we wreak havoc in our bodies—all the while believing that we have done something very beneficial for ourselves by eating the fish.

The problem, as it was with the cows, is *what the fish are eating*. Tilapia are incredibly hardy, which means that you can feed them just about anything as a fat source. What we're feeding them is corn oil, or soy, or whatever the cheapest commodity is at the time, packed with short-chain omega-6 fats that they convert to the dangerous long-chain omega-6 fats. Normally herbivore fish eat algae, which contain short-chain omega-3 fats that they convert to the very beneficial medium-chain omega-3s. Carnivorous fish then eat those fish as their source of omega-3 fats. Humans eat both types of fish.

In the best-case scenario—if we were eating wild fish, like our ancestors would have—eating fish would provide us with by far our richest source of health-giving bioactives, long-chain omega-3s. But if the fish we're eating have been raised on corn or other omega-6-rich oils, or if the fish we eat have eaten fish raised on these, then one of our healthiest foods becomes a major health problem.

All this is taking place unbeknownst to the consumer. Without knowing which fish to avoid, the general population is likely to purchase the fish (a) that is most readily available at the supermarket, or (b) that costs the least. Farmed tilapia, unfortunately, dominates both categories. Since 2000, shipments of frozen tilapia fillets from China to the United States (representing 66 percent of imports) have risen from 4 million to 140 million pounds. These Chinese tilapia fillets averaged $1.38 per pound in 2006, about even with the previous 2 years. Of course, convenience and price are important drivers in the marketplace, but the drastically different nutritional profiles are creating an absolute disaster for our health, especially when we subscribe to the widely held belief that eating any fish is beneficial.

HOW GENE SMART CAN HELP YOU GET THE OMEGAS YOU NEED

As I mentioned above, we are always doing studies on fatty acid ratios in my labs. When study participants walk in for the first time—and these are healthy people!—their omega-6 to omega-3 ratio is typically about 15:1. If we can get that ratio closer to 5:1, we can markedly change gene expression in a way that is very protective against inflammation. A ratio that's even closer to 2:1 would be ideal.

So we have to adjust our omega-fat ratios by reducing the number of omega-6 fatty acids in our diets, and increasing the number of omega-3 fatty acids. This is precisely what you will do on Gene Smart.

Reduce omega-6s. The amount of meat we eat in this country has increased precipitously. On Gene Smart, we'll taper back to a more reasonable level.

We're also going to help you make smarter choices about the meat you *do* eat. Remember, we're not just what *we* eat, but what we *eat* eats. The food that the animals we eat are fed has a direct impact on their nutritional content. A grass-fed cow, for instance, makes for a steak with a dramatically different fatty acid ratio than his corn-fed cousin—and those differences speak directly to our master health regulators in very important ways.

So although those two hamburger patties might look the same, they're vastly different from a nutritional perspective, and choosing the right one can affect your inflammatory profile. That's what you'll be doing on Gene Smart. By showing readers how to make smart choices about protein, the Gene Smart Diet will dramatically lower circulating levels of arachidonic acid from an average of 20:1 to 5:1.

Increase omega-3s. We're also going to increase the very good long-chain omega-3s.

At the World Congress of Cardiology in 2006, World Heart Federation President Valentin Fuster said Spanish researchers are making rapid progress toward development of a "polypill," a medicine combining three generic drugs to be taken by individuals with heart disease. If shown to be effective in clinical trials, the inexpensive, easy-to-administer pill could dramatically reduce premature death.

As I read this statement, I thought about the incredible power of long-chain omegas as combinational therapies. In short, I believe we already have a polypill, a natural one with very few side effects, in these unbelievably potent, health-promoting, long-chain omega-3 fats.

Overall, the long-chain omega-3s are the most well studied and proven bioactives for the prevention and treatment of many of our most devastating human diseases. The tragedy is that we're not yet taking full advantage of these wonder drugs. First of all, we need to eat more fish. It is estimated that only 18 percent of Americans will take oily fish products (whether fish or supplements) because of their taste and smell. The recipes in this book—quick, simple, delicious—will hopefully open your eyes to how tasty and easy fish dishes can be.

You'll also be making better fish and supplement choices. In all of these studies, long-chain omega-3 PUFAs such as eicosapentaenoic acid (EPA), docosapentaenoic acid (DPA), and docosahexaenoic acid (DHA), have been determined to be the primary bioactive components that account for many of the health benefits of fish. So these are bioactives that we're going to be adding to your diet at levels we know to be heart-healthy and anti-inflammatory.

One of the major mistakes that have been made with fish oils is not getting high enough dosages into the diet. For the typical supplement serving size, two capsules have approximately 400 mg of these bioactives. The typical fish has less than 200 mg of these bioactives in a 4-ounce serving. So one serving per day of these typically won't get you into the dose range that has been shown to be effective in the vast majority of clinical trials.

CHAPTER FIFTEEN

GENE SMART SOLUTION #5: INCREASE YOUR POLYPHENOLS

SOME ORGANIC FOOD *is* better for you—but not for the reasons you may think.

As it turns out, pesticide poisoning may be a comparatively minor problem (from a health perspective, anyway—the environment is another story). The real problem is that fruits and vegetables bred for uniformity and protected from environmental threats contain very little of precisely the things that make them good for us!

Unfortunately, the factory farms and aquaculture we discussed in the last chapter are not the only shifts in our food supply to detrimentally impact the types and amounts of bioactives we eat. There have been radical shifts in the way our fruits and vegetables are produced as well, which have led to radical shifts in their nutritional power, and a terrible impact on our health and weight—something else that we'll correct on Gene Smart.

But before we look at what's gone wrong, let's look at why it matters. There is some very exciting science demonstrating the health benefits to be gotten from the powerhouse polyphenols found in fruits and vegetables.

THE POLYPHENOL PRESCRIPTION

The polyphenols are present in our food in very small quantities—one of the reasons they've slipped under the radar for so long.

Small quantities or not, the polyphenols have a tremendous biological scope. They perform a wide number of functions in order to protect the plants in which they occur, and early evidence would seem to suggest that they have an equally far-reaching effect on animal cells and in intact animals.

We have strong epidemiological evidence of the power of the overall class of polyphenols on human health. Unfortunately, we have little interventional clinical data in humans, so we don't know as much about the specifics of which ones are most important and what it is that they do exactly. But they are absolutely worth inclusion at this juncture, in my opinion, because what we do know is so very compelling. Indeed, the studies that we do have (many appearing in the most prestigious journals, including *Science* and *Nature*) indicate the polyphenols are likely to be our most powerful bioactive source in the future.

The science is in its earliest stages, but what we know is exciting indeed. Most importantly, there is strong evidence for the ability of polyphenols to control gene expression, *specifically the genes that control inflammation.*

> **The polyphenols control the genes that control inflammation.**

There is, for instance, quite a lot of early evidence to suggest that certain polyphenols affect the master gene regulator NF-κB, which directs many of the genes that control inflammation. It is likely that this central control point plays a key role in how these compounds, even in such tiny quantities, combat inflammatory disease.

The potential scope of polyphenols is very wide-reaching—and it includes some of our most terrible diseases. For instance, I feel very comfortable saying that combinations of polyphenol-rich foods, especially when taken together with other potent bioactives such as long-chain omega-3 fats, are likely to play a key role in preventing and improving cardiovascular diseases including heart attack and stroke. For example, the polyphenols have been shown to effectively lower blood pressure. They appear to be important to glucose regulation, which plays a role in diabetes. They can be instrumental in weight control; more specifically, some of them actually appear to heighten metabolism and burn fat—a dieter's dream! There are data that certain polyphenols may protect our bodies from cancer, and slow tumor growth in people who have it. Those are only some of the claims.

That is why I think of these compounds as nature's pharmaceuticals, and why it is so disturbing that there are fewer of them in our food supply than there have ever been before. When scientists truly understand enough to harness all of the potential of these polyphenols, I believe they will have the power to protect us from many of our most devastating diseases and markedly increase human life spans. For now, I believe we know enough about these wildly powerful tools to use them to substantively improve our health.

I have to say, this part of the diet is not only scientifically exciting to me, but exciting for the palate as well. As a colleague in my lab once commented, "The benefits are impressive, and you can't beat the delivery systems!" She was alluding to the fact that these powerful bioactives are found not only in fruits and vegetables, but in traditional diet "no-no's" like red wine—and even chocolate!

Like the omegas, the correct polyphenols *at the correct dosages* must be utilized. This is especially true because we are focusing on those polyphenols that impact gene expression, as opposed to the thousands of polyphenols that merely have antioxidant activity. Gene Smart is the very first diet to take this important distinction into account.

WHAT THE POLYPHENOLS CAN DO FOR YOU

Resveratrol, which is found in red wine, peanuts, blueberries, as well as in other fruits like cranberries, raspberries, and plums and in supplement form too, is, by far, the most studied of the polyphenols.

In a few very interesting studies, resveratrol was shown to improve the health and survival of obese mice, and may also increase the aerobic capacity of mice.

One study, out of the lab of Harvard Medical School researcher David Sinclair, PhD, demonstrated a 30 percent increase in life span when mice were fed resveratrol with a high-calorie, high-fat (60 percent of total calories) diet. The mice still got fat, but they didn't suffer any of the negative physiological effects usually associated with being fat, such as a reduction in life span.

Another study, published in *Cell*, found that mice fed resveratrol for 15 weeks had two times the treadmill endurance of a control group. And a Finnish study examining those mice born with certain increased types of the specific gene SIRT1 (the proposed master gene regulator that resveratrol activates) found that they had faster metabolisms, helping them to burn

Two for One

Red wine contains *two* classes of polyphenols that have the potential to initiate an adaptive stress response and thus markedly improve health: resveratrol and the anthocyanins. These have powerful effects, working in many of the same areas as the bioactives on this diet:

- Epidemiological, case-control, and randomized clinical trials show that alcohol consumption at the level prescribed in Gene Smart in the form of red wine increases HDL "good" cholesterol by 20 percent.
- By treating yourself to that glass of red wine at dinner per Gene Smart's recommendation, you can reduce your risk of heart attack by more than 30 percent on average.
- Alcohol consumption (a glass of red wine with dinner) at the level prescribed in Gene Smart reduces levels of the inflammatory messenger C-reactive protein by 15 percent on average.

It is, of course, important always to drink in moderation. And people with a history of problems with alcohol should not drink at all, regardless of the health benefits of the bioactives found in red wine.

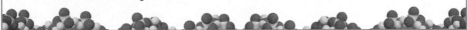

energy more efficiently—indicating that the same pathway shown in the lab mice likely works in humans, too.

Cool stuff! So why not recommend resveratrol as a supplement? Someday soon I hope that we will know enough about the dosages necessary to achieve these results, and about the absorption and metabolism of resveratrol in humans, to make general recommendations. (There are high-dose supplements available, but they are unregulated.) For now, we can't be certain of the dose ranges necessary.

So on Gene Smart you'll be getting your resveratrol the old-fashioned way—through foods and red wine. If you want to enhance the amounts, more concentrated forms are available as dietary supplements.

Resveratrol gets a lot of press, but there are a number of other polyphenols that have shown great potential to control gene expression and to impact the disease process, including ellagic acid, the anthocyanins, the catechins, and epicatechin.

Again, the science is very new. But, as you'll see, researchers are very excited about the potential of this category of bioactives to affect heart disease, as well as other inflammatory conditions.

The Polyphenols and Your Heart

The epidemiological studies are clear: There is an inverse relationship between the intake of fresh fruits and vegetables and the risk of cardiovascular disease, including heart disease and stroke. That's hardly news. But the more we find out about the polyphenols, the closer we get to knowing why.

Certainly it is true that the more fruits, vegetables, and tea (especially green tea) you consume, the less likely you are to have heart disease, which is why one of our foremost priorities on Gene Smart is to increase the amounts of the right types (those that contain high concentrations of one of the polyphenols listed above) of fruits, vegetables, and tea you consume. I have already talked extensively about the "French paradox" in this book, which credits the comparatively low rate of cardiovascular disease in French people—despite a high-fat diet—to their high consumption of polyphenols. Recently, Bauer E. Sumpio, MD, PhD, and colleagues at the Yale School of Medicine coined the term "the Asian paradox" to explain another scientific mystery.

Asian people have very low rates of cardiovascular disease. This is surprising, considering that an astronomical number of people in the countries surveyed are heavy smokers. I probably don't need to tell you that evidence strongly associates cigarette smoking with a number of detrimental effects leading to atherosclerosis, including increases in levels of fatty acids and LDL (especially small LDL particles, which are highly dangerous), and a decreased turnover of HDL cholesterol. Smoking has also been identified as aggravating hypertension, promoting platelet aggregation, and worsening the performance of the vascular system. To put it another way, cigarettes are your heart's worst nightmare.

But despite the high use of tobacco, China and Japan in particular have among the lowest incidences of arteriosclerosis and lung cancer per capita. Why? Researchers believe it has a great deal to do with the very high consumption of polyphenol-rich green tea.

Legends from China and Japan tell us that tea has been used for thousands of years for medicinal purposes—to reduce inflammation, improve bloodflow, treat infectious diseases, purify the body, and maintain mental equilibrium. In these countries, tea is not just a simple beverage, but a social custom woven into the very fabric of the culture. Approximately 3 billion kilograms of tea are produced and consumed annually (it is second in popularity only to water), and the primary tea consumed is green tea (as opposed to black, which is favored in most Western countries).

It is now believed that tea's popularity is the explanation for this paradox, and several studies support this conclusion. For example, a Japanese epidemiologic study involving 1,371 men over age 40 reported an association between the consumption of more than 10 cups (1,500 milliliters) of green tea a day and decreased blood concentrations of total cholesterol, LDL, and triglycerides, as well as an increased concentration of HDL. Pretty impressive! A recent meta-analysis involving 17 studies reported an 11 percent decrease in heart attack when three cups of tea (in this study, the tea type was not specified) were consumed daily. And in a study of 340 people, heart-attack risk declined by 44 percent in those drinking 1 cup (237 milliliters) or more of tea per day compared with nondrinkers.

It makes sense, given what we know about how the polyphenols act on a number of other important biomarkers of stroke and heart disease. For instance, they have been shown to:

Reduce platelet aggregation. One of the real biomarkers of heart disease is platelet aggregation, the so-called "sticky platelets." Here, certain polyphenols appear to help. Platelets isolated from healthy human subjects showed decreased aggregation when pretreated with red wine, grape juice, or resveratrol-enriched grape juice. (White wine had no effect.) Flavonol—found in red wine and the green and black teas you'll be drinking on Gene Smart— was reported to be the most effective inhibitor of platelet aggregation.

Improve blood lipids. Your doctor takes your blood lipid profile—your LDL cholesterol, HDL cholesterol, and triglycerides—at every visit. Obviously, high total and LDL cholesterol and low HDL are among the signature biomarkers for heart disease. So can the polyphenols help you improve this profile?

The research is not conclusive, but it looks good. In a review of animal studies, Drs. Vanessa Crespy and Gary Williamson cited five studies in which catechin/epicatechin and related molecules altered plasma lipids in a positive manner, meaning that total cholesterol went down, LDL and triglycerides went down, and HDL went up. And indeed, most human studies have shown beneficial effects (albeit modest) of polyphenols on the lipid profile in humans. Red wine consumption resulted in a modest (11 to 16 percent) increase in HDL (good) cholesterol. The use of a concentrated red grape juice by healthy subjects and hemodialysis patients for 14 days resulted in a small but significant decrease in LDL cholesterol and increase in HDL.

Improve endothelial cell function. One of the most important things when you're talking about cardiovascular disease is the proper functioning of the cells that form the veins and arteries (this is also called endothelial cell function or vascular reactivity). If these cells aren't working properly, then bloodflow is restricted, and restricted bloodflow is what leads to high blood pressure, stroke, and heart attack. Anything that makes the blood vessels more open and pliable is extremely desirable. In addition, measuring endothelial cell function is very easy (your cardiologist puts a device around your arm), so it's one of the most important biomarkers of heart disease and stroke that we have.

Here, it appears, the polyphenols can help. In patients with documented cardiovascular disease, the consumption of a grape-seed extract for 3 weeks, or purple grape juice or red wine for 14 days, improved endothelial cell function.

In addition to these clinical intervention studies, which used grape-derived products, other studies using polyphenol interventions have also demonstrated improved function. These include black tea, a cocoa drink, a fruit/vegetable juice, and a Mediterranean diet.

Reduce blood pressure. This, for me, is one of the most exciting claims the polyphenols can make. Cardiologists call untreated high blood pressure "the silent killer." It affects one in three Americans, a third of whom don't know they have it. It's also a leading independent risk factor for heart attack and stroke (the number-one and number-three leading causes of death), and a contributor to coronary artery disease, aneurysm, kidney failure, and dementia.

This is one area where the science is very sound: The polyphenols can play a major role in reducing elevated blood pressure, striking a blow against heart disease and stroke in the process.

I haven't even gotten to the best part. *The polyphenols responsible for this effect are the ones you find in chocolate.* That's right. Numerous human studies, including one published in *JAMA* in 2007, have shown that dark chocolate (as opposed to milk chocolate) reduces blood pressure and improves insulin sensitivity in humans. And not by a little, either. Studies show that the dark chocolate concentrations prescribed in the Gene Smart Diet *reduce high blood pressure in an at-risk population by an average of 18 percent.*

These effects are similar to those associated with common blood pressure–lowering medications such as beta-blockers and ACE inhibitors.

Imagine trading in your beta-blocker for a bar of chocolate! Like long-chain omega-3s and statins, this is an example of how a natural product can effectively compete with our largest-selling drugs. Applied to the population as a whole, researchers estimate that the blood pressure–lowering effect associated with cocoa could be expected to reduce the risk of stroke by about 20 percent, coronary heart disease by 10 percent, and death from all causes by 8 percent.

> **Cocoa, in the dosages found in Gene Smart, has been estimated to reduce the risk of stroke by about 20 percent, coronary heart disease by 10 percent, and death from all causes by 8 percent.**

The Polyphenols and Other Inflammatory Conditions

There are also other areas—many of them linked to inflammation—where the polyphenols can significantly contribute to our overall health.

Diabetes: Diabetes is one of the most devastating of the inflammatory diseases, not least because it puts you at risk for so many others.

> **The data to date suggest that the polyphenol profile and concentrations prescribed in Gene Smart may help to stabilize blood sugar levels and increase insulin in people with diabetes.**

As we have discussed, diabetes results when our cells can't recognize insulin. Insulin promotes the uptake of glucose (sugar from the foods we eat) into many tissues, helping to maintain blood glucose concentrations within certain parameters. Lacking this vital control mechanism, people with diabetes see their glucose levels swing wildly. Unfortunately, the consequences of persistent, uncontrolled high blood glucose are the many vascular and neural complications that contribute to diabetes-associated illness and death. So controlling blood glucose is considered to be an essential part of diabetes management.

High blood glucose levels are an important risk factor for diabetes. In rodent studies, a number of the polyphenols recommended in Gene Smart (including resveratrol, EGCG, monomeric and polymeric catechins [procyanidins], and anthocyanidin-containing extracts) reduced blood glucose levels after a glucose tolerance test in both nondiabetic and diabetic animals. These polyphenols also reduced elevated blood glucose concentrations in diabetic animals when given long-term and when administered immediately before a meal. Together, these studies are proof that test animals metabolize glucose—a crucial step in blood sugar regulation—better after polyphenol treatment.

A recent study compared the ingestion of wine, dealcoholized wine, and juice from muscadine grapes in people with diabetes. The study, which lasted 4 weeks, demonstrated that dealcoholized wine lowered plasma insulin. In addition, there was a trend toward lower fasting blood glucose and glycated hemoglobin levels in all the groups, suggesting an improvement in glycemic control. (Individuals with poorly controlled diabetes show increases in these glycated hemoglobins.) In another clinical study, catechin supplementation increased plasma insulin levels in healthy men after 12 weeks.

Although it is clear that we need more clinical data in this area, I think it's very encouraging news.

Arthritis: Animal and isolated cell studies are very encouraging regarding the influence of the polyphenols on arthritis. Several of the polyphenols, for instance, have been shown to block processes in individual cells that we know drive arthritis. Other studies have shown that some of them, including the ones you'll be eating on Gene Smart—quercetin, catechins, resveratrol, caffeic acid, and anthocyanins—reduce signs and symptoms of arthritis in animal models.

First, quercetin, catechins, resveratrol, and anthocyanins may improve the function of cells that cause rheumatoid arthritis in the joint. Chondrocytes are the only cells found in cartilage; obviously, they are critical for joint health, and are dramatically altered during arthritis. When human chondrocytes are pretreated with quercetin, an anthocyanin-enriched extract, or a wine extract rich in procyanidins, they produce lower levels of a number of inflammatory messengers.

In animal studies, researchers have found that polyphenols have a strong preventive effect. Mice given green tea are much less likely to develop osteoarthritis (only 44 percent compared to 94 percent of those who did not get green tea). Moreover, the mice who were treated with green tea but still ended up with arthritis suffered from a much less severe form. And administration of resveratrol decreases cartilage degradation in a rabbit model of osteoarthritis.

These studies haven't yet been done in humans, but they certainly will be.

Bone density: A study published in 2000 in the *American Journal of Clinical Nutrition* examined the relationship between tea drinking and bone mineral density—a predictor of osteoporosis, especially in women—in over 1,200 older women in England. (Tea drinking, you may have heard, is common there.)

The results were impressive. The tea drinkers had significantly greater (5 percent) bone mineral density, leading the researchers to conclude that tea drinking may protect against osteoporosis in older women.

Cancer: Epidemiological studies are equivocal with respect to the ability of flavonoid-containing diets to influence the risk for the development of cancers in humans. Different outcomes may be due to numerous factors, including the populations studied, the method of diet analysis used, and the type of cancers evaluated. One thing is clear, and proven without doubt: The populations that eat the most (polyphenol-containing) fruits and vegetables are also the ones with the lowest incidence of cancer.

The literature is filled with studies examining the effects of polyphenol extracts or purified compounds on cancer in cultured cell systems, and what we've seen there is very encouraging indeed. Several polyphenols—such as anthocyanins, ellagic acid, procyanidins, and trans-resveratrol—appear to be able to inhibit the growth of certain kinds of cancer cells in test-tube experiments.

What about in humans? Although intervention studies are few and involve small numbers of patients, what little has been done suggests that certain polyphenols can be beneficial in altering the disease course in cancer patients.

For instance:

- A combination of quercetin and curcumin has been shown to reduce the number and size of tumors in a small number of patients with familial adenomatous polyposis, an inherited colorectal cancer.

- A study using pomegranate juice, which is rich in ellagic acid and ellagitannins, showed that daily consumption was beneficial for prostate cancer patients with rising prostate specific antigen (PSA). (Rising PSA levels indicate a worsening disease state.) The pomegranate juice didn't stop PSA levels from rising, but it did slow the process considerably; study participants saw their PSA levels double in 54 months, compared to 15 months pre-treatment. The highest levels of ellagic acid are found in raspberries, strawberries, and pomegranates—all foods you'll eat regularly on the Gene Smart Diet.

More work is under way. In 2007, human clinical trials were initiated to examine the anti-cancer effects of black raspberries and cranberries on tumors in the esophagus, prostate, and colon. We'll have those results in the next 2 years.

THE POLYPHENOLS PROMOTE WEIGHT LOSS!

"It's my metabolism," dieters often say—and in fact, they're right. Our genes play a strong role in how much energy we expend over the course of the day, even down to how much we fidget. And the people who expend the most energy are the slimmest. The body seems to be pretty finely calibrated; even when we start exercising and watching what we eat, we find a way to sneak those calories back in.

We haven't been very successful at finding many things that really have a significant impact on metabolism—until now.

> **Certain of the polyphenols have been found to increase metabolism, enhancing our ability to lose weight.**

Specifically, the polyphenols and caffeine in green tea have been proposed as a strategy for weight loss and weight maintenance, since they may increase energy expenditure and counteract the decrease in metabolic rate that is present during weight loss. This is incredibly exciting news for those trying to slim down.

This research has been done, for the most part, in mice. Leptin is a hormone that has been correlated with decreased obesity, and polyphenol administration to mice decreases leptin expression. Although not observed in all studies, animals receiving a tea-derived catechin supplement with a high-fat diet tended to gain less weight than animals eating the high-fat diet alone. And they weren't burning muscle, but fat; there was a decrease in adipose mass, especially subcutaneous fat, but *not* in lean body mass. Both tea- and grape-derived extracts have been shown to inhibit fat-cell maturation, which in turn decreases fat accumulation in cells.

The effect of catechins on fat is not limited to animals. A number of studies indicate that the consumption of green tea components has an effect on body weight and on fat mass distribution. In a non-placebo-controlled trial, Pierre Chantre, PhD, and Denis Lairon, PhD, observed that consuming 375 milligrams of green tea over a 12-week period had pretty impressive results in moderately obese subjects. Doing nothing else, the subjects lost 4.6 percent of their body weight. That's 11.5 pounds for a 250-pound guy! And they lost 4.5 inches off their waistlines.

Another study, done in Thailand and published in 2007 in *Physiology and Behavior*, showed that the addition of green tea capsules to a controlled Thai diet increased energy expenditure by about one-third what you'd expect to see with moderate exercise—and resulted in a weight loss of over 10 pounds in 8 weeks.

In an important paper in the *American Journal of Clinical Nutrition*, green tea was reported to have important thermogenic (fat-burning) properties: It increased energy expenditure by 4 percent over a 24-hour period. Part of this is attributable to the caffeine in green tea, but the researchers confirmed that the results they saw went beyond what caffeine can do on its own.

One of the most important observations was that the polyphenols in green tea targeted fat. The weight people lost wasn't lean muscle mass, but adipose tissue—fat. So once again, these bioactives appear to be real precision instruments, with much more specific and finely tuned effects than those we'd be able to see without them.

THE CASE OF THE MISSING BIOACTIVES

Given the terrific potential of these bioactives for weight loss and management, as well as on a tremendous variety of chronic, potentially life-threatening human diseases, it's very important that they be present in our food supply. The problem? They're not—or not in the quantities we believe they need to be.

During my lectures, this is usually where someone pipes up to point out that we eat lots more vegetables than our hunter-gatherer ancestors did, primarily because more are available year-round, shipped from the farthest corners of the earth for our delectation during the cold winter months.

GAIL WALKER

AGE: 61

STARTING WEIGHT: 158 pounds

LOST: 21 pounds, 7 percent of body fat, 7 inches from waist, 6 inches from hips

CHANGES IN KEY BIOMARKERS AFTER 8 WEEKS ON GENE SMART

BMI: –3.5 points

BLOOD PRESSURE: –8 mm/Hg systolic

RESTING HEART RATE: –42 beats per minute

CIRCULATING WHITE BLOOD CELLS: 48 percent reduction

TOTAL CHOLESTEROL: –24 points

LDL CHOLESTEROL: –24 points

CRP: –32 points

IL-6: 91 percent lower

FASTING LEPTIN: 79 percent lower

IL-8: 85 percent lower

❝ As far as I'm concerned, participating in this study literally saved my life. I'd never even heard of CRP, but mine was astronomical. I was literally on a crash course for a heart attack or a stroke. And I didn't even realize it.

I got involved with the program because the whole maternal side of my family—most recently my mother—has been diagnosed with diabetes, and I'd been craving sugar and sweet stuff all the time. That really scared me, and I thought, 'You know what? You're going down that path. If you're going to do something to turn this around, you've got to do it now.' I'd been a little short of breath, and my heart had been racing, but I had no idea my CRP was as high as it was, or that I was in such danger.

They're right—we probably do eat more fruits and vegetables than our ancestors did. But there has been yet another major series of changes in our food supply since the Industrial Revolution, having to do with the way our fruits and vegetables are produced.

There's no denying it: The produce section at your friendly neighborhood supermarket is quite a sight to see. There are pyramids of perfectly formed, symmetrical cucumbers. Enormous, plump, blemish-free berries, no matter

I have always been a yo-yo diet person; I can lose the weight, but it always comes back because food is an emotional issue for me. But I've kept the weight off on this program. It's something I feel that I can live with for a lifetime. There's a great deal of variety, and I eat enough fiber to feel full. I've done low-carb diets before, but I missed the fruit! I've loved being able to eat the berries and the melon and all the delicious fruits on this diet.

The exercise was a big change for me. I'm usually an active person; I have a lot of family responsibilities, and I teach first grade. But I hadn't been focused on exercise as part of taking care of myself. I'll be honest: When I went out to join a gym, I really didn't know where the energy to do a workout was going to come from. I thought I'd have to drag myself in there. But I was really serious about it; I was there 4 days a week, sometimes 5. I know I'm not the first person to make this observation, but I was just shocked at how much energy I had after I started working out. It is so ironic, but it really is true.

The fish was another major change for me. I love fish, but I hadn't been eating as much of it as I should have been, or the right kinds. That was very revealing to me. If you're going to eat fish, you need to eat the kind that's going to give you the most omegas for your buck, or for your bite! I probably eat four or five fish meals a week now. It tastes good, and it's good for me.

I didn't know anything about polyphenols at all; most people don't. I learned that I get headaches from red wine, so I got most of my polyphenols from this muscadine extract I found, and from pomegranate juice and tea. I ate a lot more fruits and vegetables, too. At the school where I teach, there's always coffee everywhere. I felt like I was addicted to it, even the decaf. So it fit right in to replace all those cups of coffee and cream with plain green tea. I think that's made me feel a lot more peaceful and calm.

I give thanks and grace to God for everything that happened to me on this diet. I really do think it probably saved my life.**"**

what the season. Red peppers, all exactly the same size and hue, sitting politely in shrink-wrapped trays. And the tomatoes! Bright red, perfectly round, without the slightest mark or discoloration anywhere.

They look beautiful, to be sure. But a great many of us find that the tomatoes don't taste like the ones of our childhood. Those tomatoes may not have been as pretty to look at, and they certainly weren't available year-round. Bursting with flavor, we picked them when they were ripe—and ate them the same day, before their soft flesh turned mushy and the fruit flies descended. They may not have been built to last, but they were delicious!

As it turns out, taste wasn't the only casualty of their makeover. Scientists now believe that the fruits and vegetables filling our supermarkets have considerably fewer of these bioactive compounds that our bodies need to function at an optimal level.

> When food producers select for those characteristics that will make a fruit or vegetable most appealing to a consumer, they eliminate the very things that will make it best for our bodies.

Some of what's been lost is a function of the selection process. Today's growers focus more on cosmetics and durability than on other concerns. It used to be hard enough to get those farmstand tomatoes home from the fields without splitting them, much less shipped across the country in giant crates with thousands of others.

There's another crucial ingredient that the farmstand tomatoes of 40 years ago had but the supermarket tomatoes of today are missing: stress.

Yes, it's our old friend, adaptive stress, again. We believe that many of these bioactive polyphenol compounds are created as part of the fruits and vegetables' own adaptive stress response—a very similar mechanism to the one in humans that I described in Chapter 4. In that scenario, severely restricted calories provide precisely the kind of environmental stress that kicks your regulators into high gear in order to protect you.

Plant biologists have demonstrated that there is a similar response in plants. When a plant has to struggle to get enough water or nutrients, or when it finds itself "under attack" from pests or bacteria, it produces bioactive compounds to help protect itself. These act as natural pesticides and antimicrobial agents. The more stress the plant has, the more bioactives it produces.

What's fascinating is what happens when a human eats a plant that has been under that kind of stress. A theory put forth by Konrad T. Howitz, PhD, of BIOMOL Research Laboratories and David Sinclair, PhD, of Harvard called the xenohormesis hypothesis, states that some organisms have actually developed to sense stress-signaling molecules *from other species* in their environment. Because they can shift into survival mode defensively—and in advance of the threat—this gives these organisms a strong survival advantage.

The good news is that we think humans—among other animals—are designed to take advantage of such early alerts. Where's our information coming from? The polyphenols.

Plants make certain of the polyphenols only when they are being stressed by lack of water or specific nutrients or by starvation, or when they're under attack by predators such as insects or fungus. They protect the plant from a wide variety of insults and stressors by changing their responses to light, providing pigmentation to various parts of the plant, and altering the feeding behavior of insects. It has been hypothesized that resveratrol and other classes of polyphenols act as stress-signaling molecules in plants, coordinating sirtuin-mediated defenses in those plants during times of stress, much as they do in humans.

Our bodies respond to the presence of those bioactives, almost as though the plants were signaling us, saying "I've been under a lot of stress—and it is likely that you soon will be, too. Prepare yourself by activating your master health regulators to go into optimal maintenance." Drs. Howitz and Sinclair have proposed that animals have retained their ability to recognize and respond to certain plant stress molecules because these provide a useful advance warning of a deteriorating environment or food supply. The idea that we developed in such a way that allows us to receive warning signals from the plant kingdom is incredibly neat. It tickles my fancy to imagine my body receiving signals from the bell pepper on my plate.

But we're not finding these bioactives in modern fruits and vegetables in anywhere near the concentrations we should be, in part because modern farming practices have eliminated most of the stressors that a plant in the wild might have to contend with. Plants are watered regularly, and sprayed with pesticides. We no longer build concrete bomb shelters to protect us from the Red Menace; why would a plant squander its resources to protect itself against a threat that doesn't exist?

> **Plants need certain kinds of stress to produce bioactive compounds. They don't get that stress in the high-yield, low-risk greenhouses favored by agribusiness.**

That may be why a recent study from the University of California, Davis, discovered that levels of two types of flavonoids—quercetin and kaempferol, some of the bioactives we've been talking about—were substantially higher (79 and 97 percent, respectively) in organic tomatoes than their conventional counterparts. In this case, the researchers believe that yet another technological innovation—the use of inorganic nitrogen in conventional fertilizer— is responsible, since flavonoids are produced to protect the plant when not enough nitrogen is available. Conventional tomatoes don't have to "worry" about having enough available nitrogen, and so they never armor up. But we end up the real losers.

Pesticides and synthetic nitrogen are just the tip of the iceberg. Another technological advance is robbing our foods of the bioactive compounds we need to fine-tune our bodies. Fruits and vegetables are perishable—a problem when they have to be picked, crated, shipped across the country, unloaded, unpacked, and then sold. The food industry's solution is to pick fruits and vegetables long before they're technically ripe. Instead of vine-ripened, most of the fruits and vegetables we eat are crate- or counter-ripened.

Truthfully, we don't know the full ramifications of this—or even, to be honest, what fruits and vegetables are most likely affected. But there has been a great deal of research in grapes. As grapes ripen, we see powerful changes in bioactive content. Evidence to date suggests that the bioactives in grapes are primarily found in the skins, and that allowing the grapes to ripen on the vine creates striking changes in bioactive content, specifically a real increase in anthocyanins and other so-called aromatic polyphenols. These are the very bioactives that have been demonstrated to have the most profound effect on the master health regulators.

I feel fairly comfortable extrapolating that something similar happens in other fruits as they ripen. For one thing, it has been scientifically proven that the polyphenol content increases as fruits get darker—as most of them do as they ripen. It makes intuitive sense as well; if polyphenols are natural pesticides, it seems likely that they'd show up when they're most needed—at the height of deliciousness, or when the fruit is ripe.

So we're not necessarily eating *fewer* fruits and vegetables than our grandparents were—but those we are eating have many fewer of the bioactive compounds that activate the master health regulators. What we've gained in uniform size and unblemished skin, we've likely lost in polyphenols, and many of the other valuable bioactive compounds that give us all that bang for our vegetal buck.

HOW GENE SMART CAN HELP YOU
GET THE POLYPHENOLS YOU NEED

With Gene Smart, you'll be adding more fruits and vegetables to your diet. The critical advantage of the Gene Smart Diet over all other diets to date is that it pays close attention to the *concentrations* and *total amounts* of bioactive polyphenols that the scientific literature has deemed most important. As my father used to say to me often, "You can't dance at every wedding"; with polyphenols, this has never been truer. In particular, I will focus on trans-resveratrol, the anthocyanins, the catechins, and ellagic acid within foods.

There are several thousand polyphenols, each with its own antioxidant and gene altering properties. I will focus on those that have been shown to alter both gene expression and inflammatory disease in animals and humans. It does little good to simply generalize and then eat food categories; the very fact that it is so much more complicated than that explains why so many of our diets fail.

For example, ordinary red wine contains between 0.1 and 6.0 milligrams per liter of resveratrol, depending on the grape variety. Muscadine wines, commonly found in the American Southeast, have been reported to contain much higher levels. By contrast, white wine has 10 to 100 times *less* because white wine is fermented after the skin has been removed, and most of the resveratrol is in the skin. So all wine is not created equal—not by a long shot.

This is one of the key advantages of recognizing that the health benefits come from specific bioactive compounds *within* the food, and not the food itself. In the case of polyphenols, the food is simply the delivery system for the bioactive, and it's the concentration of the bioactive that must be taken into account. But it does make life beautiful when the delivery system is a spicy pinot noir!

Some fruits and vegetables have a higher content of the polyphenols that we are aiming for than others; in Part 4, you'll find common fruits and vegetables divided into groups of "high" and "low" polyphenolic content, enabling you to shop and choose the best foods for you with ease. I recommend that you incorporate "high" fruits and vegetables into your diet whenever possible.

CHAPTER SIXTEEN

WHAT GENE SMART CAN DO FOR YOU

GENE SMART IS A ONE-STOP SOLUTION. This diet stands alone because it harnesses the power of the adaptive stress response and the master health regulators behind it—the body's natural defense system—against threats both external and internal. By doing so, it will enable you to do what would once have been thought impossible: to help direct your biological destiny.

Gene Smart is the best that science can provide at this time in calorie restriction mimetics, because it uses a combination of strategies to attack chronic, full-body inflammation. And the best news of all is that you don't have to go hungry. In fact, quite the opposite. Gene Smart simply puts you back in touch with your body's natural survival system. In this section, you'll find everything you need to know to do the diet. But before we get to the nuts and bolts, let me quickly recap what you can expect from Gene Smart—and show off a little with some of the great results we've gotten so far!

REVERSING THE DAMAGE

We've seen how many of the environmental (diet and lifestyle) elements we take for granted in modern life suppress the adaptive stress response that activates the master health regulators. Our hunter-gatherer ancestors ate only whole grains, because they were all that was available. They didn't have to choose (or pay extra for!) organic vegetables or "wild" fish; in the hunter-gatherer days, all vegetables were organic, and all fish wild. All of these factors positively impacted their health regulators.

In other words, there was a fundamental synchrony between the way our ancestors' bodies were designed and the way they were used and fed—a synchrony that supported their master health regulators, and that naturally resulted in optimal health for the conditions that hunter-gatherers faced. That's why many scientists believe that if our ancestors had antibiotics and better slingshots, they would have lived longer than we do—and in much greater health.

> In the primordial forest, our master health regulator pathways got exactly what they needed to set the dial for survival and maximum health.

But while much may have changed in how and what we eat, what has remained constant and intact is the feedback loop between food, lifestyle, and the health regulators. If our physiology is most ideally suited to the diet and lifestyle of a hunter-gatherer, then every substantial change in our food supply, lifestyle, and dietary habits—aquaculture and agribusiness, the striking increase in calories, the severe reduction in physical activity, the prevalence of refined flours, a reduction in concentrations of bioactive compounds, and a shift in omega fatty acid ratios, to mention only a few—has stretched the rubber band of our bodies' tolerance a little further.

Increased caloric intake induces a caustic wave of pro-inflammatory events; changes in the fat-based bioactives we consume cause increases in cardiovascular disease and diabetes; a reduction in dietary fiber intake reduces our ability to control our weight and blood glucose. A reduction in physical activity produces more pro-inflammatory and fewer anti-inflammatory signals, and eating fewer bioactive compounds in the form of polyphenols fails to stimulate a beneficial adaptive stress response. The result? The wrong signals are sent to the body's natural survival switches, resulting in chronic inflammation, weight gain, the diseases associated with obesity, and premature aging.

Thankfully, there is a great deal of give in the rubber band; our miraculous bodies have taken in stride many of the changes that have come about as a result of industrialization. But clearly, the pandemic of obesity and inflammatory diseases has come from stretching that rubber band too far.

There is hope. Now that we understand some of the central mechanism behind the epidemic of epidemics, *we can do something about it*. Fortunately, an intervention is not only possible, but immediately available to us. Without it, modern life will continue to scramble the messages we send this essential system, setting our course for premature aging, overweight, illness, and an early death.

For us to experience a significant reduction in whole-body inflammation with a resulting change in aging and disease, we must systematically address each issue. Addressing each individually may have a small effect, but to have a dramatic effect, you need to address all of them, which is precisely what Gene Smart does.

Let me summarize some of the measurable benefits you can expect to see once you begin the Gene Smart Diet.

1. GENE SMART HELPS PREVENT AND REVERSE CARDIOVASCULAR DISEASE

An analysis of data from 10 studies with over 300,000 individuals shows that the fiber dosages prescribed in Gene Smart dramatically reduce heart disease as measured by a number of important risk outcomes, including decreasing the risk of death from heart disease by an average of 40 to 60 percent.

The fish oil recommendations also provide a powerful defense against cardiovascular disease, as shown by the fact that they alone reduce average risk of nonfatal heart attacks by 27 percent and risk of stroke by 12 percent. Another study showed that consuming one small serving of fish a day translates to a *35 percent reduction in fatal coronary heart disease*. You actually get the equivalent of three meals of fish a day on Gene Smart, combining both the diet and supplements.

And the red wine recommendations alone have been demonstrated to reduce heart attack risk by more than 30 percent, on average.

But we don't just have to depend on other people's studies. In our own, 8-week-long Hillsdale Study, we saw reductions in all major heart disease risk factors, including resting heart rate, blood pressure, LDL cholesterol (an average of 10 milligrams per deciliter), triglycerides (an average of 20 milligrams per deciliter). We also saw dramatic changes in markers of diabetes, fasting insulin, HOMA indices, hemoglobin A1c, and SCD1 activity, which all contribute to the risk of diabetes. And we saw marked drops in the markers and gene expression associated with whole-body inflammation: The worse off the patients were when they started, the better the change they saw.

The protocols recommended in Gene Smart are so potent that I believe them to be more effective than any single conventional pharmaceutical at reducing independent risk factors for cardiovascular disease and heart attack—and with none of the negative side effects! If your blood work and other assessments have shown that you are at high risk for heart disease, you can expect to see significant favorable improvement in your test numbers in as little as 8 weeks.

Change your omega-3 index. Research indicates that the percentage of omega-3 fats in your blood cells rivals C-reactive protein levels as a predictor of heart attack. The Gene Smart Diet is tailored to increase your omega-3 index, thereby reducing your chances of heart attack and sudden death by more than 50 percent, on average. In the Hillsdale Study, there was a greater than 50 percent increase in long-chain omega-3s on average (in individuals who had not been taking them at the beginning of the study).

Lower high triglycerides. In people with high triglycerides, the concentrations and duration of fish oil prescribed in Gene Smart have been proven to reduce triglyceride levels by an average of 20 to 30 percent, on average.

Lower elevated resting heart rate. In people with elevated resting heart rates—an independent predictor of cardiovascular disease and sudden death—the fish oil concentrations and duration prescribed in Gene Smart have been shown to reduce heart rate by 2.5 beats per minute, or over 10 million fewer heartbeats in an 80-year lifetime—which translates to significant benefits for cardiovascular health. We saw approximately the same reduction in the Hillsdale Study.

Lower LDL (bad cholesterol). The fiber dosages recommended in Gene Smart have been shown to reduce LDL cholesterol by an average of 10 to 15 percent. We saw an average loss of greater than 10 milligrams per deciliter in 8 weeks in the Hillsdale Study.

Raise HDL (good cholesterol). Epidemiological, case control, and randomized clinical trials show that alcohol consumption at the level prescribed in Gene Smart in the form of red wine increases HDL "good" cholesterol by 20 percent.

Reduce arachidonic acid. The foods and supplements prescribed in the Gene Smart Diet mirror studies proving that you can dramatically lower circulating levels of arachidonic acid and shift the omega-6 to omega-3 ratios from an average of greater than 15:1 to less than 5:1. That's certainly what we saw in the Hillsdale Study participants—particularly heartening, given that high levels of AA (resulting from typical American diets!) have been shown to increase an inappropriate inflammatory response—a contributing factor in a host of crippling chronic conditions.

Lower CRP. The inflammatory marker CRP is now heralded as the single most predictive factor in heart disease risk, and studies show that exercise protocols like the one in Gene Smart can help reduce CRP by 50 percent. Alcohol consumption (a glass of red wine with dinner) at the level prescribed in Gene Smart reduces CRP by 15 percent, on average.

Emerging data reveal a strong inverse correlation between fiber concentrations as recommended in Gene Smart and circulating CRP levels; one study showed that CRP concentrations were 63 percent lower in participants who consumed the most fiber.

Participants in the Hillsdale Study lowered whole-body inflammation more than 35 percent in 8 weeks. The critical markers that dropped most in our study were important ones: leptin and interleukin-6. We saw a 35 percent reduction in circulating leptin levels, the pro-inflammatory protein produced by fat cells, and a greater than 90 percent reduction in IL-8 gene expression, a cytokine that controls the movement of inflammatory cells into tissues.

Lower high blood pressure. Studies—most recently in *JAMA* in 2007— show that the dark chocolate concentrations prescribed in the Gene Smart Diet *reduce high blood pressure in an at-risk population by an average of 18 percent.* "The silent killer"—affecting one in three Americans, a third of whom don't know they have it—is a leading risk factor for heart attack and stroke (the number-one and number-three leading causes of death) and a contributor to coronary artery disease, aneurysms, kidney failure, and dementia. The Hillsdale participants had a 6 mm/Hg drop in systolic blood pressure.

Prevent a second heart attack. A large clinical trial—conducted with over 11,000 patients—showed that fish oils of the sort and the concentrations prescribed in Gene Smart can reduce sudden death *by an average of 45 percent.* Why is this important? According to the American Heart Association, one out of four men and one out of three women who live through a heart attack will die of sudden heart attack within the following year. The science in Gene Smart cuts this horrifying statistic by almost half.

Note: Current estimates attach a price tag of $550 billion to the global pharmaceutical dollars spent on cardiovascular drugs. Gene Smart offers a nonmedical intervention without any of the side effects, and at a fraction of the cost!

The exercise protocol alone has been revealed to add 4 years to your life.

2. GENE SMART SPEEDS WEIGHT LOSS AND GIVES DIETERS AN EDGE

- Studies have shown that over 12 weeks, dieters enjoyed a 7- to 10-pound weight loss, even without reducing calories, just by adding fiber and exercise to their diets in the concentrations prescribed in Gene Smart.

- Additional studies show that adding fiber to calorie-reduced diets (in the concentrations recommended in the Gene Smart Diet) facilitated the loss of 28 percent more weight than calorie reduction alone. There is a strong and proven inverse correlation between high fiber consumption of the type recommended in Gene Smart and obesity; in other words, the more fiber you eat, the less likely you are to be obese.

- Studies reveal that overweight individuals who supplemented their diets with omega-3 fatty acids at the levels recommended in Gene Smart burned 26 percent more calories *from fat*, on average, and reduced their insulin levels by 50 percent, on average. In the Hillsdale Study, we saw dramatic reductions in fasting insulin levels—an average of 33 percent in just 8 weeks.

- The fish oil concentrations prescribed in the Gene Smart Diet have been proven in studies to increase weight loss by an average of 24 percent in obese women on calorie-reduced diets.

- In one study, the addition of green tea at the levels recommended in Gene Smart resulted in a weight loss of over 10 pounds in 8 weeks.

- The exercise protocols in Gene Smart will increase strength by greater than 35 percent, on average. Omega-3 fats reduce body fat and promote muscle by improving the flow of blood to muscles during exercise.

Taken together, this easily explains why participants in the Hillsdale Study told us things like, "I lost more weight than I meant to lose," and "The pounds just seemed to fall off me!" We saw weight loss of between 1.5 and 2 pounds a week—over 600 pounds lost amongst all 57 study participants in just 8 weeks. And their body composition changes were even more dramatic, including an average of one-half inch of waist circumference, and almost one-half of a percent of body fat *per week*.

3. GENE SMART WILL HELP STABILIZE BLOOD SUGAR LEVELS

- Studies show that by following the dietary recommendations for fiber and whole grains outlined in the Gene Smart Diet, individuals can reduce their risk of becoming diabetic by 35 percent.

- Gene Smart is great news if you are diabetic. Clinical trials proved that an exercise regimen like the one offered in Gene Smart conducted on individuals with type 2 diabetes improved insulin control by 23 percent on average and prompted a whopping 40 percent reduction in CRP.

- Our Hillsdale Study participants saw serious reductions in many of the biomarkers associated with insulin resistance, metabolic syndrome, and diabetes, including: fasting insulin, HOMA (an indicator of insulin resistance), and others like hemoglobin A1c and SCD1.

- Most impressively, Gene Smart reduced fasting insulin levels (a sign of insulin resistance and the beginning of type 2 diabetes or metabolic syndrome) by 33 percent, on average.

4. GENE SMART CAN HELP YOU FROM HEAD TO TOE

Because Gene Smart reaches behind the control panel to turn off inflammation at the very source—your genes—it has an incredible ability to address all kinds of inflammatory conditions. For example, it can:

Slow cognitive decline. In studies where individuals consume fish oil according to protocols outlined in Gene Smart, older subjects were seen to have fourfold less cognitive decline over a 5-year period than the control group. (Conversely, studies in the elderly show that when the ratio of omega fatty acids does not follow the balance prescribed in Gene Smart—specifically, when omega-6s are consumed in higher amounts than permitted on Gene Smart—there was a 76 percent increase in cognitive loss.)

Stave off depression. Epidemiological studies show an inverse correlation between depression and fish consumption, and six out of seven clinical trials showed that the EPA levels prescribed in Gene Smart significantly improved depressive symptoms. We are currently examining this in monkey models to test the effectiveness of omega-3s in preventing depression.

Treat asthma. Consuming fish oils at the dosages and duration prescribed in Gene Smart has been scientifically proven in studies to improve lung function in response to exercise by greater than 69 percent and dramatically reduce mediators of inflammation in respiratory fluids (leukotrienes by over 70 percent, prostaglandins by greater than 90 percent, and cytokines by greater than 70 percent). Although not statistically analyzed, several participants in the Hillsdale Study reported getting off their asthma medications during the study.

Improve the symptoms of rheumatoid arthritis. Increasing fish oil and borage oil consumption—as outlined in Gene Smart—has been clinically

Good News for Men!

By preventing or reversing cardiovascular disease, you not only improve heart health, but often affect other health problems you may not immediately associate with cardiovascular function—like erectile dysfunction! Just one of the possible collateral benefits of Gene Smart.

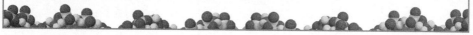

proven to relieve symptoms of RA. Those with RA use fewer nonsteroidal anti-inflammatory drugs (NSAIDs) and report a decrease in morning stiffness and in the number of painful joints.

Additional evidence exists to support the protocols recommended in Gene Smart as part of an overall strategy to prevent arrhythmia, COPD, osteoporosis, osteoarthritis, Crohn's disease, IBS, psoriasis, and certain cancers. And the exercise protocol in Gene Smart has been proven to extend life by nearly 4 years!

EFFECTIVE ALONE, UNBEATABLE TOGETHER

It's a staggering line-up of measurable benefits—and those are just the individual components! What Gene Smart does is put them together, so that they're working *synergistically* to speed weight loss, beat back inflammation, and turn back the hands of time. It is a terrible combination of factors that have made us so very sick; now it's time to harness the explosive power of Gene Smart to reverse the trend.

Let's look at CRP as an example: This is a direct measure of chronic, low-level, whole-body inflammation. We know that the exercise similar to that prescribed in Gene Smart can reduce CRP by up to 50 percent. Drinking a glass of red wine with dinner can reduce CRP by 15 percent, on average. We also know that increasing fiber has a powerful effect on CRP, lowering it as much as 50 percent in some studies. So what we have is not one, not two, but three arms of the Gene Smart program working together to fight chronic, low-level, full-body inflammation.

Are these additive? Probably not. But will it be more effective to deploy *three* separate strategies that have been scientifically proven to lower levels of this inflammatory molecule, as opposed to just a single one? You can bet on it. I don't believe there has ever been a diet which gathered so many strands of cutting-edge science together into one, simple, easy-to-follow program. Each arm of Gene Smart is powerful; working together, it's nothing short of a revolution.

And no, you don't have to return to the primordial forest! You can keep your computers, your antibiotics, the conveniences and creature comforts—and yes, even many of your favorite foods. Using nothing more complicated than ordinary table foods, you can reset the master health regulators by changing the signals you send them, neutralizing the impact of the environmental threats that scramble the regulators' health promoting signals.

For the first time, *all* the essential elements are in place. We've seen high-fiber diets before; we've seen diets that emphasize fish oils, and even ones that talked about polyphenols—even if they didn't know that's what they were doing. But for the first time, we are not talking about broad classes of bioactives, in broad classes of food. Technological changes have taken our food supply too far out of line to make these generalizations possible. Each day, Gene Smart gives you specific dosages and specific types of bioactives—and tells you the exact foods necessary to obtain the bioactives that match up with the science.

Gene Smart uses everything we know—all the scientific knowledge at our disposal—to help these factors work together, reversing the tide of aging and disease.

THE KEYS TO YOUR SUCCESS

"I thought this was my destiny;
I thought I had no choice. I thought
I had no control over my body."

—A HILLSDALE STUDY PARTICIPANT

Until you understand the key driver behind your weight problem—your genes—getting to and maintaining a healthy weight *is* out of your control. Left to fend for ourselves in this overabundant society, our willpower stands no chance.

With Gene Smart, you'll finally have the weapons you need to fight back against these strong biological forces. But much will be required of you, as well. I think of the struggle to lose weight as a triangle. On one side, you have diet and lifestyle. These old habits are hard enough to change—but it's made even harder by your biology, which makes up the second side of the triangle. Your hormones and other signals given by your hunter-gatherer genes control everything, from your appetite, to satiety, to how much energy you have, to how fast you will put on or burn fat. And your biology, I'm sorry to tell you, doesn't want you to lose weight. In fact, every ancestral survival gene within you is telling your body to do exactly the opposite, as protection against a famine that's not coming in 21st-century America.

"I feel like an addict," one of the participants in the study confessed to me before we began. And that's not a specious comparison; in fact, your brain activity is very much like one of an addict—your genes are sending signals that look very much like the signals in an addict's brain, and to many of the same sites. Brain activity in the addiction regions of the brain will be dramatically increased until you eat. And, without help, that's precisely what's going to happen.

And, I'm sorry to say, your body doesn't particularly want to experience beneficial adaptive stress. This beneficial stress system was put there to protect us before we reproduced; from nature's perspective, we're just taking resources that could be used by those who can reproduce (assuming that we're beyond our reproductive years, as most of us are).

That's why the challenge that you have been given is difficult. It's certainly why most commercial diet programs fail so miserably in a very short period of time. It reminds me of nothing so much as the ancient Greek myth of Sisyphus. Punished for defying the gods, he was doomed to push a heavy rock up a mountain—forever. Once at the top, the rock would roll down to the bottom again, for all eternity. This ceaseless, pointless toil is a good metaphor for the dieting/weight-gain seesaw that so many of us find ourselves on. Without a strategic plan that addresses the root causes of our problem—our genes—we have a fate that is no less burdensome than the one shouldered by Sisyphus. And that's why we feel so out of control.

It's also why the third side of our triangle is "willpower." But willpower is no match for our genes. So *how do we win this epic battle?*

Two ways: First, we must use an approach that works with our genes, instead of against them. That's what Gene Smart is designed to do. And we must use a holistic strategy to optimize our success. In our Hillsdale Study, the participants identified several additional lines of attack that I believe made their experience so incredibly successful.

Next are several of the *critical* concepts and components that I believe made the Hillsdale Study and make the Gene Smart program so successful:

Improve your self-esteem and perception. As I have said before, the vast majority of us are in this situation *not* because we're lazy, pathetic, or weak, but because we're genetically programmed to do what we're doing, even though it's making us terribly sick. Hearing this for the first time can be freeing; it certainly was for many of the Hillsdale participants. And I count how much better they felt about themselves as our greatest success.

You are a good and strong person struggling with something that's been out of your direct control. This is something you're going to have to tell yourself, loud and often, because what you'll hear from society (and probably, from yourself) is something different. Even worse, this line of thinking can lead to a mini-rebellion on your part—"I'm weak and bad? Oh, I'll show you how weak and bad I can be—by eating the entire box!"

Don't allow yourself to become overwhelmed, or to get bogged down in feeling out of control, or as if the problem has no solution. There is a solution—in fact, Gene Smart offers you five of them! This is how you were programmed. Your reaction is a natural one. It is not, however, a healthy one. But there are positive, rational, and easily implemented steps you can take to reverse that biology.

Hold yourself accountable. Willpower alone is not enough to bring about this change. You're going to have to marshal your resources—and you start by realizing that you can't do this alone.

If you have compulsive eating habits, you may want to stop by a meeting for people who struggle with similar issues; the 12-step format has helped millions of people with a wide range of dependency problems, including with food.

If you are a person of faith, we encourage you to use your spirituality to help you change. In virtually all religions, participants are encouraged to keep their bodies healthy, as well as their souls and their minds. Perhaps your relationship with a higher power will help you to recognize your body as a temple, and to treat it as such.

Rally your community. Tell two close friends what you are doing, give them your starting weight, and tell them to hold you accountable. Clean out the kitchen and get the whole family involved. Find a "program partner," someone who will go through the program with you, and work through it together. My wife and I work out together—and you can't imagine the trash we talk to each other, in the interests of motivating one another.

Keep a record. This is, of course, another form of accountability. A recent study suggested that the most important determinant of compliance to a diet was whether the individual on the program documented their food intake. I suggest you keep food and exercise logs. They're very satisfying to look back on—and good motivation when you feel yourself starting to slip.

Finally, I have given you the very specific tools in this program to reduce calories without being hungry. I don't honestly know what parts of the diet and/or exercise program are responsible for the satiety factors responsible for this effect (although I suspect fiber and exercise are a powerful one-two punch), but I can tell you that over 80 percent of our participants reported not being hungry even when reducing calories. As far as you are concerned, it really doesn't matter what's driving the effect—simply that you have been given a set of specific tools that allow you to reduce calories, dramatically lower markers of inflammation, and markedly improve energy metabolism. *Use them!*

PART FOUR

The Gene Smart Diet

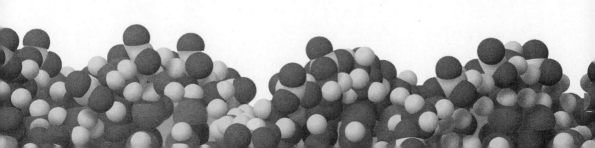

CHAPTER SEVENTEEN

STARTING GENE SMART

I BELIEVE THAT IT IS ABSOLUTELY IMPERATIVE that every one of us makes a radical shift in what and how much we eat, because most of the calories we currently consume are suppressing our bodies' natural ability to defend themselves. This has disastrous implications for our health. Indeed, some of the foods we currently think of as "healthy" choices, like certain types of fish, can be very poor choices indeed.

In addition to signaling the regulators to optimize health generally, the Gene Smart Diet can help us muffle the alarm bells that trigger the aging process. These master health regulators can help us to prolong the period of peak cellular maintenance, even as we pass out of our chronological youth. With some simple interventions, we can enlist the regulators so that we slow the activation of the internal trip wire of inflammation that leads to the degeneration and decline we once associated with "normal" aging.

> Fighting obesity and slowing the aging process may be as elegantly simple as tricking our bodies into believing that they're still in their reproductive prime—which is exactly what the master health regulators can help us to do.

As long as the regulators receive the correct signals from us—as they will on the Gene Smart Diet—we can slow down (or even turn back) many aspects of the aging clock. Gene Smart can help you enjoy more prime years, regardless of how many candles there are on your cake.

CHANGING THE WAY YOU EAT

Gene Smart will require that you change the way you eat. I know that's not easy. Eating when, what, and how we like makes up some of our most ingrained habits, and I understand that changing those habits, especially over the long term, can be a real challenge.

Lots of things interfere with our best intentions: work and sleep and family schedules, personal preferences, budgetary constraints, time, allergies and intolerances, and level of culinary ability. Not to mention that excessive appetite during periods of abundance—always, in other words—is likely a trait that we developed in order to protect us. The problem is that the famine never comes.

But you can do this; you simply must.

Some of us may already be highly motivated because we're in extreme pain, or living with life-threatening illness. But this plan is one that must be adopted by all of us, whether we're currently coping with a chronic inflammatory condition or simply in line for one. We must realize that we are eating not only to get nutrients, but to engage our adaptive stress response, the body's best natural defense. We can do so by giving our bodies the foods that contain the right bioactive compounds, and engaging in the right types of exercise in the right amounts, to protect us against aging, obesity, and disease.

THE RIGHT PLAN

Want two good ways to fail with a diet? Here's one: Go with a plan that's too rigid. Here's another: Choose a plan that's so far away from what you've always eaten that you might as well be on the moon. With either approach, failure is almost guaranteed. So how can we help you adopt the Gene Smart Diet without failing? Well, we need to start realistically with where you are with your eating, and figure out how to make some simple changes.

> **Your body will change with even the simplest of adjustments in your eating habits.**

The good news is that you don't have to do a lot to reap big changes in the way you look and feel. The more you do, the more progress you'll see.

And, although I'm very interested in what's *in* your food, I never forget that food is food, not just bioactives. I'm a guy who likes to eat, and I promise what you'll find in this plan will not only make you feel good, it'll taste good, too. Designing these delicious menus was not, in all truth, a very difficult task, considering how amazing the foods are that we had to work with.

A hamburger made with grass-fed beef tastes better than its feedlot counterpart; in my opinion, a piece of hearty, nutty multigrain toast blows white bread right out of the water. And I don't care how embarrassed it makes my kids—I'm the guy at the farmers' market who's eating that perfect, sun-warmed, heirloom German Johnson tomato out of my hand like an apple. I love the way a glass of red wine enhances a gorgeous meal, and I don't mind finishing it off with a complex and delicious square or two of dark chocolate.

Those are some of the changes you'll be making in what you eat. But another way to ensure your success—and maximize the pleasure you get from Gene Smart—is to use this plan as a reason to start thinking about *how* you eat, as well.

Much has been made of late of the "French" way of eating. But as someone who grew up on a farm in the Deep South, eating whole, good foods, thoughtfully prepared and gratefully received, I'm not so sure what's French about it. We ate what we could grow, and we canned the rest. Our fruits and vegetables were always picked at the peak of ripeness. Only small portions of meat were eaten, and our meat consumption typically coincided with specific times of the year—late fall, when the animals were slaughtered. Clearly, my parents, raised as they were in the Depression era, made the most of what we had, and we enjoyed every bite.

Here's what you won't find in Gene Smart: *diet foods*. That's usually what nutritionists push on people who struggle with weight issues. In my opinion, all that does is feed into our value-sizing mentality, what I consider to be the country's obsession with "more." But more low-calorie "fake food" isn't better—and it's certainly not better for your health.

Let's make every bite count. Remember, the bioactives in these delicious foods are how we're reaching behind the panel and controlling our very genetic destiny!

Will It Cost More?

I'm not going to sugarcoat it (or whatever the low-glycemic version of sugarcoating might be): Fresh and wild fish, grass-fed beef, and fresh fruits and vegetables cost more than the foods you may be used to piling into your shopping cart. Eating this way will also require that you spend a little more time thinking, planning, and preparing your food.

But that doesn't necessarily mean that this diet is more expensive, in the long run. Spending more money and time on eating better is considerably cheaper than purchasing the over-the-counter medications and prescription drugs that you'll need later as an antidote to those so-called less expensive food choices.

The prestigious *New England Journal of Medicine* just published a review on the cost of health care per person in this country. The states that had the highest rates of obesity are, not coincidentally, the states where individuals spend the most on health care. The choice is yours: Pay now or pay later.

And the choice to consume drugs over whole foods comes with multiple unwanted side effects. In Europe, they don't use the term "side effects"; they don't differentiate between the primary and secondary effects of pharmaceuticals. Our strategy, of course, has always been to take a drug—and then another one to mask the side effects caused by the first one.

That said, there are many ways to tend to your pennies on this eating plan. Here are some:

- Buy fresh fish when it is on sale, and freeze it for later use. Ask your fishmonger to wrap it in freezer paper in individual portion sizes (or do it yourself when you get home).

- In most of the recipes, you can easily substitute one fish for another, based on what's on sale at your fish market—or on hand in the freezer. Feel free to do so after you consult our fish list (pages 217–218) to ensure that you're getting the same long-chain omega-3 content.

- Don't be afraid to try something new in place of a more expensive fish (again, make sure you consult our fish chart on pages 217–218);

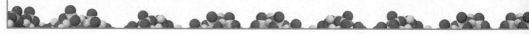

THE GENE SMART APPROACH: THREE PHASES

The Gene Smart approach combines what we know about ancestral diets, together with modern discoveries about the nutritional control of human genetics—now called nutrigenomics. So how do we get you there from here?

Gene Smart has three phases: The Adaptive Response Phase, the Preconditioning Phase, and the Optimal Maintenance Phase. Here's an overview.

just buy it in a smaller quantity and test out a recipe. I tried smelt for the first time earlier this week, and it was delicious.

Fresh produce can also be expensive, especially when you're eating out-of-season items that have been shipped in to your grocery store from around the world. In my experience, these foods tax not only my wallet, but my tastebuds, too. Of course, you don't have to stick to what's available at the farmers' market all year long; this isn't *Little House on the Prairie*, and you'd never stay on a diet that asked you to eat root vegetables all winter. Here are some alternatives:

- Eating foods seasonally and purchasing them at your local farmers' market is an excellent choice—one that supports your local economy and the environment, and will ultimately deliver better nutritional quality. So I do recommend doing that, especially in the summer and fall.

- Buying your favorite fruits and vegetables in large quantities is cost-effective (by the end of the summer, my neighbors are desperate to give their zucchini and tomatoes away), and canning or freezing them yourself makes them even less expensive. Your local county agricultural extension agency will have a food preservation expert, equipment for borrowing, and classes to help you learn new skills.

- It is not only cost-effective but appropriate, from a bioactive perspective, to incorporate more frozen fruits and vegetables into your diet. They can be purchased in large quantities at stores like Sam's Club and Costco. These foods have been unfairly vilified, considering that most are packed at the peak of their freshness and ripeness. So-called "fresh" produce, by contrast, is often picked in an unripe and nutrient-poor state and then shipped for days (weeks, sometimes!). Not surprisingly, the nutrient content—and the flavor—suffers dramatically.

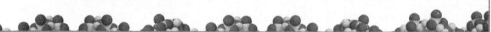

Phase I: The Adaptive Response Phase

This is the most rigorous stage of the program. Thank goodness it lasts for just a short 3 weeks for most folks!

In my experience, it's good to have a little rigor up front. First of all, it gets you in the right state of mind. Most of us have gotten pretty badly off track. We eat junk, and too much of it; we exercise half-heartedly, if we do it at all.

Sometimes it takes a little rigor to make a real break with that unhealthy past; I think of it as pressing a "reset button" in my brain.

But that reset button isn't just for your brain. There's a physiological explanation for why I have designed the first 3 weeks of this program to be more demanding than the ones that follow.

Remember, the point of the program is to activate an adaptive stress response. Because of our habits and environments, we've unwittingly been doing exactly the opposite, which is to say that the majority of the choices we make every day depress our bodies' natural survival switch. In order to turn things around, I believe we have to power that survival switch back up, and the only way to do that is with some of that benevolent stress. Your attention in this early phase ensures that your body will make the transition to "survival" mode in the quickest and most efficient way possible. In so doing, we'll maximize the early activation of the master regulators controlling gene expression that we have talked about throughout this book.

STEP #1: CUT CALORIES

Our first step has to be to "put out the fires"—to quell the low-pressure systems that are causing our perfect storm. For all the reasons we have already explored, the first and most important thing we can do is cut calories.

A Note for the Significantly Overweight

We recommend reducing your calories for the first 3 weeks, which should be enough to kick-start the adaptive stress phase of the diet.

As you'll see, it's also a pretty effective way to lose weight, which—as you well know by this point in the book—is the most significant thing you can do to improve your health and your inflammatory profile. So if you are overweight, and are motivated to continue in this first phase of the diet for longer than 3 weeks, I urge you to do so. You can lose all the weight that you need to, in a safe, healthy manner, by using the Adaptive Response Phase of the diet.

I urge you to use the tools you'll find here to take control of your own health at this important juncture in your life. If you are overweight or obese, following the Adaptive Response Phase for longer periods will only make you healthier, as evidenced by those folks who have followed this diet for years.

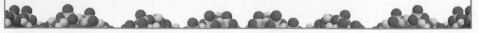

Gene Smart Diet

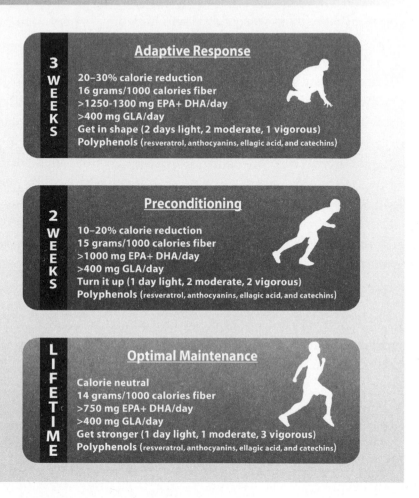

Adaptive Response

3 WEEKS

20–30% calorie reduction
16 grams/1000 calories fiber
>1250-1300 mg EPA+ DHA/day
>400 mg GLA/day
Get in shape (2 days light, 2 moderate, 1 vigorous)
Polyphenols (resveratrol, anthocyanins, ellagic acid, and catechins)

Preconditioning

2 WEEKS

10–20% calorie reduction
15 grams/1000 calories fiber
>1000 mg EPA+ DHA/day
>400 mg GLA/day
Turn it up (1 day light, 2 moderate, 2 vigorous)
Polyphenols (resveratrol, anthocyanins, ellagic acid, and catechins)

Optimal Maintenance

LIFETIME

Calorie neutral
14 grams/1000 calories fiber
>750 mg EPA+ DHA/day
>400 mg GLA/day
Get stronger (1 day light, 1 moderate, 3 vigorous)
Polyphenols (resveratrol, anthocyanins, ellagic acid, and catechins)

Is it calorie restriction? No. In the 3-week Adaptive Response Phase of the Gene Smart Diet, you will reduce your calories by 20 to 30 percent. Now, this is nowhere near what your hunter-gatherer ancestors might have experienced during a famine—or, for that matter, the 40 percent calorie restriction that we often use in laboratory animals. Is it calorie reduction? It sure is. Reducing the number of calories you eat is the only way to lose weight, and doing so by 20 to 30 percent will rapidly move you into an adaptive stress response in a manner that you can endure for 3 or more weeks.

Let me say that this is not easy. I understand that. But there is no easy way to correct the disconnect between genes and lifestyle that your body has experienced throughout your entire life. Think of it as preseason practice, getting your body ready for a better life; I know you can do it, and I know you'll feel the difference immediately.

The human data suggest that restricting calories by 20 to 30 percent will accomplish two objectives: First, it will activate those master health regulators that occur as a result of the stress response. Science has not yet shown us the minimum degree of restriction, or the minimum time necessary to activate the master regulators in humans. However, numerous studies have demonstrated that losing weight alone markedly reduces the body's levels of inflammatory messengers. And, the more weight you lose, the better off you are. For example, a 10 percent weight loss has been shown to decrease levels of CRP by 26 percent, while a 15 to 16 percent weight loss has been shown to decrease these levels by 32 to 34 percent.

> **Gene Smart will help you to lose weight more effectively and with greater ease than any other diet you've ever been on. When you do, you will dramatically reduce your production of inflammatory messengers.**

From studies such as these, together with an understanding of what a person can realistically be expected to do—one that comes from carrying out 2 decades' worth of human studies with controlled diets—I believe that a 20 to 30 percent calorie reduction as the initial activator of the stress response makes a lot of sense.

What if you're one of the lucky ones who doesn't need to lose a pound? I suggest reducing your calorie intake by 10 to 20 percent as described anyway. You won't lose more than you can easily make up, and I think the benefits of kicking your body into an adaptive stress response in this way outweigh the downside. Please note: If you are underweight at the start of this diet, you *should not* further restrict your calories.

But for the majority of us, this first phase is a tremendous opportunity to trim some of the excess weight we've been carrying around, as well as put our bodies on high alert.

STEP #2: INCREASE INSOLUBLE AND SOLUBLE FIBER

In addition to cutting calories by 20 to 30 percent, you will increase your daily intake of insoluble and soluble fiber (a 70:30 ratio) to 16 grams of fiber for every 1,000 calories that you consume. So if you eat 1,800 calories a day, you'll need to get 29 grams of fiber a day. Aside from all of fiber's health benefits—and, as you'll remember from Chapter 13, there are many—this is a good example of how Gene Smart supports your efforts to lose weight. Increasing fiber is, in itself, an incredibly useful strategy to help people reduce calories. This step alone was the key to weight loss in the Hillside Study.

I know, because it's what I do, too! Recently, I let myself go for a couple of months—too much work, too much of what I call "convenient eating" (eating what's around), and not enough exercise. Sure enough, I gained almost 15 pounds. I increased my fiber content and exercised more . . . and sure enough, the magic formula works! When I increase the fiber in my diet, I feel fuller, which means that I eat less—and more responsibly. You know you're not making good choices when you're so ravenous you can't see straight. Quiet your appetite, and it suddenly becomes much easier to choose the right snack, as opposed to the "right-now" snack. Add a little exercise and voilà! Weight is gone.

One of the biggest downsides to some of the major diets out there, including South Beach and Atkins, is their poor fiber content. Frankly, it is no wonder that folks have a hard time following them over the long term. I would starve to death—or at least feel like I was—if I had to reduce calories without increasing fiber.

STEP #3: MORE POLYPHENOLS, PLEASE!

Third, we will increase your polyphenol intake by emphasizing foods that contain high amounts of four classes of polyphenols: the anthocyanins, ellagic acids, catechins, and trans-resveratrol.

As I have said, the science is far from complete here. We are not sure which polyphenols best activate the master health regulators, or how the various classes of polyphenols are absorbed and metabolised. Further, there is a great deal missing in the data when you go looking for the actual content and amounts of specific polyphenols in fruits and vegetables. That

A Note about Fish Oil Safety

Unlike most dietary supplements, fish oils have been extensively studied for safety and efficacy.

It is very important to consult your physician before taking fish oil if you have a bleeding disorder; if you consume more than 3 grams a day of long-chain omega-3 fatty acids from fish or fish oil; or if you plan to combine omega-3s with other drugs that affect responses like bleeding. Consumption of more than 3 grams per day has been shown to increase the risk of bleeding in some cases, but there's little evidence of significant bleeding risk at lower doses.

Very high intakes of fish oil have been suggested to increase the risk of hemorrhagic (bleeding) stroke, primarily because they can decrease platelet aggregation, prolong bleeding time, and break down blood clots.

Your risk of bleeding may be elevated if you take fish oil supplements with certain medications. These include aspirin, blood thinners such as warfarin (Coumadin) or heparin, anti-platelet drugs such as clopidogrel (Plavix), and nonsteroidal anti-inflammatory drugs such as ibuprofen or naproxen.

Omega-3 fatty acids have many of the same anti-platelet activities as aspirin, so combining them magnifies this effect. Compared to aspirin alone, the combination of aspirin with omega-3 fatty acids markedly reduces platelet aggregation and blood platelet count, and prolongs bleeding time.

Omega-3 fatty acids significantly lower triglyceride levels, so they may add to the effects of triglyceride-lowering medications such as niacin, fibrates such as gemfibrozil (Lopid), or resins such as cholestyramine (Questran). Because omega-3 fatty acids can slightly increase levels of LDL "bad" cholesterol, they may counteract the LDL-lowering effects of statin drugs such as atorvastatin (Lipitor).

Minor side effects of omega-3 fatty acids may include gastrointestinal upset such as bloating, nausea, and diarrhea.

Because omega-3 fatty acids have the potential to interact with many medications, talk to your doctor before you start to take any fish oil supplement. If you're on any medication that affects blood coagulation, it's especially imperative that you first consult your physician.

No one should ever take high doses of omega-3 fatty acids without medical supervision.

Should young children take fish oil supplements? I think we have enough scientific evidence at this point to say yes, but there are not enough studies with regard to dosage. There is a huge difference between the ability of young children and adults to digest omega-3 fatty acids. In our laboratory, we've found that children require a far lower concentration of fish oils to achieve the same blood levels of omega-3 fatty acids as adults.

So while I believe that parents should feed their children "oily" fish, I recommend that children under 18 *not* take fish oil supplements, except under the direction of a pediatrician.

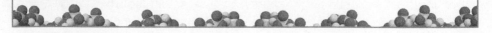

Where's the Wine?

No red wine is offered during the first 5 weeks of the plan, as it often can stimulate the appetite and cause a person to overeat at a time when caloric reduction is the goal. There are a few dark chocolate desserts and snacks built into the Adaptive Response menus, but as with red wine, dark chocolate can add calories at a time when calorie reduction is the goal.

So you have something to look forward to! And not just something delicious and relaxing, either; according to studies, by treating yourself to that glass of red wine at dinner per Gene Smart's recommendation, you can reduce your risk of heart attack by more than 30 percent, on average.

Obviously, if you don't drink wine, you can still do Gene Smart by adding nonalcoholic beverages with similar polyphenol profiles to your diet. Whether you're living in sobriety, don't like the taste, or simply prefer not to, I hope you'll investigate the delicious, high trans-resveratrol juices and supplements available at specialty food stores.

said, I believe that we can provide enough of the polyphenol classes that have shown the most promise, both in regulating gene expression and in influencing disease models in animals and humans, to further induce a stress response. The evidence at this time best supports the controlling effects of trans-resveratrol—the family of anthocyanins, ellagic acids, and catechins—on gene expression, so we will add high amounts of these in the form of whole fruits and vegetables, green tea, and dietary supplements that contain concentrated amounts of the polyphenols. (For more on the polyphenols, visit www.genesmart.com.)

If you remember those mice that stayed lean despite higher-fat diets and were able to exercise twice as long as a control group, you know that this aspect of Gene Smart will likely support your efforts as well.

STEP #4: ADD THE OMEGAS

In the Adaptive Response Phase, you will increase your intake of long-chain omega-3 fatty acids to 1,250 to 1,300 milligrams per day, and increase medium-chain omega-6s such as gamma-linolenic-acid (GLA) to between 400 and 500 milligrams per day.

These are the concentrations of long-chain omega-3s and short-chain omega-6s that the scientific literature has shown to reduce inflammatory messengers, lower blood lipids, and prevent and treat a number of inflammatory diseases. Even better, they're the numbers that my laboratory has shown to markedly reduce inflammatory gene expression. Also, increasing these fatty acids will shift your circulating ratios of long-chain omega-6s to long-chain omega-3s from greater than 15:1 to less than 5:1. Again, these ratios are well within the American Heart Association guidelines in terms of concentrations of omega-3s. Further, new studies that identify omega-3 levels as a predictor of heart disease suggest that a 5:1 ratio like this would reduce heart attack rates by more than 50 percent.

And don't forget—studies have shown that the combination of omega-3s and calorie reduction has been shown to enhance weight loss. It's a little free speed, so enjoy that turbo boost!

In the Adaptive Response Phase, 400 to 500 milligrams of the long-chain omega-3s you eat every day will come from whole foods, primarily fish. The remainder of the long-chain omega-3s, together with the short-chain omega-6s, will come from dietary supplements. The omega-6s you need are simply not present in high enough quantities in our food supply to get from whole foods, so you must take dietary supplements.

STEP #5: JUST ADD EXERCISE!

Finally, the Gene Smart plan is going to ask you to add exercise, moving you from a comparatively sedentary "modern" lifestyle to a much more active one. (If you are already active, you will increase your level of activity in order to increase the adaptive stress response.) Now, exercise will certainly help you to achieve your weight-loss goals. Not, perhaps, as quickly or easily as the gym ads would have you believe, but then, they're not talking about how good that treadmill is for your inflammatory profile!

To the best of our knowledge, this Adaptive Response Phase of the Gene Smart Diet mimics that of our hunter-gatherer ancestors in a number of important ways. It delivers a reduction in calories; an increase in fiber, polyphenols, and exercise; and an adjustment in omega-6 to omega-3 concentrations and ratios.

> The Adaptive Response Phase of Gene Smart attempts to
> mimic the diet and lifestyle your hunter-gatherer ancestors
> would have experienced.

Phase II: The Preconditioning Phase

I recommend that you follow the Adaptive Response Phase for a minimum of 3 weeks. (Ideally, you'll stay in that phase of the diet until you're at a weight that is healthy for you.)

Once you've arrived at your optimal weight, you'll move to the 2-week-long Preconditioning Phase.

It's called Preconditioning because it's "conditioning" you to what your diet should be for the rest of your life. You'll be happy to know that this phase is a little less stringent than Phase I. Most importantly, you are moving to a 10 to 20 percent reduction in calories; you're also reducing your fiber and the long-chain omega-3s. You will continue to consume high quantities of polyphenols, and you will actually increase your physical activity as you continue to "get into shape."

Phase III: The Optimal Maintenance Phase

Given the available science, I believe this phase of the Gene Smart Diet is likely to continuously activate those master health regulators responsible for optimal cellular and whole-body maintenance.

The goal in this phase is to be isocaloric, which is just a fancy way of saying that the calories you take in balance the number of calories you burn. But don't worry! You can still get many of the benefits of calorie restriction, even without restricting or reducing calories. The polyphenols and the long-chain omega-3s are maintained at a high level so you get all the benefits, without any of the suffering. (To optimize heart health, we'll be keeping your long-chain omega-6 to omega-3 ratios well below 5:1.) And you'll be further "stressing" your body and activating all those anti-inflammatory gene pathways with the described exercise program.

You won't find two important polyphenolic sources—dark chocolate and red wine—in the earlier phases of the diet because of their caloric impact and their potential effects on appetite. Congratulations—graduating to the Optimal Maintenance Phase of this diet means that you can begin to add these in.

CHAPTER EIGHTEEN

FOLLOWING GENE SMART

WHAT GENE SMART GIVES YOU, the consumer, are choices as to how you want to proceed with this plan. That's why you should think of what follows as suggestions within guidelines. I want this to be a plan that you can follow for the rest of your life—and I personally always prefer to focus on what I *can* have, rather than what I can't. And the good news is that the foods you can eat on the Gene Smart Diet are delicious ones indeed.

One particularly fascinating recent study looked at the advantage of the "polymeal," which used foods from seven basic groups every day: fruits, vegetables, garlic, almonds, fish, wine, and dark chocolate. The study authors concluded that participants eating from these groups daily would reduce their cardiovascular events by 76 percent, potentially extending their lives an extra 4.8 to 6.6 years. Many of these same food groups are now better defined and expanded upon within the Gene Smart Diet.

What is most exciting about this for me is that these foods can create the basis of an extremely pleasant and livable diet: one that your whole family can enjoy for a lifetime, one that can be incorporated into eating out, and, perhaps most importantly, one that I believe gives you all the health-promoting, life-extending benefits of calorie restriction, without leaving you starving.

In fact, it is one of the few diets that actually allows you to have your chocolate cake and eat it, too!

Gene Smart Diet System

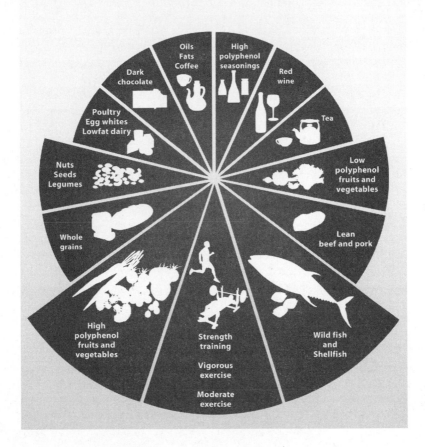

FISH RECOMMENDATIONS

The Adaptive Response Phase of the diet has the goal of increasing your intake of long-chain omega-3 fatty acids (EPA [eicosapentaenoic acid] + DPA [docosapentaenoic acid] + DHA [docosahexaenoic acid]) to a target of 1,250 to 1,300 milligrams per day. As with all bioactive classes, the *types* and *dosages* of the omega-3 fats are absolutely critical here.

We have designed the diet so that you take in an average of 400 to 500 milligrams of EPA and another 200 to 300 milligrams of DHA + DPA per day in the form of whole foods using fish that have high levels of long-chain omega-3s in their tissues.

Before You Begin

Before you begin, it's a good idea to take an inventory of your kitchen. If nothing else, this exercise will require a good, honest look at what your eating habits really are. It might be time to reorganize; I certainly find that ease and convenience affect my food choices, particularly when I'm in a rush. Making sure that my healthiest choices are front and center helps. These don't have to be big changes—for instance, a Tupperware dish filled with chopped vegetables in the crisper, frozen berries high in transresveratrol and anthocyanins thawing on the top shelf of the fridge (my favorite for breakfast), or a fruit bowl filled with the bounty of the season on the counter—but you'll see they make a big difference.

Get rid of tempting foods. You might have bought those cookies for your kids, but if they're going to cause a problem for you during a weak moment, they have to go. (They're no good for your kids anyway!) But that doesn't have to mean leav-ing the larder bare; it just means that it's time to restock with the good stuff.

Start by preparing a grocery list for the week. (We've included a sample pantry list on pages 255–257.) Review the food you'll be eating in the first week, and look at weekly grocery flyers for any fish specials. Make any minor substitutions for foods that you know you won't consume, figure out how many people you are feeding for the week, and then scale the grocery list to your needs.

People who have lost weight and kept it off all say the same thing: The key is in the preparation. When do you make poor choices? I make them when I'm starving, or when I'm already 15 minutes late, or when the demands of others are taking precedence over what's best for my body and my inflammatory profile. On page 258 I've provided some plan-ahead tips that will simplify your prep work. Use them: Spending a little extra time up front will speed your journey toward better health.

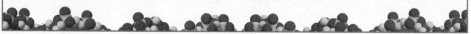

The following categories of fish will help you maximize your fatty acid intake. But because the Adaptive Response and Preconditioning Phases of the diet require you to reduce your calories, it is nearly impossible to meet the overall goals of 1,250 to 1,300 milligrams of EPA + DHA per day without using supplements, so these are especially important at first.

By the time you reach the Optimal Maintenance Phase, you should be able to taper off to slightly lower doses of supplements, predominantly by including great fish in your diet.

Similarly, short-chain omega-6s like GLA cannot be found in higher doses in our food supply. Consequently, they must be provided as dietary supplements.

What follows are lists of commonly eaten fish, categorized according to our best data on their fatty acid profiles. You may notice that these lists differ slightly from those shown in my previous book *Inflammation Nation*. The values in that book were obtained from the USDA database, not from actual studies published by my laboratory or others. Most notably, farmed Atlantic salmon has now been included in Category 2.

Much of this information appeared in an article by my laboratory that was published in the *Journal of the American Dietetic Association* in 2008, and I believe this list represents the latest status of the fatty acid content of fish in this country. Using the list will make it easy for you to grocery shop—or to order when you're dining out. Simply choose Category 1 fish whenever possible.

Category 1 Fish Suggestions

These fish contain over 500 milligrams of long-chain omega-3s per 3.5-ounce serving, and a very favorable ratio of long-chain omega-6 to omega-3 fatty acids.

Please note: These are likely not all the Category 1 fish that nature provides; they are simply the ones that my laboratory has directly analyzed to ensure their content.

Mackerel	Canned wild Alaskan salmon
Coho salmon	Canned sardines
Sockeye salmon	Canned gourmet salmon,
Copper River salmon	prime fillet
Trout	Canned skinless pink salmon
Canned albacore tuna	

Category 2 Fish Suggestions

These fish contain between 150 and 500 milligrams of long-chain omega-3s per 3.5-ounce serving and a favorable ratio of long-chain omega-6 to omega-3 fatty acids.

Haddock	Perch
Cod	Black bass
Hake	Swordfish
Halibut	Oysters
Shrimp	Alaskan king crab
Sole	Farmed Atlantic salmon
Flounder	

Category 3 Fish

These fish are a good low-calorie protein source, but contain little (< 150 milligrams) of the beneficial long-chain omega-3s.

Mahi-mahi

Skate

Bluefin tuna

Monkfish

Red snapper

Wahoo

Grouper

Corvina

Tuna

Category 4 Fish

These contain little or no long-chain omega-3s and detrimental long-chain omega-6 to omega-3 ratios. These fish are not recommended if you have an inflammatory disorder.

Tilapia

Farmed catfish

WHOLE FOOD OR A PILL?

With the exception of the omegas, the bioactives we are looking at most closely exist in nature and in whole foods, and are best consumed that way for a variety of reasons.

The pith of an orange contains the best source of flavonoids in the orange. When we remove the pith to make juice, we deny ourselves some of those benefits. Could we add it back in? Probably. But in order for those polyphenols in the pith to be made available to our bodies, we need to have healthy microflora flourishing in our gut. That is something that can only happen when fiber is consumed—something that will happen naturally if you eat an orange.

You might be able to get all the best nutrients from a pill or supplemental beverage or other delivery device, and certainly the manufacturers of these products would have you believe that's true. In reality, eating whole foods is the best and most satisfying way to get all this into our systems.

That said, I know we live in the real world. I work long hours, and I travel a great deal, and sometimes I fall a little short. Additionally, many of the bioactives eaten by our hunter-gatherer ancestors are no longer in the modern food supply. For example, it is difficult to get enough long-chain omega-3s, especially when you're watching calories—unless you eat fish at every meal. There are populations that do this as a matter of course, but unless you're Inuit, you'll probably want to add supplements containing fish oil to your diet. Short-chain omega-6s like gamma-linolenic acid (GLA) are no longer present in large amounts in our food supply. Consequently, GLA must be obtained from a supplement of borage oil.

While the Gene Smart diet focuses on whole foods, supplements are recommended when it is not practically possible to fulfill our bioactive criteria with whole foods.

Taking Supplements

Several studies have analyzed the contents of fish oil supplements. The good news is that they contain few calories (about 9 calories per capsule), low amounts of arachidonic acid (about 5 to 15 milligrams per gram of oil), and almost no mercury.

The bad news is that many fish oil supplements don't contain as much EPA and DHA as advertised. In one study published in the *Journal of Food Science*, researchers analyzed 20 different fish oil supplements. They found that the EPA concentration was typically 50 to 75 percent lower than stated on the label. Only one product had a concentration above 100 percent.

The researchers also found that the EPA content per gram of oil had an extremely wide range: from 62 to 256 milligrams.

Another study found that the EPA concentration in fish oil supplements was 20 to 30 percent lower than stated on the label. While this is somewhat more favorable, it still underscores the need to improve the quality of dietary supplements on the market in this country.

My recommendation is to buy fish oil supplements that contain an EPA concentration between 150 and 450 milligrams per capsule (typically 1,000- or 1,200-milligram capsules). This relatively high concentration will minimize the number of gel capsules you need to take each day.

As mentioned above, the certainty of ingredients can be an issue with any dietary supplement. For more on selecting the right supplement, go to www.genesmart.com.

GLA

GLA is the only dietary supplement that is an essential component of the Gene Smart Diet. When I say essential here, I mean that it can't be gotten from foods. Studies from several labs, including my own, suggest that when GLA is taken with EPA from fish or fish oil, it maximizes the program's anti-inflammatory benefits. Because GLA has largely been eliminated from our food supply, the only way to get it is from dietary supplements containing either borage-seed oil or evening primrose oil. The Gene Smart Diet recommends at least 450 to 550 milligrams of GLA a day from supplements. (Unfortunately, compared to fish oil supplements, there isn't a great deal of research on the content of borage-seed oil or evening primrose oil, so it's more difficult to know exactly how much active GLA is in these supplements.)

Borage-seed oil is the richest source of GLA, with concentrations ranging from 20 to 26 percent. For evening primrose oil, the typical GLA concentration is 9 percent.

When choosing a borage-seed oil supplement, it's best to pick one that contains 200 to 300 milligrams of GLA per gram of oil.

Borage-seed oil hasn't been studied as extensively as evening primrose oil.

How to Take Oil-Based Supplements

It's very important to always take fish oil or GLA supplements with your meals. If you take your supplements between meals, they won't be properly digested and you won't reap their anti-inflammatory benefits.

When you eat food and are digesting fat, it stimulates your pancreas to release bile salts, which are needed to emulsify the fatty acids in dietary supplements so they can get into your bloodstream. In short, it enhances the supplements' bioavailability.

As the popularity of omega-3 fatty acids has increased, many manufacturers are now adding low concentrations of them to breads, health bars, and other food products. Such manufacturers are obviously hoping to appeal to people who dislike the taste of fish and fish oil.

We don't yet know how well the fatty acids in these foods are absorbed. What we do know, however, is that the omega-3 is often alpha-linolenic acid from flax seed, which is very inefficiently converted to long-chain omega-3s in humans (see pages 162–163 for more about this). Further, the concentrations are almost always too low to have a therapeutic effect.

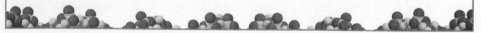

Although borage seeds contain a small amount of liver toxins called pyrrolizidine alkaloids, tests have shown that these toxins are not present in borage-seed oil. Minor side effects from borage-seed oil may include bloating, nausea, indigestion, and headache.

Case reports suggest that evening primrose oil can increase the risk of seizure in some people, so it should not be taken if you have a history of seizure disorder. Evening primrose oil also may increase the risk of seizure if you take medications for the treatment of mental illness such as chlorpromazine (Thorazine), thioridazine (Mellaril), trifluoperazine (Stelazaine), or fluphenazine (Prolixin). Minor side effects associated with evening primrose oil may include headache, abdominal pain, nausea, and loose stools.

I'd like to emphasize that you should *never* take GLA supplements unless you also get sufficient amounts of EPA, either from fish or fish oil supplements. Clinical trials in my laboratory show that borage-seed oil taken alone causes a marked increase in blood levels of AA. This effect is greatly reduced when GLA is taken in combination with EPA.

As with fish oil supplements, I strongly recommend that GLA supplementation be supervised by a physician.

POLYPHENOL RECOMMENDATIONS

The polyphenols are amongst our most powerful bioactives. Luckily for us, their delivery systems—chocolate, red wine, and the delicious fruits of the season—are easy pills to swallow!

Dark Chocolate

Yes, that's right—chocolate is an essential part of Gene Smart.

But not all chocolate is equal. Milk chocolate consists of about 33 to 45 percent cacao, the seed from which chocolate is made. Mid-dark chocolates (often with other sweet additives like toffee, nuts, or fruit) are in the 45 to 60 percent range. Bars labeled "dark chocolate" are often 60 to 80 percent cacao, with baking chocolate at the far end of the spectrum. How will you know what percentage you're getting? Unlike milk chocolate, dark chocolate often specifies the cacao content on the label. Certainly, you'll be able to find bars that do at gourmet groceries and health food stores.

A general rule of thumb? The darker the chocolate, the higher the poly-phenols. Furthermore, the most convincing studies showing the lipid (i.e., total cholesterol and LDL) lowering effects of chocolate have been carried out using dark chocolate. So I'd like you to stick with chocolate that is over 60 percent cacao, preferably one in the 70 percent area.

The recommendations you'll find in Gene Smart are based on the current science. The idea is to eat enough dark chocolate to see a positive effect, with-out going overboard and exceeding your caloric load or saturated fat limits. As it turns out, that's less tricky than it seems. As you know, chocolate bars and cocoa do contain fat. However, the amount of fat in a dark chocolate candy bar is small, and well worth it, considering that the polyphenol profile has been shown to lower blood lipids and blood pressure, decrease platelet and plaque formation, increase arterial vasodilation (which in turn reduces blood pressure), and decrease other body inflammatory responses.

Unfortunately, there are no definitive studies that set an optimal amount for dark chocolate consumption. So, for the optimal maintenance phase of the Gene Smart Diet, we recommend that you try to fit in up to 3.5 ounces per day, with 1.5 ounces per day minimum, especially if you are hypertensive. Research has shown a beneficial effect on hypertension among people who consume dark chocolate every day. Studies vary widely in the amount of chocolate—and even those that do reveal how much dark chocolate was consumed don't tell us what percentage of that chocolate was cacao. A significant reduction in sys-tolic and diastolic blood pressure has been seen with daily consumption of a 1.5- to 3.5-ounce portion of dark chocolate over about 2 weeks.

To help gradually increase your cacao intake, you might try bars that con-tain other ingredients. Choose those that have high polyphenolic additives—ingredients like currants, raspberries, orange peel, blueberries, and cranberries—as opposed to ones made with flaked coconut, toffee, or "fruit flavoring." Bars with nuts like almonds and walnuts will be better for you, because of the healthy fats they contain, but they will also be higher in calo-ries, so that's something you're going to want to keep an eye on. Bear in mind that fillers like these take away from the amount of dark chocolate you actu-ally consume.

One caveat: Chocolate consumption has been reported to interfere with nonheme iron absorption. If you take an iron supplement in the form of a pill, or rely on getting iron from iron-rich plant foods like spinach salad, wait at least 2 hours after consuming your chocolate to take the supplement or eat that salad. You might want to consider getting your chocolate first thing in the morning, while taking your iron supplement at lunch or later in the day.

Red Wine

The rich tradition of drinking wine with meals dates back as far as written history, and it is a pleasure shared across a great many cultures. It's not hard to see why: For those of us who enjoy it, a glass of wine enhances not only the flavors of food, but the mood as well, creating a very pleasant dinner environment. Ironically, though, wine—at least from a nutritional perspective—has been one of the least researched aspects of our dinner fare. When you consider the long history of wine consumption, it's odd that we're only just now tapping into its capacity to deliver health-giving polyphenols.

Still, at this point, we don't know much with regard to the polyphenols that are most potent in regulating gene expression or the specific polyphenol content of each wine. Bioactive content—especially trans-resveratrol and the anthocyanins—is influenced by any number of factors, including vintage, weather, sunlight, ripening, and processing, all of which are variable to some degree in the making of the wine.

Choose a wine. Most of the available studies have looked at the difference between white wines and red or rosé wines. In these studies, red wines are the clear winners, meaning that they typically have 10 to 100 times more of the critical polyphenols (trans-resveratrol and the anthocyanins) than rosés or white wines.

The few studies completed to date that quantify the polyphenol content of the different grape varietals within the larger category of "red wine" have concluded that pinot noirs offer the higher polyphenol levels, closely followed by egiodola, the syrahs, the cabernet sauvignons, and then the merlots.

French wine also appears to have a bit more of a phenolic effect than the California varietals. This may be due to the fact that the French red wines tested were very likely aged in wood barrels and made with yeast-derived phenolics, while the California types were fermented in stainless steel. That said, as a consumer of many delicious California wines, I don't find the current data compelling enough to switch to either one exclusively.

Don't be intimidated! Experts speculate that one reason Americans drink less wine than Europeans do is the intimidation factor. European children grow up seeing their parents drink wine at dinner, and are often encouraged to sniff—if not taste—the wine for themselves. By the time they're old enough to drink it with dinner, they know what they like and don't like.

Selecting a wine can be daunting, and for people on a budget, the idea of spending money on a bottle of wine that may or may not be good on your palate is a risk. There are some things you can do to make this process a little more pleasant for yourself.

The first is to get recommendations! Ask friends what they like, find a small, knowledgeable wine store with a helpful staff, or go to wine tastings (bring a designated driver to the event). You may also want to learn some basic wine vocabulary—old world versus new world, fruity versus earthy, light versus heavy, sweet versus dry—so you can be specific about what you enjoy (or not) about the wines you're trying. If you find something you like, write it down lest you forget it next time you are at the store. If you really like it, buy a case of it. Many stores offer a "case price discount."

Lastly, learn some wonderful toasts, and share what you've learned with friends, as the sharing of a fine wine is like the sharing of a happy life.

Salud!

Gene Smart recommendations: The Gene Smart Diet recommends a

Proceed with Caution!

There is, of course, ethanol in wine, which can lead to inebriation; as with everything else, moderation is key.

It's worth noting here that polyphenols are always secondary in importance to a person's ability to responsibly handle the alcoholic beverages they consume. I have personally lost family members to alcoholism and know firsthand its potential devastation. If you have a physical, emotional, or religious reason for abstaining from alcohol, then please disregard the recommendation to consume red wine.

As I have mentioned before, if you're not able to consume wine, there are several nonalcoholic juices high in trans-resveratrol and anthocyanin at specialty-food stores, as well as a number of high-purity trans-resveratrol supplements.

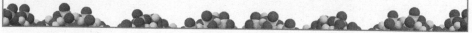

3- to 6-ounce glass of red wine 3 to 6 times a week. That's a glass with dinner, a few times a week.

How much you initially include in your diet depends on how many extra calories you can handle, and whether or not consuming alcohol encourages your appetite. Sometimes having a glass of wine, especially prior to dinner, can inhibit your ability to self-regulate your food intake. If that's the case, you may want to pre-proportion your dinner, or enjoy your glass of wine later, "after the kitchen has closed."

Tea

Brewed tea has long been known to decrease risks associated with certain cancers (including lung, stomach, esophageal, colon, and bladder), coronary heart disease, and stroke. Tea is rich with flavonoids that are not destroyed by the brewing process or in the presence of acid (as with the addition of lemon juice.) The reason that tea is thought to be so high in these beneficial polyphenols is because they are found in the plants, in the leaves and stems, and they are stimulated by sunlight. Catechins are the main class of flavonoids in tea and constitute about 25 percent of the dry weight of fresh tea leaf, although total catechin content varies widely depending on type of tea, growing location, light variation, and altitude.

The exception to these beneficial effects of tea, according to current research, is that they are limited to brewed teas and not reconstituted or bottled tea beverages. Some companies are adding back antioxidants as supplements to their bottled tea beverages; my advice is to save money by drinking the brewed kind.

Teas with the highest catechin content are the green teas, which are closely followed by the black teas, with oolong, Earl Grey, Ceylon, and Darjeeling leading the pack. (Technically, oolong is a third category of tea, but from a polyphenolic perspective, it goes with the black teas.) There is not much information about white teas at this time, but considering what we know about the development of polyphenols and the fact that white tea is really "baby" tea and has not spent as much time in the sun as its more mature black and green cousins, it may lack some of their beneficial polyphenols. Don't avoid white tea if you enjoy it; it's still a better beverage than any soda on the market. But try to develop a taste for the green or black teas.

You can boost your polyphenol intake and variety for the day by brewing standard tea and then adding in 2 ounces of fruit juice—fresh if you can find it, bottled if you can't. Some of the best include any of the following, alone or in blended combinations: pomegranate, cranberry, blueberry, cherry, orange, unsweetened apple, cider, or Concord grape. Congratulations—you've just added resveratrol, anthocyanins, and ellagic acid! Juice is caloric, so don't forget to figure it into your daily calculations. You can also dilute the brewed tea to weaken the flavor—1 cup of tea in 2 cups of water, for example.

What about caffeine? Not surprisingly, recent studies suggest that certain genetic differences determine how different people react to caffeine. That's why one person gets the shakes from the vestigial amount left in decaffeinated coffee, while someone else can swig back a whole pot of "the hard stuff" without so much as a jitter.

In general, I believe that caffeine has gotten a bad rap. It is a diuretic, but most people can readily adapt to a typical caffeine load; it's only when someone consumes caffeine in an amount greater than they can metabolize that the diuretic effect really kicks in. So if you normally drink two to three caffeinated drinks per day and then decide you really need some extra, you may find yourself taking a few more trips to the restroom.

The good news for the caffeine-sensitive is that decaf teas also contain protective levels of catechins. Tea can be decaffeinated by two different processes. If the label on your tea doesn't specify which method is used, you can be fairly sure that it was done using chemicals and not water distillation. Choose water-distilled teas if you can.

Some of the herbal teas are high in polyphenols, but there are brand-specific data and there is a huge variability in herbal tea blends, so I won't make any recommendations regarding these.

Gene Smart recommendations: I suggest drinking at least 2 to 3 cups of tea per day, or more if you can do so without exceeding your fluid needs or caffeine thresholds. The right amount for you depends on your size, your activity level, and the temperature/humidity of the environment you live in. For most people, this recommendation means not drinking in excess of 3 or 4 cups of caffeinated tea per day, and before switching over to decaffeinated tea, and not consuming more than 8 to 12 cups over the course of a day.

A Note about Coffee

The coffee bean does not have a high polyphenol content compared to, say, green tea. That being said, coffee is often the number-one source of polyphenols for Americans, simply because we drink so much of it. Coffee provides the average American with almost 1,300 milligrams of polyphenols daily.

From the available science, I'm not sure a strong argument can be made that coffee has the types of polyphenols that are bioactives, so please don't substitute coffee for your fruits and vegetables. On the other hand, there is no reason not to enjoy your morning cup of brew when you're doing Gene Smart. Do try not to doctor it up with excess fat and sugar calories if possible, although you may want to take advantage of the fact that having your chocolate and coffee together can be a delicious way to get your Gene Smart chocolate portion in. Use cocoa powder, the artificial sweetener of your choice (if you choose to sweeten), and—if you wish—some skim milk in your coffee.

Fruits and Vegetables

I have divided fruits and vegetables into two categories: those high and low in polyphenol. Based on the data to date—which, bear in mind, are not extensive at this point in time—I believe the best evidence for bioactives and their particular effects on gene expression favors fruits and vegetables that are rich in anthocyanins, trans-resveratrol, catechins, and ellagitannins. Consequently, high-polyphenol fruits and vegetables are ones that have been shown to contain high levels of those phytonutrients.

Another caution: Despite the distinction I've made, *all* fruits and vegetables are recommended as part of a healthy diet, and *all* of them contain some of the thousands of known polyphenols. A "low" vegetable is better than a slice of white bread any day.

But you'll want to get the most polyphenolic bang for your buck. Fruits and vegetables aren't widgets; their polyphenol concentration levels are widely variable.

Here's why: Polyphenols are found in the leaves and stems of plants. They are stimulated to develop when a plant is exposed to sunlight as well as when it's under stress (the adaptive stress response). Different concentrations of polyphenols can be found in different fruits of the same tree, depending on each fruit's exposure to the sun throughout the growing season. That's why I choose frozen fruits in winter—they were picked at the peak of ripeness, as opposed to the "fresh" fruits at the grocery store, with their heavily stamped passports.

These certainly are not the only variables: Fruits and vegetables can vary in their polyphenol content depending on several other factors, such as the amount of rainfall. Even size matters: Since most polyphenols are concentrated in the skin, leaves, and stems, a small cherry tomato has a higher concentration of polyphenols than a large tomato because it has a higher skin-to-interior plant ratio. Curly kale will have more polyphenol content than a flat-leaf lettuce like romaine.

Another factor that determines polyphenol content is the degree of ripeness at picking, storing, and processing of the produce.

Here are some things that you can do to ensure that the fruits and vegetables you're eating are really delivering what your body needs:

Leave the skins on! Peeling produce can diminish its polyphenol content. That vibrant purple or red color that you often see in fruit and vegetable skins indicates the presence of one of the three bioactive polyphenol families we're targeting: anthocyanins, trans-resveratrol, and ellagitannins.

Cook carefully. Cooking methods can also affect the polyphenol content of produce. The worst cooking methods, the ones that leach out the most bioactives, include boiling and microwaving. The best cooking techniques to preserve these nutrients are flash stir-frying and steaming.

Ideally, I'd suggest that you serve and eat produce in as minimally processed a manner as possible. Gene Smart isn't a raw-food diet; in fact, many foods, especially some vegetables, are more digestible in cooked forms than they are raw. But there's a difference between something that's cooked and something that's been obliterated. Overprocessing destroys most of the beneficial polyphenols. The grinding processes used to make "breaded veggie sticks" or processed cold cereals can also destroy these natural components, but they are usually added back in by enrichment or fortification. The making of juices and jellies can also destroy polyphenol content.

Choose local and organic when possible. Eating as seasonally, locally, organically, and sustainably as possible is very important. When possible, eat foods that are ripe, and were ripened on the tree. They've gotten more sun exposure, and more polyphenols have developed as a result.

Fruits and vegetables grown according to organic standards have long been known to be better for the earth, and there's now evidence that they're better for you. Not for the obvious reasons; in fact, there's very little to suggest that synthetic pesticides are harmful to humans. But fruits and vegetables grown organically develop more polyphenols as natural pesticides (again—that's our old friend, the adaptive stress response at work) than those grown using chemical pesticides.

Produce is also more nutritious if it is harvested locally, where it can often be allowed to ripen on the vine. This also increases polyphenol content via sunlight exposure—as opposed to being boxed unripe and shipped for days.

Look for heirlooms. If you visit your farmers' market regularly, you may have noticed some unusual-looking vegetables there: odd-looking (and sometimes quite ugly!) tomatoes in an incredible variety of colors, sizes, and shapes, with fanciful names like Brandywine, Jubilee, German Johnson, and Mortgage Lifter, and melon and eggplant varieties you've never seen before.

These are heirloom vegetables. You know how there are a variety of types of squashes, so that a recipe might call for butternut, acorn, or spaghetti squash? Well, imagine a world in which there were *thousands* of different varieties of squash—and of other fruits and vegetables as well. You actually don't have to imagine it: That's the way it was, before the widespread adaptation of industrial agriculture. To give another example, most of us are familiar with five or six different types of apples, but our ancestors would have had many, many more.

Heirloom plants, which have been rapidly increasing in popularity across the United States and Europe, are grown from saved seeds. There is reason to believe that these fruits and vegetables are considerably richer in polyphenols. They are varieties that are more susceptible to stress and disease. They disappeared largely because farmers could grow more resistant varieties, with the assurance that they would be able to survive almost any season. However, as we know from Chapter 15, stressing plants markedly increases the content of key bioactives such as trans-resveratrol, because these are natural protectants for the plants.

Heirloom fruits are less resistant to disease and not as "pretty," which is one of the reasons farmers have not brought them back in a widespread way. I believe that is about to change. My former house was on a small farm, and I grafted and grew about 30 heirloom varieties of apples as a hobby. They were hard to keep healthy but once you had one of those apples, there was nothing on this planet that tasted better.

To take the risk, the farmer has to be properly rewarded. But with more people wanting fruits and vegetables that taste like something—not to mention our growing awareness of how much better these heirloom varieties are for our health—I believe that we have reached that balance point. I believe that the growth of heirloom fruits and vegetables will be explosive in the next decade—or at least I *hope* so.

Gene Smart recommendation: Because there are so many different chemicals in this category—the isoflavones in soy products, resveratrol in red wine, hydroxybenzoic acids in tea, and anthocyanins in fruits and vegetables, just to name a few—it's difficult to know with any precision what intake is optimal. In all phases of the diet, it would be wise to consume more of the higher-content polyphenolic fruits, vegetables, nuts, and seeds.

Below, I have listed foods likely to be beneficial based on their polyphenol content.

High-Polyphenol Fruits

Apple cider and juice
Apples, green (with skin)
Apples, red (with skin)
Apples without skin, apple
    butter, or applesauce
Apricots
Blackberries
Blood oranges
Blueberries
Cherries, sweet or sour
Chokeberries
Cranberries
Currants, black or red
Dates
Elderberries
Gooseberries
Grapes, red or purple
Kiwifruit
Lemons

Limes
Lingonberries
Mangoes
Marionberries
Nectarines
Oranges: navel, tangelos,
    tangerines, etc. (the white
    pithy stuff is flavonoid-rich)
Peaches
Pears
Plums and prunes (dried plums)
Pomegranates
Quinces
Raisins
Raspberries
Rhubarb
Strawberries

High-Polyphenol Vegetables

Artichokes

Broccoli

Cabbage, red

Celery (particularly the hearts)

Corn

Eggplant (aubergine)

Fennel

Garlic

Greens (like kale and turnip)

Kohlrabi

Leeks

Lovage

Onions, red and yellow

Parsnips

Peppers, small, spicy

Pumpkins

Rutabagas

Scallions

Shallots

Spinach, raw

Sweet potatoes

Tomatoes, cherry or grape

Watercress

Legumes, Nuts, and Seeds

Almonds

Cashews

Chickpeas

Dried beans—black beans,
red kidney beans, pinto beans,
black-eyed peas

Fava beans

Flax seeds

Hazelnuts

Lentils

Nut butters

Peanuts

Peas, English

Peas, green

Pecans

Pistachios

Pumpkin seeds

Snap beans

Sunflower seeds

Walnuts

Dark Chocolate

> 60 percent cacao dark chocolate

Red Wine

Pinot noir, cabernet, merlot

Tea

Brewed green tea, black tea,
oolong tea, green decaf tea, or
black decaf tea served hot or
cold and flavored with lemon,
if desirable

Herbs, Spices, and Seasonings

Basil

Capers, red or green

Chives

Cinnamon

Curry

Dill weed

Horseradish

Ketchup

Oregano

Parsley

Rosemary

Sage

Tarragon

Thyme

Vinegar

Low-Polyphenol Fruits

Avocados

Bananas

Figs

Fruit jellies and jams

Grapefruits

Pineapple

Processed juices and juice drinks

Low-Polyphenol Vegetables

Bell peppers, green or red

Bok choy

Brussels sprouts

Cabbage

Carrots

Cauliflower

Cucumbers

Endive

Mushrooms

Potatoes, white

Pumpkin

Spinach, cooked

Squash, yellow

Tomatoes, canned

Tomatoes, large fresh

Zucchini

THE GENE SMART EXERCISE PLAN

We've known that exercise is good for us since the dawn of time—definitively and scientifically, since the 1940s. Then how come most Americans spend their weekends doing everything *but* getting enough exercise?

Seven out of ten American adults don't exercise regularly despite the overwhelming evidence of health benefits. Clearly, we have to reverse this trend.

I think that one of the reasons we've been so loath to do it is that we don't see the return we're led to expect. As we saw in Chapter 12, exercise isn't the magic weight-loss bullet all those gym ads would have you believe. I've found that unhitching exercise from weight-maintenance or weight-loss goals has been very freeing. Personally, I find it much more motivating to know that I'm working out to combat inflammation and a variety of other maladies than to lose weight—especially because I know I'm having an astronomical impact on my inflammatory profile, if only a so-so impact on my waistline.

Exercise Guidelines

So you don't forget how incredibly important exercise is to your new lifestyle, you will see reminders of the recommended exercise routine on each day of the diet in Chapter 19.

In the first phase of the diet (Adaptive Response), you will begin with 2 days of light circuit training, 3 days of light-to-moderate exercise, and 2 days of rest per week. We will work from that baseline. The chart below shows you your progression through the Adaptive Response and Preconditioning Phases.

OVERVIEW OF EXERCISE PLAN

WEEK	SAT	SUN	MON	TUES	WED	THUR	FRI
1	Light Exercise 30 min.	Light Circuit 15/20/15	Moderate Exercise 30 min.	Rest	Moderate Exercise 30 min.	Light Circuit 15/20/15	Rest
2	Light Exercise 30 min.	Light Circuit 15/20/15	Moderate Exercise 30 min.	Rest	Moderate Exercise 30 min.	Light Circuit 15/20/15	Rest
3	Light Exercise 30 min.	Moderate Circuit 15/35/15	Moderate Exercise 30 min.	Rest	Vigorous Exercise 15 min.	Light Circuit 15/20/15	Rest
4	Light Exercise 30 min.	Moderate Circuit 15/35/15	Moderate Exercise 30 min.	Rest	Vigorous Exercise 15 min.	Moderate Circuit 15/30/15	Rest
5	Light Exercise 30 min.	Vigorous Circuit 15/45/15	Moderate Exercise 30 min.	Rest	Vigorous Exercise 20 min.	Moderate Circuit 15/30/15	Rest
6 and beyond	Moderate Exercise 30 min.	Vigorous Circuit 15/45/15	Moderate Exercise 30 min.	Rest	Vigorous Exercise 20-30 min.	Vigorous Circuit 15/45/15	Rest

If you are one of the 70 percent of Americans who does not exercise regularly, the Adaptive Response Phase will introduce you to exercise and then gradually move you into an exercise regimen that will "get you into shape" over a 3-week period. According to research, that's all it takes to begin to see some impressive changes, both in your body and in your inflammatory profile!

The Preconditioning Phase will then increase the amount you exercise slightly, over a 2-week period. We will then move you to the Optimal Maintenance Phase. By that point you'll know everything you need to know in order to exercise healthily—and for the maximum adaptive stress benefit—for the rest of your life.

If you're just beginning an exercise program, or haven't been anywhere near a gym for a few years, this is going to require not only willpower, but intelligence. Too much too soon is a good way to sideline yourself with an injury. Start doing something and push yourself to do more—gently! If what we suggest initially is too difficult, please back it down in terms of minutes and level of activity. This balance is critical.

It's traditional at this point to suggest that you see a doctor before starting a fitness regimen. If you're healthy and have no chronic diseases, you

What You'll Need for Your Gene Smart Workouts

Don't tell the athletic gear companies, but you really don't need too many accessories to get a good workout. You'll need some way to get your heart rate up—whether that's the elliptical machine at the gym or the hill outside your door (both work equally well)—and you'll need some hand weights. The type of mat used for yoga and Pilates can also be helpful if you like a little padding when you stretch. An exercise ball and exercise bands are helpful as well.

If you prefer to work out at home, I suggest that you keep your eye out for yard sales and ads on Craigslist (www.craigslist.org), where home workout equipment (often barely used!) is often available at bargain-basement prices. And while a fancy outfit isn't necessary, I do strongly recommend that you invest in good-quality, properly fitted sneakers.

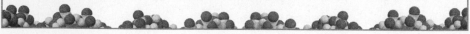

may not need to. However, if you want to engage in vigorous exercise and you are a male over age 45, with two or more cardiac risk factors (e.g., you have high cholesterol, high blood pressure, or diabetes; you're a smoker; or one of your immediate relatives died from heart disease), then you should absolutely talk to your physician first. She will most likely want to do some stress-testing prior to signing off. And I would suggest caution in general; if there's anything in your medical or family history that makes you think you should visit your physician prior to starting a fitness plan, schedule that appointment today.

Aerobic Activity

Many of my recommendations specify "moderate" or "vigorous" aerobic activity. But what does that really mean?

The beauty of Gene Smart is that it's tailored for you, and it's designed to be the kind of program that you can integrate fully and successfully into your life—not something you have to quit your job to do.

Below you will find some acceptable forms of both types of exercise, along with the number of calories you can expect to burn doing them, depending on how much you weigh.

MODERATE EXERCISE (30 MIN)	130 LBS (KCAL)	180 LBS (KCAL)	230 LBS (KCAL)
Walking, 3.0 mph	103	142	182
Cleaning, vigorous	133	184	235
Mowing lawn (push mower)	163	225	288
Bicycling, 10-11.9mph	177	245	313
Ballroom dancing, fast	163	225	288
Golf, pulling clubs	147	203	260
Swimming, leisurely	177	245	313
Aerobics, low impact	147	203	260
Calisthenics, light (beginning yoga)	133	184	235
Racquetball, casual	207	287	366

VIGOROUS EXERCISE (30 MIN)	130 LBS (KCAL)	180 LBS (KCAL)	230 LBS (KCAL)
Jogging	207	287	366
Running, 12-min. mile	235	326	416
Hiking, rigorous	177	245	313
Shoveling snow	177	245	313
Basketball	235	326	416
Tennis, singles	235	326	416
Skiing, cross country	265	367	470
Aerobics, high impact	207	287	366
Bicycling, 12-13.9 mph	235	326	416
Calisthenics, vigorous (push-ups)	235	326	416

You'll notice that the calorie values are for 30 minutes, as the program does not recommend that you do any of these activities (aside from the circuit routines) for more than a half-hour at a shot. Why? The latest data reveal that it is not the *amount* of time you exercise that is critical, but the *level of intensity* at which you work.

The best gauge of intensity is something called target heart rate. The American Heart Association recommends that you should aim within 50 to 85 percent of your maximum heart rate. The following chart shows estimated target heart rates for different ages.

Note: A few high blood pressure medications lower the maximum heart rate and thus the target zone rate. If you're taking such medicine, call your physician to find out if you need to use a lower target heart rate.

How Should I Pace Myself?

When starting an exercise program, aim for the lower end of your target heart rate zone (50 percent) during the first few weeks. Gradually build up to the higher end of your target zone (75 percent). When I say "moderate" on the exercise charts above, this means working at between 60 and 75 percent. When I say "vigorous," this means working between 75 and 85 percent. Again, you won't start at that level, but you will work up to it.

AGE (YEARS)	TARGET HR ZONE 50–85 PERCENT (BEATS PER MINUTE)	AVERAGE MAXIMUM HR 100 PERCENT (BEATS PER MINUTE)
20	100–170	200
25	98–166	195
30	95–162	190
35	93–157	185
40	90–153	180
45	88–149	175
50	85–145	170
55	83–140	165
60	80–136	160
65	78–132	155
70	75–128	150

Circuit with Strength Training

Strength training is defined in this book as working 8 to 10 muscle groups using weights heavy enough to result in substantial fatigue within 8 to 12 repetitions. Again, how heavy those weights are will depend on you and how strong you are—and you should expect to see that change as you make your way through the program.

Recovery is when your muscles rebuild, so I recommend that you leave a day or two of rest in between strength-lifting sessions, so that muscles can recover before the next bout. I personally train almost every day, but focus on different muscle groups: If I do back, biceps, and quads on Monday, I'll do chest, triceps, and hamstrings on Tuesday.

It is recommended that people doing strength training move to a heavier weight once they're able to easily perform 10 to 12 reps at their current weight. This is a rule you shouldn't ignore. If it feels too easy, it is too easy. And don't get hung up on the numbers! If you can easily do a set with 10 pounds, then it's time to move up to 12, or you'll stop seeing the benefits. I've seen far too many people who don't push themselves to lift or move a weight because they perceive that it is too heavy. You don't have to start

Help! It Hurts!

Exercise is, to my mind, the best possible illustration of an adaptive stress response. No matter what level of activity you have been doing, you will immediately begin to enter an adaptive response phase as soon as you start to increase your activity. If you've been inactive for quite some time, you'll definitely feel "different"; just don't expect to feel better right away! Moving and strengthening muscles might create some new aches and pains, and these may not go away for a bit as your body "adapts" to its more active lifestyle.

I personally like the feeling of a little warmth and stiffness in my muscles, and I know I'm not alone in this, as weird as it might sound. Because I know how good exercise is for me and my inflammatory profile, a little tightness acts almost like a positive biofeedback throughout the day: "You did good this morning, Ski!" At any rate, you can take solace in knowing that the stiffness you feel means you're doing it right!

And it won't last forever. The length of this exercise-based Adaptive Response Phase may feel like it is extending beyond the initial 3 weeks, well into your Preconditioning Phase. By the same token, your Preconditioning Phase may feel like it is going on longer than the 2 weeks allotted to it. Don't worry! It's all relative to the level of intensity you are trying to perform. Listen to your body. Don't get caught up in the numbers or even my program; find the balance between overdoing it and giving up.

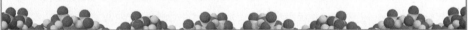

powerlifting—in fact, it's safest to increase the amount of weight you lift in low increments—but don't stagnate.

If you have never lifted weights before, I would recommend that you find a professional at your fitness center or take a class from a certified trainer in order to learn how to do the exercises properly and to create a plan for your particular needs and goals. You can also get references from friends and physicians.

One more note, especially for women: Contrary to a still prevalent myth, weightlifting will not bulk you up, especially when doing large numbers of reps. Trust me, it's not that easy! There is, hands down, nothing better for increasing your metabolic rate, or for helping it to stay up. In my opinion, strength-training is an essential part of a successful anti-inflammation plan.

Here is a complete, full-body, circuit weight-training session, perfectly customizable to you, according to the amount of weight you can comfortably handle.

Chest—Bench Press: Start on your back on a flat bench or floor. Hold weights straight up over your chest with hands a few inches wider than shoulders and your elbows soft. Inhale as you lower the weights down to your chest, exhale as you press them back up to the starting position. Do not arch your back and make sure your feet are flat on the floor at all times.

Shoulders—Lateral Raise: Stand with feet hip-width apart and hold weights at your sides. Keeping elbows slightly bent, inhale as you lift your arms straight up to the sides, stopping at shoulder level, and exhale while lowering the weights back down to starting position. Keep elbows bent, and do not go above your shoulder level.

Back—Rowing: Stand in wide stance, holding the weights at your sides. Bend knees and tilt torso (back straight/abs in) forward about 45 degrees, straightening the arms so the weights are at the sides of your knees. Exhale as the weights are pulled upward, bending elbows and squeezing back to bring weights toward your waist; inhale as you slowly lower weights to starting position.

Biceps—Hammer Curls: Stand or sit while holding weights at sides with palms facing up or at sides. Exhale while bending the elbows and raising the weights toward the shoulder in a bicep curl, making sure not to move the elbows. Inhale while lowering the weights to starting position. You can also alternate your arms so one is coming up as the other is going down.

Triceps—Kickbacks: Stand with feet shoulder-width apart, holding weights at sides with palms facing in. Bend knees and tilt torso (back straight/abs in) about 45 degrees, keeping your back and head in neutral position. Bend both of your elbows toward the ceiling, and exhale as you straighten arms back behind you, squeezing the back of your arm without moving your elbow. Inhale as you return your arm to the starting position. You can do both together, or alternate your arms.

Glutes, Hamstrings, and Quadriceps—Squats: Stand with feet hip-width apart, abs in, holding weights in hands. Inhale as you bend your knees and hips while keeping your head up and back flat, stopping when knees and hips are at 90 degrees, and your thighs are parallel to the floor. Pretend you are sitting back into a chair (stick your rear end out) and keep your knees *behind* your toes; you should be able to see your toes at all times. Exhale as you straighten your legs and hips, pushing through the heels, and squeeze the butt to lift back to standing position. Arms can be straight down at sides or on shoulders, holding weights.

Glutes, Hamstrings, and Quadriceps—Lunge: Stand with feet in a split stance, right leg in front, left leg in back. Holding weights at sides, inhale as you bend both knees and lower into a lunge, keeping front knee behind the toe and knees no lower than a 90-degree angle. Exhale as you squeeze through the heel to raise back up to starting position. Do a full set of reps, and then switch legs.

Abdominals—Crunches: There are many variations for this exercise; use your favorite, or try this traditional situp.

Start flat on your back with knees bent and both feet flat on the floor; place your hands across your chest, with your fingertips on opposite shoulders. Exhale as you slowly pull your head, neck, shoulders, upper back, and lower back off the floor (in that order). Slowly return to the starting position by placing your lower back, upper back, shoulders, neck, and head back on the floor (in that order). Inhale as you near the starting position.

Circuit Training

Combining aerobic activity with weight training is called circuit training, and it's the best way to get the best of both worlds. I recommend three separate circuit-training programs, outlined in full below.

THE 15/20/15 WORKOUT

Light Circuit Training

Warmup

Start your exercise program with 15 minutes of light aerobic activity such as walking, cycling, or jogging, followed by some light stretching exercises (after the muscles have been warmed up) to gently increase the range of motion before beginning your weightlifting program.

Light Weight Workout

One set of 10 to 12 reps of the weight program found on pages 259–261. (Beginners start with light weights, and rest 2 minutes between each exercise.)

Finish your workout with an additional 15 minutes of light aerobic activity. Stretching after your weight workout is optimal for flexibility and preventing exercise injuries. Vigorous stretching to increase flexibility should be done only after your complete workout when the muscles and joints have been thoroughly warmed up.

Toward the end of the first 3 weeks of this training, begin to increase your weights, shooting for 10 repetitions at 80 percent of your effort—80 percent of the weight that you can accomplish in 10 repetitions.

THE 15/35/15 WORKOUT
Moderate Circuit Training

Once you have moved through 2 weeks (2 times a week) of the light circuit training, I will begin to move you to moderate circuit training. Begin with 15 minutes of light aerobic activity such as walking, cycling, or jogging, followed by some light stretching exercises (after the muscles have been warmed up) to gently increase the range of motion before beginning your weightlifting program. Then you will begin your weight training, using 80 percent of the weight that you can lift for 10 repetitions. Additionally, I want you to increase to 2 sets (10 to 12 reps) for each exercise. You now may rest 1 minute and 30 seconds between each set and 2 to 3 minutes between each exercise.

Finish your workout with an additional 15 minutes of light aerobic activity. Stretching after your weight workout is optimal for flexibility and preventing exercise injuries. Vigorous stretching to increase flexibility should be done only *after* your complete workout when the muscles and joints have been thoroughly warmed up.

How Should I Start?

Assess where you are right now. Keep a 3-day log of all your activity, noting 30-minute blocks (or 10-minute blocks, if you are on the go all the time). Include 2 typical workdays and 1 day "off" in your diary so you can see how your activity changes on nonworkdays. Then add up how much time is spent on moderate activity.

Is it 30 minutes a day or less? If so, then you're going to work up to the workout by walking. Walk as much as you can comfortably, and then work toward increasing this a little bit every day. Start to incorporate other moderate activities into your day, and keep increasing the blocks daily until you come up to the recommended aerobic activity guidelines.

Don't overdo it. It's tempting to be overzealous at the beginning of a plan, when you're high energy and highly motivated, but it can actually be quite destruc-

tive. The more exercise you get in, the better you will start to feel. But if you push yourself too hard too soon, you run the risk of injury or backsliding.

As the gyms that run ads every January know, it's one thing to start an exercise regimen—and another to keep it up.

Need help getting motivated? Here are some tips:

- Get an exercise partner. Make your workouts dependent on each other; one suggestion I've heard is to swap shoes at the end of the workout, so that each of you has to show up the next time. Just make sure it happens!

- Tap into some of the great new exercise plans that can be downloaded to your digital player.

- Join a gym and take a class. Try a yoga, tai chi, or ballroom-dancing

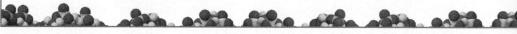

THE 15/45/15 WORKOUT

Vigorous Circuit Training

Now it's time to really have fun!

When we've worked you through the Adaptive Response and Preconditioning Phases of the Gene Smart diet and exercise program, your body and mind will be ready for this workout. Take pride in what you've accomplished—you've earned it! This will be your Optimal Maintenance workout. You will do it twice a week, and you can use it for the rest of your life—or until you want to challenge yourself further with newer and more rigorous activity.

class and see what you like—you won't know until you try.

- Exercise on vacations, or as part of a vacation. I think my family's favorite activity in the world is beach football. Our neighbors go skiing every weekend in the winter, and often plan their summer vacations around cycling or hiking. Just because it's fun doesn't mean it's not good for you!

- Start to work on projects in and around the house that include lifting and moderately vigorous activities. Your housemates and neighbors may thank you for your efforts.

- Walk the dog more—you know Fido won't mind!

- Take your kid—or borrow one—and go play on the playground. Keeping up with an active 4-year-old can be a real eye-opener, and playground equipment is perfect for strength training; this is when I do my chin-ups!

- Put up a badminton net or some soccer goalposts in the backyard and challenge your kids and neighbors.

Soon you'll find—as I do—that exercise is really essential time for my brain to relax while I'm doing something with my body. Rollerblading around an empty parking lot, lap swimming, or jogging on a track can be just as good as meditating. Often, it's during a workout that I come up with some of my most interesting ideas.

Most importantly, have fun being active. It is one of those things that can take on a life of its own once you find out what you like to do. I won't say the phrase, but you know it—just get out there and move.

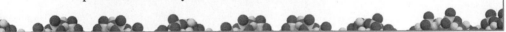

You'll do light aerobic training for 15 minutes, followed by light stretching. Then, we will move to three sets of each exercise at 85 to 90 percent of the weight that you can handle for 10 repetitions. You can rest 1 minute between each set and 2 to 3 minutes between each exercise.

Finish your workout with an additional 15 minutes of light aerobic activity and vigorous stretching.

CHAPTER NINETEEN

LOSING WEIGHT ON GENE SMART

AS YOU HAVE READ THROUGHOUT THIS BOOK, caloric restriction is a surefire way to keep your cells from aging more rapidly, but the main reason we know that people restrict their calories is to promote weight loss.

Why? It's the only thing that works. To lose weight, you have to affect the equation between energy intake and energy expenditure.

> **There's no successful diet on the planet that doesn't come down to this basic energy equation: Burn more than you consume.**

If your energy intake is greater than your energy expenditure, you have a positive energy balance, and you gain weight. If you spend more than you take in, you lose weight. Fat stores in the body are converted to energy to be used, thereby shrinking fat cell size and body appearance.

> **In order to lose weight, you've got to reduce your calorie intake.**

When you follow the Gene Smart Diet you can choose the level of caloric reduction you want by restricting your portion sizes.

Reducing calories on Gene Smart will be easier than on other diets you've tried for one reason: The level of fiber we recommend is much, much higher than on other plans.

| **The more fiber you eat, the less hungry you are.**

It's that simple. You'll be getting an additional boost from the increased amount of omega-3s in your diet. Omega-3 fats have the potential to influence fat storage and loss because of the way they activate gene expression through master regulators. Essentially, long-chain omega-3 fats can effectively mediate a shift in fuel metabolism, so that you're not storing fat, but burning it. Several animal studies have shown a reduction in fat mass after supplementation with omega-3 fats.

There haven't been a lot of studies looking at the omegas found in fish oils and weight loss in humans. Very recently, though, Dr. Alison Hill and colleagues at the University of South Australia at Adelaide demonstrated that omega-3 fats reduce body fat by improving the flow of blood to muscles during exercise. Specifically, 68 overweight and obese people were monitored over a three-month period. They were divided into four groups. One group took daily doses of omega-3s in the form of fish oil, while another was given sunflower oil with no other alteration to their normal diet. Both groups undertook moderate exercise programs (a 45-minute walk or run three times a week), while another two groups received either fish oil or sunflower oil but did no exercise.

The group that took sunflower oil and exercised did not lose any weight. But the group that took the fish oil doses and exercised lost an average 4.5 pounds in only 3 months. So although exercise may not be the most efficient way to lose weight, the fish oils do appear to work synergistically with exercise to increase its effectiveness. In addition to weight loss, omega-3 consumption from fish oil significantly impacts both metabolic syndrome and type 2 diabetes by reducing circulating lipids (particularly elevated triglycerides) and platelet aggregation.

HOW MANY CALORIES DO YOU NEED?

How many overall calories should you take in? Dietitians have used numerous calculations to determine a person's basal metabolic needs, which is the number of calories a person burns a day at rest. With this number in hand they then estimate an activity level and factor that in to determine the average number of calories needed per person per day.

The problem is that these calculations are, at best, an average estimate. There are two standardized calculations that are most often used to determine basal energy expenditure (BEE)—the Harris Benedict method or the Mifflin–St. Jeor (MSJ) method. Studies have shown that the better calculation to use for both overweight and normal-weight persons is the MSJ calculation. The Harris Benedict calculation tends to overestimate caloric needs of overweight and obese persons.

First, you'll need to find your weight in kilograms and your height in centimeters. These calculations should help. (You can also use the interactive calculator at www.genesmart.com.)

Height in inches × 2.54 = height in centimeters
So someone who is 5' 9", or 69", is 175.3 centimeters.

Weight in pounds ÷ 2.2 = weight in kilograms
So someone who weighs 180 pounds weighs 81.8 kilograms.

Then you will need to calculate your BEE:

**For men: BEE = (10 × weight in kg) + (6.25 × height in cm)
– (5 × age in years) + 5**

**For women: BEE = (10 × weight in kg) + (6.25 × height in cm)
– (5 × age in years) – 161**

However, if your BMI is over 30, then you may have to do the MSJ calculation with an adjusted body weight (ABW) and not your actual body weight. This is because excess adipose (fat) tissue is not as metabolically active as muscle and organ tissues in the rest of the body. In other words, adipose cells use significantly fewer calories than other tissues so it is important to adjust for this difference in calculating a person's metabolic needs. So, again, only use the ABW if your BMI is over 30, and this is due to being overweight and not to being excessively muscular.

The ABW calculation is different for men and women because they have different levels of lean tissue to fat tissue even when overweight.

To do this calculation you need to find your ideal body weight (IBW) in relation to your gender and height. (You can find that information at this link: http://healthlinks.washington.edu/nutrition/section12.html#e)

Then use your IBW to find your ABW:

For men: ABW = IBW + .38 × (Actual weight – IBW)

For women: ABW = IBW + .32 × (Actual weight – IBW)

And finally, to get your total energy expenditure you need to include an activity factor. This is a number based on your daily activity level:

1.1 = Sedentary, just performing typical daily activities (TDA)

1.25 = Low activity, TDA plus 30 minutes of walking 3 times per week

1.4 = Active, TDA plus 45 minutes of moderate exercise 3 times per week

1.6 = Moderately active, TDA plus 60 minutes of vigorous exercise 4–5 times per week

1.75 = Very active, TDA plus 60 minutes of vigorous activity or heavy work every day of the week

Multiply your activity factor by the MSJ BEE to get your total energy expenditure per day.

Let's determine your BEE using the Mifflin–St. Jeor calculation. You can consult one of the many websites that will provide you with personalized daily calorie requirements like the one in the calculator menu at http://www.freedieting.com/calorie_needs.html. Then just enter your height, weight, gender, age, and average activity level. Or if you want to actually measure your BEE there are new handheld devices (the BodyGem is one brand name) that measure your actual caloric usage levels. These machines measure your lung output and then calculate your caloric needs. The test is best done first thing in the morning after a 15-minute rest period and before you have had any stimulants such as coffee or tea and before you have exercised or eaten anything. You can find a health provider to administer this test at many of your local hospital outpatient clinics and some gymnasiums.

After you have this number, you can decide how low you want to reduce your calories. As an example I will use a person whose BEE was calculated at 1,450 calories per day and activity level is moderate, which means on average they burn 2,320 calories per day. If you drop this level by 20 percent (464 calories) as suggested in the Adaptive Response portion of the diet, you would need to consume 1,856 calories per day. This taken together with an increase in exercise load will efficiently move you to your desired weight.

This kind of restriction is great to get you jump-started and will work—but then there will be the inevitable plateau and you will have to switch gears. The plateau will occur for different people at different times but, in general, it usually happens in the 3- to 4-week range, which is why the Gene Smart Diet has an initial 3-week phase before changing the routine and then a final shift into permanently changed eating habits. But again let me emphasize, if you need to lose more, extend the Adaptive Response portion of the diet. You can work through the plateaus.

As you can see from our example above, we don't recommend that your caloric intake ever drop below your original BEE number. Because when you go below your BEE, you will experience a sudden drop in energy and a total reshifting of your metabolic rate to an even lower number. This can cause weakness, a lightheaded feeling, and lack of energy to get your exercise routine done. As you add in some isometric/weight-lifting activity and build your muscle mass, your metabolic rate will actually increase and you will lose inches and weight faster than ever, even after the initial 3-week change-over phase.

THE RIGHT CALORIE FIT *FOR YOU*

Gene Smart is a personalized diet, meaning that you figure out what your body's specific caloric requirements are.

Now, the first two menus (Adaptive Response and Preconditioning) do require that you reduce your caloric load. But you'll have to do a little work to make sure that the diets given here are tailor-fitted to your particular caloric requirements.

The programs are based on a person whose BEE is 2,000 calories (kcal)/day. Based on that, the Adaptive Response (AR) menus average 1,600 kcal/day over the course of a week, the Preconditioning (PC) menus have 1,800 kcal/day, and the Optimal Maintenance (OM) menus become calorie neutral—meaning that the person is eating the BEE recommendation of 2,000 kcal/day.

Now, you almost certainly require a different caloric level than what's suggested in the menus in this chapter, depending on your own personal BEE

What about Diet Sodas and Artificial Sweeteners?

I can anticipate the letters now: "I can't believe that a scientist would recommend artificial sweeteners in a book that's supposed to be about better health." But it's a classic risk-benefit equation: I believe that the benefits of losing weight—which artificial sweeteners can help you do—outweigh the risks of these products.

Let me tell a story, by way of illustration. A man at one of my kids' events recently asked me for advice. He's about 300 pounds and can't seem to get his weight down; he has an arthritic knee and is beginning to have some lung problems, together with signs of metabolic syndrome—all the things we would expect from someone of his size. We talked about his diet for a bit, and one thing popped out at me immediately: He consumes about four big soft drinks—or about 800 empty calories—every day.

Ideally, he'd replace all of those with water and unsweetened green tea. But it was clear from talking to him that going cold turkey simply wasn't an option; sodas are his Achilles' heel. So we spent a little time discussing some compromises. He did think that he might be able to switch to iced tea with Splenda and to diet soda (starting with half diet and half regular, and then moving to entirely diet), so that's what I recommended he do. I'm going back to his home city in 3 months, and I fully expect to see that he's shed 25 pounds by doing nothing more than dropping his sugar-drink habit.

There is very little hard science to suggest that artificial sweeteners are bad for you. That may not be satisfying to everyone—it's not particularly satisfying to me, to be honest—but I'm a realist. One day I may be able to recommend a no-calorie natural sweetener (and stevia is certainly showing promise in that regard). Until then, considering how much evidence there is of the harmful effects of obesity, I advise people to choose artificial sweeteners when the alternative is sugar or high-fructose corn syrup.

If my new friend doesn't lose weight, it is guaranteed that he will face serious, life-threatening, obesity-related diseases very soon, and he's only 38 years old. So for me, being able to get a handle on his weight problem far outweighs whatever risks he might court by drinking a diet soda or two.

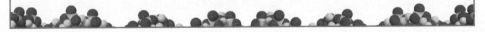

equation, which you calculated on page 246. How will you adjust the diet to fit your needs? By adjusting portion sizes.

For example, if you need to consume 2,500 kcal/day, according to your BEE calculation, you will need to increase the proportion of everything in all the menus by 2,500/2,000, or 25 percent. In contrast, if your BEE is 1,750 kcal/day, you will need to decrease the proportion of everything in your menus by 1,750/2,000, or 12.5 percent.

CUTTING CALORIES ON GENE SMART

In the Optimal Maintenance portion of the Gene Smart Diet we are going to allow you to include some foods that you might not ordinarily associate with losing weight, like 4 to 6 ounces of red wine and 1 to 3 ounces of dark chocolate.

It's true that these foods do add calories. If you're trying to lose weight, you may want to use low-fat or fat-free products in other areas of the diet in order to compensate.

Do what you can. For instance, if you like half-and-half in your coffee, you might want to switch to the reduced-fat version. You can always use reduced-fat or fat-free cream cheese in recipes, and I think you'll find that reduced-fat sour cream will hardly be a change you will notice.

People traditionally have a hard time changing from whole milk straight down to fat-free or 1 percent milk; they always tell me drinking fat-free milk is similar to drinking white water. It doesn't bother me, and in fact, it's the only kind of milk we have in my house, but I don't want you to do something that doesn't work for you. Whole milk is about 3.5 percent fat, so switch first to 2 percent and then after you have adjusted to that, move down to 1 percent. If even those changes are too radical, try mixing higher-fat milk equally with the next fat level down in a 50/50 ratio until you can move to the next level.

Remember: Slow change is better than no change at all—and much better than the backlash that comes when you give in and revert to milkshakes!

FASTING: A TURBO CHARGE

One thing you may consider to boost your entry into the diet is a once-a-week soup fast day.

What? Did you read that correctly? In a book that promises all the benefits of calorie restriction without calorie restriction, do I actually have the audacity to start this program off with a *fast?*

Hold on—let me explain. I know that this is unconventional, but it's not quite as terrible as you think. First of all, it is commonplace in many cultures to incorporate a periodic day of fast, and it is something that has been done since the beginning of time. I personally do it a few times a year. Why? I find that it does more than anything else to press the reset button I mentioned earlier.

For me, the benefits are as much spiritual and emotional as they are physical. For instance, I find that a day without solid food tremendously increases my mindfulness about food—something I can periodically use when it feels like I'm in a cycle of eating most of my meals in front of a keyboard or behind the wheel. I enjoy the mental clarity I get when I'm fasting, as well as simply knowing that I can do it, and the reminder that a day without solid food doesn't kill me.

Second of all, it's not a true fast. You'll be eating helpings of nutritious, delicious soup throughout the day. This will help you to avoid hunger and keep your energy level up—it really is a much gentler way to fast.

I know that a soup fast won't be right for everyone. But I hope that if you've ever been even a little curious about what it would be like to go a day without food, you'll give it a try.

There are some pretty good reasons to do so. First of all, several studies in the scientific literature have demonstrated that fasting can have the same effects on a number of the master regulators and biological endpoints as traditional calorie restriction. Consequently, this is another means to induce an adaptive stress response—the kind of kick-start your body can really benefit from.

The other main purpose of the fast day is to readjust your palate and stomach to a new load of food. The food you will eat on the Gene Smart Diet has a high satiety level due to the fiber. But a day of fasting will also reduce your need for food—the way you feel after a bout with the flu. You will actually feel full on less food, more so than if you go right from a high-caloric and fat-gram–heavy meal intake to a more fiber-filled whole-foods diet.

Drinking the recommended soups will also give you a slight diuretic effect and cause you to lose some water weight. While this is not "real" weight loss, in the sense that fat cells have not shrunk permanently, we all feel better when we see the numbers on the scale go down and our waistbands feel a little looser. Water loss can be an instant motivator. While too much lost water is not healthy, some initial water weight loss is fine, especially if it helps you get moving more or encourages you to stick to a new and more healthful eating strategy.

There are three soup choices for the fast day depending on what you like. You can choose a hot or cold soup, and you can choose a vegetable: leeks, cucumber, or celery. (The recipes can be found on pages 260, 267, and 275.) They need to be made from scratch. You can purchase a comparable ready-made processed version if you need to, but chances are high that it will contain excess amounts of sodium and fat. Homemade soups can be prepared the morning of the fast or the day before and then consumed every 2 to 3 hours depending on hunger levels. You are also able to drink tea or water between your soup meals.

A note: Although I do think this is a great way to kick your body into high gear, know when to say when. I do not suggest fasting more than a day or two, as this is not the goal of the diet, and I do not believe that *prolonged* fasts are a part of any healthy diet.

This fast is also not intended to "cleanse" body systems as this has not been proven to be healthy or an effective means of permanent weight loss.

MENUS

The menus in the first two phases (Adaptive Response and Preconditioning) feature reduced calories. You almost certainly require a different caloric level than that suggested based on the BEE equation you calculated in the previous section. The diets given here are based on a person whose BEE is 2,000 kcal/day. Based on that, the Adaptive Response (AR) menus average 1,600 kcal/day over the course of a week. Accordingly, the Preconditioning (PC) menus have 1,800 kcal/day over the week and then when a person moves to Optimal Maintenance (OM) menus, the levels become calorie neutral at the 2,000 kcal/day energy allotment.

Remember, you will have to adjust your portion sizes based on your BEE. As noted above, if you need to consume 2,500 kcal/day according to your BEE calculation, you will need to increase the proportion of everything in all the menus by 2,500/2,000, or 25 percent. In contrast, if your BEE is 1,750 kcal/day, you will need to decrease the proportion of everything in your menus by 1,750/2,000, or 12.5 percent.

The Adaptive Response menus include one Soup Fast day during the week. Again, I strongly recommend that you do the Soup Fast, but if you choose not to, simply substitute another day of the Adaptive Response plan for the fast. No red wine is offered during the first 5 weeks of the plan, as it often can stimulate the appetite and cause a person to overeat at a time when caloric restriction is the goal. There are a few dark chocolate desserts and snacks built in the AR menus, but as with the red wine, dark chocolate adds calories at a time when calorie reduction is the goal, so if you're significantly overweight, you'll probably want to either skip these or substitute something equally caloric over the course of the day.

And just so you don't forget how incredibly important exercise is to your new lifestyle, you will see reminders of the recommended exercise routine on each day of the diet. In the first phase of the diet (Adaptive Response), you will get 2 days of light circuit training, 3 days of light to

Adding Fiber—Comfortably

Here's the good news that I will emphasize over and over: Increasing fiber virtually guarantees weight loss. As soon as you incorporate more fiber—cereals, fruits, and vegetables—into your diet, your caloric load will go down.

But if you're not used to eating fiber, you'll want to increase your fiber consumption *carefully* in order to give your stomach a chance to make some adjustments. Otherwise, you might notice some gas and bloating sensations. It's not the end of the world, considering that fiber's other side effects include lowered cholesterol and triglycerides, improved blood pressure, a reduction in the risk of heart disease, and lowered whole-body inflammation. But there's no sense in being uncomfortable, so here are some tips:

Increase the amount of fiber in your diet gradually. First, increase soluble forms of fiber and then slowly incorporate more insoluble types later on. (The menus are written this way.)

Drink plenty of fluid as you increase your fiber load—at least 8 to 12 glasses of fluid per day. (This should come from water or, preferably, brewed tea. Remember that excess caffeine can be dehydrating and so it is best to include decaffeinated brewed tea for most of your tea intake.) The great thing about increasing your fiber intake with whole fruits and vegetables is that they are loaded with water, which adds to your body's natural ability to properly digest the fiber. But don't forget to drink up, too.

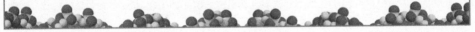

moderate exercise, and 2 days of rest per week. We will progress on from that baseline.

Everyone is starting at a different place with exercise; the best approach is to recognize that you have to crawl before you can run. The goal is to start doing something and pushing yourself, gently! If what we suggest initially is too difficult, please back it down in terms of minutes and level of activity. I have a hard time with this because I am so competitive by nature. However, my mom's old adage "those that can't hear can feel" is never more true than with exercise. Push yourself, but not too hard.

Once again, proceed with safety as your foremost goal. If you're unsure about how to do the exercises properly, check your local gym or YMCA for a certified personal trainer, and if you have even the slightest concern about your physical ability to begin an exercise program, please check with your physician first.

The first 5 weeks of the diet are geared toward adapting and preconditioning your body to reduced calories, eating more fiber and polyphenols, and balancing your long-chain omega-6 fatty acids to omega-3 ratio. To the degree that it is possible, the meals are written so that you can rely on common foods that can be found year-round. But if you are starting this meal plan during strawberry or blueberry season, by all means purchase extra and freeze them to use later. And if shrimp or wild-caught salmon go on sale, then buy extra and freeze some for later.

I have also tried to incorporate a lot of ways to cook extra and then utilize the leftovers for lunch the next day. This is especially important for those of you who don't like to cook and may see this initial phase as daunting.

Snacks should be consumed at the time of day that best works for your schedule. Midmorning is best if you eat an early breakfast and a late lunch; midafternoon is best if you have an early lunch and you don't want to arrive home starved and ready to eat anything you come across. Bedtime snacks are discouraged because often you may be trying to readjust your eating habits from a heavy nighttime meal to eating breakfast for the first time.

Make soup for the Day 1 fast and wake up the next day and start on your road to better Gene Smart health. The current plan assumes that your Soup Fast day will be a Saturday and then the meal plan follows from that basis.

As you can see, many of the lunches are made from the evening leftovers, and are meant to be easy to eat at work with the help of occasional microwaving and/or refrigeration. The weekday breakfasts are also supposed to be quicker options and may include some leftovers from the cooked weekend breakfasts.

Grocery List

Before you start the Gene Smart Diet, you may want to stock up your kitchen and pantry. The following list isn't complete, but it will give you an idea of what you'll be needing. Sometimes the amounts indicate a little extra, which you can use to feed others or carry to the next week.

PRODUCE	AMOUNT TO BUY
Apples	3 medium
Berries	2 cups or 1 bag of frozen
Cantaloupe	1
Carrots	2 large or 1 bag baby carrots
Cherries	½ cup
Dates, Medjool	4
Grapes	1 bunch
Lemons	2 medium
Oranges	2
Parsley	1 bunch
Peach	1
Pear	1
Asparagus	1 bunch
Beans, green	1 small package
Broccoli	1 small head
Cabbage	1 small head
Celery	1 bunch
Cucumber	1 small
Eggplant	1 small
Lettuce, dark green	1 head
Mushrooms	1 small package
Onions, green	1 bunch

(continued)

Grocery List (cont.)

PRODUCE	AMOUNT TO BUY
Onions, red	2 large
Pepper, green bell	1 small
Pepper, red bell	1 small
Potato, sweet	1 medium
Potatoes, purple fingerling	3 small
Snow peas	1 cup
Spinach	1 bag
Squash, yellow, or zucchini	2 medium
Tomatoes, cherry	1 pint

NUTS	
Almonds	8 ounces and save
Mixed nuts, dry-roasted	8 ounces and save
Walnuts	8 ounces and save

CANNED/BOTTLED ITEMS	
Cocktail sauce	1 bottle and save
Cranberry or pomegranate juice	64-ounce bottle and save
Jam, sugar-free, berry of choice	1 small jar and save
Tomato sauce	1 jar and save

BREADS, CEREALS, GRAINS	
Bagels, whole-wheat	1 package and freeze all but 2
Bread crumbs, plain	8 ounces and save
Bread, whole-wheat	1 loaf and freeze ¾ of it
Bun, hamburger, whole-wheat	Buy 1 in deli/bakery
Cereal, low-fat granola	1 small box and save
Cereal, Multigrain Cheerios	1 small box and save
Cereal, shredded wheat	1 small box and save
Couscous	1 pound and save
Crackers, whole-wheat, small	1 box Wheat Thins and save
Oatmeal, long-cooking	1 box and save
Pita, whole-wheat	1 package and freeze all but 2
Rice, brown	2 pound bag and save
Rolls, dinner, whole-wheat	1 package and freeze all but 2

OILS, FATS, DRESSINGS	
Cooking spray	1 can and save
Dressing, ranch, reduced-fat	1 bottle and save
Margarine, trans-free	1 pound and save
Mayonnaise, cholesterol-free	1 jar and save
Oil, canola	1 bottle and save
Oil, olive	1 bottle and save

EGGS AND DAIRY	
Cheese, feta	½ pound and save
Cheese, mozzarella, reduced-fat	8 ounces and save
Cheese, Parmesan	8 ounces and save
Cheese, provolone	1 ounce
Cottage cheese, 1%	8 ounces and save
Cream cheese, reduced-fat	8 ounces and save
Egg substitute, liquid	1 quart and save
Milk, 1%	1 quart and save
Pudding or mousse, chocolate, sugar-free	1 package
Yogurt, frozen, sugar-free, fat-free	1 cup
Yogurt, low-fat, vanilla	2 cups (16 ounces)

SEAFOOD, BEEF, CHICKEN, PORK	
Bacon	1 strip (buy 1 package; bacon freezes well)
Beef, tenderloin	6 ounces
Canadian bacon	2 ounces
Chicken, boneless skinless breast	4 ounces
Lox (Chinook salmon)	3 ounces
Mackerel, wild	6 ounces
Pork, lean chop	4 ounces
Pork, tenderloin	5 ounces
Salmon, sockeye, wild	8 ounces
Shrimp, raw or frozen	4 ounces
Trout, rainbow, wild or farmed	5 ounces

Suggested Saturday prep day activities to do while you make your soup:

1. Slice 1–2 red onions and store in a ziptop bag or reusable plastic-ware container in the refrigerator for use in cooking and salads throughout the week.

2. Cube 1–2 red and green bell peppers and store in a ziptop bag or reusable plasticware container in the refrigerator for use in cooking and salads throughout the week.

3. Cube 1–3 stalks of celery and store in a ziptop bag or reusable plas-ticware container in the refrigerator for use in cooking and salads throughout the week.

4. Chop 1 large broccoli crown into small bite-sized pieces and store in a ziptop bag or reusable plasticware container in the refrigerator for use in cooking and salads throughout the week.

5. Take a pound of organic whole carrots and cube one-third, grate one-third, and cut into sticks that last one-third; store each in its own ziptop bag or reusable plasticware container in the refrigerator for use in cooking, snacking, and salads throughout the week.

6. Blend 4–8 ounces reduced-fat cream cheese with 1–2 tablespoons mix-ins (chopped walnuts, scallions, dehydrated vegetable seasonings, diced red onion or chives, etc.) for eating on whole-grain bread or in wraps.

7. Make a batch of whole-grain or high-fiber muffins: Keep what you need and take the rest to your neighbors, co-workers, or teachers so that they can experience great health—and you don't end up with too many tempting extra muffins around. You can also freeze muffins, but there is some quality loss.

8. For the Optimal Maintenance Phase—take 3.5-ounce dark choco-late candy bars and divide each into three portions and store in ziptop bags away from heat and light; then grab one when you need to.

9. Make a large batch of brown rice, cool it, and store for use over the next 3 to 4 days. Brown rice takes twice as long to cook as white rice and nine times as long as quick rice, so if you make it in advance you won't have to wait around for dinner after work.

10. Make twice as much of something you like for Sunday breakfast (French toast, oatmeal, hoecakes, whole-grain pancakes or waffles) and save some for one or two quick and easy breakfasts later in the week.

Day 1

SOUP FAST

Take your pick from Celery Soup (below), Leek and Parsley Soup (page 267), or No-Cook Cold Cucumber Soup (page 275). Enjoy 1 to 1½ cups every 2 to 3 hours from waking until 3 hours before bedtime.

You may drink 8 ounces of green tea, black tea, or water between soup servings. You may use regular or decaf tea. Do not engage in vigorous exercise today.

Note: If you prefer not to kick-start the program with a fast day, you may skip to Day 2 or substitute an Adaptive Response menu.

Several participants in the Hillsdale program chose commercially available soups containing fewer than 140 calories per serving. If they became too hungry during the soup fast, they would have a piece of whole-grain bread with their soup. Others chose to "fast" with approximately 500 calories' worth of cereal and skim milk; this will also work to shift your body into an adaptive response mode.

CELERY SOUP

1 tablespoon olive oil

1 bunch celery, chopped (about 7 cups)

4 green onions (whites and about 3" of greens), chopped

1 medium leek, white and pale green part chopped (discard the tough dark green tops)

1 medium russet potato, peeled and cut into 1" cubes

4 cups water + 2 teaspoons salt or 4 cups low-sodium chicken broth

1 cup fat-free plain yogurt

Chopped fresh parsley

Heat the oil in a large heavy stockpot over medium-high heat. Add the celery, onions, and leek and cook, stirring occasionally, until beginning to soften, 8 to 10 minutes. Add the potato and water or broth and bring to a boil. Reduce the heat and simmer until the potato is tender, 8 to 10 minutes longer. Let cool about 10 minutes.

Stir the yogurt into the soup. In batches, transfer the soup to a blender and puree (or puree in the pot with an immersion blender). Strain the soup through a strainer. Store in containers in the refrigerator. Serve chilled or at room temperature sprinkled with parsley.

**Makes 4-6 servings
(enough for 1 day)**

EXERCISE SUGGESTION

Light exercise such as walking, stretching, housework, or yardwork for 30 minutes early in the day.

DAY 1 NUTRITIONAL VALUES

Calories: 575
Fiber: 17 grams
Percent fat: 24.6
AA: 0 milligrams
GLA: 0 milligrams
EPA: 0 milligrams
DHA + DPA: 0 milligrams
Long-chain omega-6/omega-3 ratio: 0
Cholesterol: 4 milligrams

Day 2

BREAKFAST

VEGETABLE SCRAMBLE: ³⁄₄ cup liquid egg substitute, 2 tablespoons chopped red onion, and 2 tablespoons chopped red bell pepper cooked in a nonstick skillet coated with cooking spray

- 1 slice whole-wheat toast with 1 teaspoon trans-free margarine and 1 tablespoon reduced-sugar or sugar-free berry jam
- ½ cup cherries
- 6 ounces hot or cold brewed tea blended with ¼ cup recommended juice (see page 256)
- 1 fish oil and 1 borage oil capsule
- 6 ounces hot coffee if desired (sugar substitute and fat-free milk if needed)
- 16 ounces water between breakfast and lunch

LUNCH

SHRIMP COCKTAIL: 4 ounces cooked shrimp with 2 tablespoons cocktail sauce

- ½ medium baked sweet potato with 1 teaspoon trans-free margarine

ZUCCHINI BROIL: ½ cup shredded zucchini cooked until soft in the microwave, then topped with 1 tablespoon plain bread crumbs and 1 ounce reduced-fat shredded mozzarella cheese and broiled

- 1 medium pear (or 1 serving other in-season high-polyphenol fruit of choice)
- Calorie-free drink or 6 ounces tea
- 16 ounces water between lunch and dinner

DINNER

DIJON PORK: 2 ounces cooked pork tenderloin (cook extra for the Pork Sandwich tomorrow) with 1 teaspoon Dijon mustard (or to taste)

- ½ cup cooked couscous, made with lemon juice and lemon zest
- 1 cup cooked snow peas with 1 tablespoon trans-free margarine
- ½ cup sugar-free dark chocolate mousse
- 2 fish oil capsules and 1 borage oil capsule
- Calorie-free drink or 6 ounces tea
- 16 ounces water before bed

SNACK

1 cup sugar-free, fat-free frozen yogurt

EXERCISE SUGGESTION

Light circuit training (15/20/15) as described on page 240.

DAY 2 NUTRITIONAL VALUES

Calories: 1,577
Fiber: 25 grams
Percent fat: 17
AA: 97 milligrams
GLA: 450 milligrams
EPA: 733 milligrams
DHA + DPA: 546 milligrams
Long-chain omega-6/omega-3 ratio: .08
Cholesterol: 300 milligrams

Day 3

BREAKFAST

BAGEL AND LOX: 1 medium whole-wheat bagel with 2 tablespoons reduced-fat cream cheese and 2 ounces lox (smoked Chinook salmon)

- 1 cup mixed fresh berries (or ½ cup frozen mixed berries)
- 6 ounces hot or cold brewed tea blended with ¼ cup recommended juice (see page 256)
- 1 fish oil and 1 borage oil capsule
- 6 ounces hot coffee if desired (sugar substitute and fat-free milk if needed)
- 16 ounces water between breakfast and lunch

LUNCH

PORK SANDWICH: 1 whole-wheat hamburger bun with 2 ounces cooked lean top loin pork roast and 2 teaspoons cholesterol-free mayonnaise

COLESLAW: 1 cup shredded red cabbage tossed with 1 tablespoon cholesterol-free mayo

- 2 cups cantaloupe chunks (or 1 serving other in-season high-polyphenol fruit)
- Calorie-free drink or 6 ounces tea
- 16 ounces water between lunch and dinner

DINNER

LEMON FISH EN PAPILLOTE (FISH COOKED IN PARCHMENT)

4 ounces skinless trout fillet

1 teaspoon olive oil

1 teaspoon lemon zest or lemon juice

Place the trout on one side of a large piece of aluminum foil or parchment paper. Top with the olive oil and lemon zest or juice. Fold the foil or parchment over the fish and seal the edges together.

Place the packet on a baking sheet and bake in a 350°F oven for 10 minutes, or until the fish flakes easily with a fork.

- 3 baby carrots, cut into sticks
- 12 (4"-long) zucchini sticks
- ½ cup cooked brown rice mixed with 1 tablespoon thinly sliced green onion and 1 teaspoon trans-free margarine
- 1 serving in-season high-polyphenol fruit
- 2 fish oil capsules and 1 borage oil capsule
- Calorie-free drink or 6 ounces tea
- 16 ounces water before bedtime

SNACK

- 6 small whole-wheat crackers
- 1 ounce reduced-fat cheese

EXERCISE SUGGESTION

Moderate exercise (from suggestions on page 241) for 30 minutes.

DAY 3 NUTRITIONAL VALUES

Calories: 1,575	
Fiber: 26 grams	
Percent fat: 25	
AA: 59 milligrams	
GLA: 450 milligrams	
EPA: 1,021 milligrams	
DHA + DPA: 1,479 milligrams	
Long-chain omega-6/omega-3 ratio: .02	
Cholesterol: 179 milligrams	

Day 4

BREAKFAST

- 1 cup bite-size shredded wheat cereal with ¾ cup 1% milk
- ½ cup blueberries
- ½ cup 1% cottage cheese
- 6 ounces hot or cold brewed tea blended with ¼ cup recommended juice (see page 256)
- 1 fish oil and 1 borage oil capsule
- 6 ounces hot coffee if desired (sugar substitute and fat-free milk if needed)
- 16 ounces water between breakfast and lunch

LUNCH
CHICKEN SALAD WITH CRACKERS

3 ounces chopped cooked skinless chicken breast

¼ cup chopped red onion

¼ cup chopped celery

¼ cup chopped fresh parsley

1 tablespoon cholesterol-free mayonnaise

6 small whole-wheat crackers

Mix together the chicken, onion, celery, parsley, and mayonnaise. Serve with the crackers.

- ½ cup sliced cucumber tossed with a combination of 1 teaspoon olive oil, vinegar to taste, and herbs and seasonings of choice
- 1 medium apple (with skin)
- Calorie-free drink or 6 ounces tea
- 16 ounces water between lunch and dinner

DINNER

- 3 ounces cooked lean eye of round beef, thinly sliced and served au jus

ROASTED VEGETABLES

1 cup sliced summer squash or parsnips

6 asparagus spears or green beans

¼ medium red onion, coarsely chopped

¼ cup cubed peeled eggplant

6 cherry tomatoes

1 tablespoon olive oil

In a small roasting pan, combine the squash or parsnips, asparagus or beans, onion, eggplant, and tomatoes. Drizzle with the olive oil and toss to mix. Roast in a 400°F oven for about 15 minutes, or until the vegetables are browned and tender.

- ½ medium baked sweet potato with 1 teaspoon trans-free margarine
- 1 small whole-wheat dinner roll with 1 teaspoon trans-free margarine
- 2 fish oil capsules and 1 borage oil capsule
- Calorie-free drink or 6 ounces tea
- 16 ounces water before bedtime

SNACK

- 8 ounces sugar-free, fat-free yogurt
- ¼ cup high-fiber cold cereal or granola

EXERCISE SUGGESTION

Rest.

DAY 4 NUTRITIONAL VALUES

Calories: 1,636
Fiber: 22 grams
Percent fat: 27
AA: 34 milligrams
GLA: 450 milligrams
EPA: 540 milligrams
DHA + DPA: 360 milligrams
Long-chain omega-6/omega-3 ratio: .04
Cholesterol: 173 milligrams

Day 5

BREAKFAST

- 1 medium whole-wheat bagel with 1 tablespoon reduced-fat cream cheese
- 1 medium orange
- 6 ounces hot or cold brewed tea blended with ¼ cup recommended juice (see page 256)
- 1 fish oil and 1 borage oil capsule
- 6 ounces hot coffee if desired (sugar substitute and fat-free milk if needed)
- 16 ounces water between breakfast and lunch

LUNCH

BEEF AND CHEESE PITA: 1 (6") whole-wheat pita spread with 1 tablespoon reduced-fat ranch dressing and stuffed with 2 ounces cooked lean eye of round beef (thinly sliced against the grain), 1 ounce provolone cheese, and 1 dark green lettuce leaf

SPINACH SALAD: 3 chopped cherry tomatoes, 1 cup fresh spinach, 1 chopped slice cooked lean bacon, and ¼ cup sliced mushrooms tossed with 1 tablespoon olive oil, vinegar to taste, and herbs of choice

- 1 small peach (with skin) or 1 serving other in-season, high-polyphenol fruit
- Calorie-free drink or 6 ounces tea
- 16 ounces water between lunch and dinner

DINNER

ORANGE SALMON: 4 ounces sockeye salmon (or other Category 1 fish; see page 217) poached in ¼ cup orange juice (make extra for tomorrow's salad)

GREEN BEANS ALMANDINE: 10 cooked green beans tossed with 1 tablespoon slivered almonds and 1 tablespoon trans-free margarine

- 3 small purple fingerling potatoes, cubed and cooked in a foil packet

BAKED APPLE: 1 medium apple (with skin), cored and stuffed with a mix of 1 tablespoon oatmeal, 1 tablespoon crushed walnuts, and 1 teaspoon cinnamon, then baked in a 350°F oven for 40 to 60 minutes.

- 2 fish oil capsules and 1 borage oil capsule
- Calorie-free drink or 6 ounces tea
- 16 ounces water before bedtime

SNACK

1 cup Multigrain Cheerios with ¾ cup 1% milk and ½ cup blueberries

EXERCISE SUGGESTION

Moderate exercise (from list on page 241) for 30 minutes.

DAY 5 NUTRITIONAL VALUES

Calories: 1,653
Fiber: 33 grams
Percent fat: 29
AA: 102 milligrams
GLA: 450 milligrams
EPA: 981 milligrams
DHA + DPA: 948 milligrams
Long-chain omega-6/omega-3 ratio: .05
Cholesterol: 148 milligrams

Day 6

BREAKFAST

- 1 cup mixed fresh berries (or ½ cup frozen mixed berries) blended with 4 ounces low-fat vanilla yogurt
- 1 slice whole-wheat toast with 1 ounce reduced-fat cheese
- 6 ounces hot or cold brewed tea blended with ¼ cup recommended juice (see page 256)
- 1 fish oil and 1 borage oil capsule
- 6 ounces hot coffee if desired (sugar substitute and fat-free milk if needed)
- 16 ounces water between breakfast and lunch

LUNCH

ORANGE SALMON SALAD

2 cups dark green lettuce

¼ cup grated carrot

¼ cup sliced red onion

1 teaspoon olive oil

Vinegar, to taste

Seasonings of choice

1 ounce crumbled feta or soft goat cheese

3 ounces leftover orange-poached sockeye salmon (or other Category 1 fish; see page 217)

Combine the lettuce, carrot, and onion in a large bowl. Whisk together the olive oil, vinegar, and seasonings. Drizzle the dressing over the salad and toss. Top with the cheese and salmon.

- 1 slice whole-wheat bread
- 1 cup red or purple seedless grapes

- Calorie-free drink or 6 ounces tea
- 16 ounces water between lunch and dinner

DINNER

ITALIAN PORK CHOPS: 4 ounces lean pork loin chop, ¼ cup sliced green bell pepper, and ½ chopped medium red onion cooked in a nonstick skillet coated with cooking spray, then with ½ cup prepared tomato sauce added

- ½ cup cooked brown rice with 1 teaspoon trans-free margarine
- 1 cup spinach sautéed in 1 teaspoon olive oil
- 1 medium apple (with skin)
- 2 fish oil capsules and 1 borage oil capsule
- Calorie-free drink or 6 ounces tea
- 16 ounces water before bedtime

SNACK

- 1 ounce dry-roasted nuts

EXERCISE SUGGESTION

Light circuit training (15/20/15) as described on page 240.

DAY 6 NUTRITIONAL VALUES

Calories: 1,664
Fiber: 21 grams
Percent fat: 32
AA: 25 milligrams
GLA: 450 milligrams
EPA: 990 milligrams
DHA + DPA: 1,067 milligrams
Long-chain omega-6/omega-3 ratio: .01
Cholesterol: 202 milligrams

Day 7

BREAKFAST

- ⅔ cup prepared low-fat granola cereal with ¾ cup 1% milk
- 6 ounces hot or cold brewed tea blended with ¼ cup recommended juice (see page 256)
- 1 fish oil and 1 borage oil capsule
- 6 ounces hot coffee if desired (sugar substitute and fat-free milk if needed)
- 16 ounces water between breakfast and lunch

LUNCH

PITA PIZZA

1 (4") whole-wheat pita
¼ cup tomato sauce
2 ounces diced cooked Canadian bacon
1 tablespoon chopped red onion
1 tablespoon sliced mushroom
2 ounces shredded reduced-fat mozzarella cheese

Top the pita with the tomato sauce, bacon, onion, mushrooms, and mozzarella. Place on a baking sheet and bake in a 350°F oven for 15 minutes, or until the pita is heated through and the cheese is melted.

- 1 ½ cups red or purple seedless grapes
- Calorie-free drink or 6 ounces tea
- 16 ounces water between lunch and dinner

DINNER

- 4 ounces broiled or grilled Atlantic mackerel (or other Category 1 fish; see page 217)
- 1 cup steamed broccoli sprinkled with 1 ounce grated Parmesan cheese
- ½ cup cooked brown rice mixed with ¼ cup cooked grated carrot and ¼ cup cooked green peas
- 1 small whole-wheat dinner roll with 1 ½ teaspoons trans-free margarine
- 2 fish oil capsules and 1 borage oil capsule
- Calorie-free drink or 6 ounces tea
- 16 ounces water before bedtime

SNACK

- 4 Medjool dates

EXERCISE SUGGESTION
Rest.

DAY 7 NUTRITIONAL VALUES

Calories: 1,642	
Fiber: 21 grams	
Percent fat: 25	
AA: 205 milligrams	
GLA: 450 milligrams	
EPA: 1,546 milligrams	
DHA + DPA: 2,166 milligrams	
Long-chain omega-6/omega-3 ratio: .02	
Cholesterol: 175 milligrams	

Day 8

SOUP FAST

Take your pick from Leek and Parsley Soup (below), Celery Soup (page 260), and No-Cook Cold Cucumber Soup (page 275). Enjoy 1 to 1 ½ cups every 2 to 3 hours from waking until 3 hours before bedtime. Drink 8 ounces green tea or black tea or water between soup servings. You may use regular or decaf tea. Do not engage in vigorous exercise today.

LEEK AND PARSLEY SOUP

1 tablespoon olive oil

3 medium or 2 large leeks, white and pale green parts chopped

1 bunch fresh flat-leaf parsley, stems separated and chopped (save parsley leaves for garnish)

1 medium zucchini (unpeeled), shredded with a grater

4 green onions (white parts and about 3" green parts), chopped

4 cups of water + 2 teaspoons salt or 4 cups low-sodium chicken broth

Heat the oil in a large heavy stockpot over medium-high heat. Add the leeks and parsley stems and cook, stirring, until the leeks lighten in color, 4 to 5 minutes. Add the zucchini, green onions, and water or broth and bring to a boil. Reduce the heat and simmer for 8 to 10 minutes. Let cool about 10 minutes.

Store in containers in the refrigerator and serve warm with fresh parsley leaves as garnish.

**Makes 4-6 servings
(enough for one person)**

EXERCISE SUGGESTION

Light exercise (such as walking, stretching, housework, or yardwork) for 30 minutes early in the day.

DAY 8 NUTRITIONAL VALUES

Calories: 326
Fiber: 12 grams
Percent fat: 37
AA: 0 milligrams
GLA: 0 milligrams
EPA: 0 milligrams
DHA + DPA: 0 milligrams
Long-chain omega-6/omega-3 ratio: 0
Cholesterol: 0 milligrams

Day 9

BREAKFAST

- 2 medium (6") cornmeal hoecakes (make extra for tomorrow's breakfast) with 2 teaspoons trans-free margarine, 1 tablespoon honey, ¼ cup blueberries, and 7 chopped English walnut halves
- 6 ounces hot or cold brewed tea blended with ¼ cup recommended juice (see page 256)
- 1 fish oil and 1 borage oil capsule
- 6 ounces hot coffee if desired (sugar substitute and fat-free milk if needed)
- 16 ounces water between breakfast and lunch

HOECAKES

Magnolia Cafe, Austin, TX

6 large eggs

2 ½ cups buttermilk

2 ¼ cups yellow cornmeal

1 cup all-purpose flour

⅓ cup sugar

1 tablespoon baking powder

1 teaspoon baking soda

¾ teaspoon salt

8 tablespoons (about) butter, melted

Pure maple syrup

Preheat oven to 250°F. Beat eggs in large bowl to blend. Add buttermilk, cornmeal, flour, sugar, baking powder, baking soda, and salt. Beat until smooth. Mix in 6 tablespoons melted butter.

Add ½ tablespoon melted butter to large nonstick skillet over medium heat. Working in batches, pour batter by ¼ cupfuls into skillet, spacing apart. Cook pancakes until golden brown on bottom and some bubbles begin to break around edges, about 2 minutes. Turn pancakes over; cook until bottoms are golden brown, about 2 minutes. Transfer pancakes to baking sheet; place in oven to keep warm. Repeat with remaining batter, adding more melted butter by ½ tablespoonfuls to skillet as necessary. Serve with maple syrup.

Serves 6 to 8

LUNCH

EASY CHILI

3 ounces ground beef (95% lean)

½ cup canned kidney beans, rinsed and drained

1 cup canned diced tomatoes

Chili seasoning, to taste

2 ounces reduced-fat Cheddar cheese, grated

Coat a nonstick skillet with cooking spray and heat over medium heat. Add the beef and cook, breaking up the meat with a wooden spoon, until browned, about 5 minutes. Add the beans, tomatoes, and chili seasoning and cook, stirring occasionally, until thickened slightly, about 10 minutes. Serve with the cheese sprinkled on top.

- 6 whole-wheat crackers
- 1 medium apple (with skin)
- Calorie-free drink or 6 ounces tea
- 16 ounces water between lunch and dinner

DINNER

CRAB CAKES

6 ounces Alaskan king crabmeat (or other Category 1 or 2 fish; see page 217)

¼ cup plain bread crumbs

2 tablespoons liquid egg substitute

1 teaspoon Old Bay seasoning

2 tablespoons canola or safflower oil

Mix together the crab, bread crumbs, egg substitute, and Old Bay seasoning. Form the mixture into 2 patties. Heat the oil in a small skillet over medium heat. Add the crab cakes and cook, turning once, until browned, 8 to 10 minutes.

- 1 large tomato, sliced, broiled, and sprinkled with chopped fresh parsley or thyme
- 1 cup steamed broccoli
- 2 fish oil capsules and 1 borage oil capsule
- Calorie-free drink or 6 ounces tea
- 16 ounces water before bed

SNACK

- 4 (4") celery sticks with 1 tablespoon peanut butter

EXERCISE SUGGESTION

Light circuit training (15/20/15), as described on page 240.

DAY 9 NUTRITIONAL VALUES

Calories: 1,637
Fiber: 24 grams
Percent fat: 36
AA: 102 milligrams
GLA: 450 milligrams
EPA: 1,042 milligrams
DHA + DPA: 614 milligrams
Long-chain omega-6/omega-3 ratio: .06
Cholesterol: 189 milligrams

Day 10

BREAKFAST

- 2 leftover medium (6") cornmeal hoecakes (heated in toaster), with 2 teaspoons trans-free margarine and 1 tablespoon honey
- 6 ounces hot or cold brewed tea blended with ¼ cup recommended juice (see page 256)
- 1 fish oil and 1 borage oil capsule
- 6 ounces hot coffee if desired (sugar substitute and fat-free milk if needed)
- 16 ounces water between breakfast and lunch

LUNCH

TUNA, APPLE, AND WALNUT SALAD WITH CRACKERS

3 ounces canned white albacore tuna in water, drained

¼ cup chopped apple (with skin)

¼ cup diced celery

¼ cup grated carrot

¼ cup diced red bell pepper

7 English walnut halves, chopped

1 tablespoon cholesterol-free mayonnaise

6 small whole-wheat crackers

Mix together the tuna, apple, celery, carrot, bell pepper, walnuts, and mayonnaise. Serve with the crackers.

- 1 ounce dark chocolate
- Calorie-free drink or 6 ounces tea
- 16 ounces water between lunch and dinner

DINNER

- 3 ounces baked skinless chicken breast (make extra for Chicken Salad tomorrow)
- ½ cup cooked brown rice
- ½ cup cooked green peas and pearl onions
- ½ cup cooked carrots
- 1 whole-wheat dinner roll with 1 teaspoon trans-free margarine
- 12 Bing cherries
- 2 fish oil capsules and 1 borage oil capsule
- Calorie-free drink or 6 ounces tea
- 16 ounces water before bed

SNACK

- 1 cup low-fat vanilla yogurt
- 1 medium peach

EXERCISE SUGGESTION

Moderate exercise (from list on page 235) for 30 minutes.

DAY 10 NUTRITIONAL VALUES

Calories: 1,626
Fiber: 19 grams
Percent fat: 25
AA: 43 milligrams
GLA: 450 milligrams
EPA: 738 milligrams
DHA + DPA: 910 milligrams
Long-chain omega-6/omega-3 ratio: .03
Cholesterol: 217 milligrams

Day 11

BREAKFAST

BAGEL AND LOX: 1 medium whole-wheat bagel with 2 tablespoons reduced-fat cream cheese and 3 ounces lox (smoked Chinook salmon)

- 6 ounces hot or cold brewed tea blended with ¼ cup recommended juice (see page 256)
- 1 fish oil and 1 borage oil capsule
- 6 ounces hot coffee if desired (sugar substitute and fat-free milk if needed)
- 16 ounces water between breakfast and lunch

LUNCH

CHICKEN SALAD

3 ounces chopped baked skinless chicken breast

1 tablespoon reduced-fat mayonnaise

1 teaspoon yellow mustard

2 dark green lettuce leaves

6 cherry tomatoes, each cut in half

Mix together the chicken, mayonnaise, and mustard. Line a plate with the lettuce and top with the chicken salad. Sprinkle the tomatoes on top and serve.

- 1 cup red grapes
- Calorie-free drink or 6 ounces tea
- 16 ounces water between lunch and dinner

DINNER

- 4 ounces cooked beef flank steak, thinly sliced against the grain (make extra for the steak salad tomorrow)

BROILED TOMATOES PARMESAN: 2 plum tomatoes, split open, sprinkled with ½ ounce grated Parmesan cheese, and broiled until the cheese is lightly browned

- 1 cup cooked brown rice mixed with 1 cup cooked spinach, ¼ cup sliced red onion or scallions, ½ cup cooked sliced mushrooms, and 1 ½ teaspoons olive oil
- 1 small whole-wheat roll with 1 teaspoon trans-free margarine
- 2 fish oil capsules and 1 borage oil capsule
- Calorie-free drink or 6 ounces tea
- 16 ounces water before bed

SNACK

- ½ cup reduced-fat ricotta cheese
- ½ small apple, diced and sprinkled with 1 teaspoon cinnamon and/or nutmeg

EXERCISE SUGGESTION

Rest.

DAY 11 NUTRITIONAL VALUES

Calories: 1,643
Fiber: 21 grams
Percent fat: 29
AA: 115 milligrams
GLA: 450 milligrams
EPA: 696 milligrams
DHA + DPA: 649 milligrams
Long-chain omega-6/omega-3 ratio: .08
Cholesterol: 289 milligrams

Day 12

BREAKFAST

- 1 multigrain English muffin with 2 teaspoons trans-free margarine and 2 tablespoons reduced-sugar or sugar-free berry jam
- ¾ cup 1% cottage cheese
- 1 cup strawberries
- 6 ounces hot or cold brewed tea blended with ¼ cup recommended juice (see page 256)
- 1 fish oil and 1 borage oil capsule
- 6 ounces hot coffee if desired (sugar substitute and fat-free milk if needed)
- 16 ounces water between breakfast and lunch

LUNCH

STEAK AND ORANGE SALAD

2 tablespoons unsweetened orange juice

1 tablespoon peanut oil

Vinegar, to taste

Seasonings of choice

2 cups dark green lettuce or baby spinach

¼ cup mandarin oranges

¼ cup grated carrot

¼ cup sliced red onion

2 ounces cooked beef flank steak, thinly sliced against the grain

Mix together the orange juice, peanut oil, vinegar, and seasonings. In a serving bowl, toss together the lettuce, oranges, carrot, and onion. Lay the steak slices on top of the salad, drizzle with the dressing, and serve.

- 6 small whole-grain crackers
- Calorie-free drink or 6 ounces tea
- 16 ounces water between lunch and dinner

DINNER

6 ounces baked sockeye salmon (or other Category 1 fish; see page 217)

½ cup cornbread stuffing, prepared from mix

½ cup cooked English peas

APRICOT CRISP: 2 apricots, halved, topped with 1 tablespoon oats, 1 teaspoon crushed pecans, and 1 teaspoon trans-free margarine, then baked in a 350°F oven for 14-16 minutes, or until flaky.

- 2 fish oil capsules and 1 borage oil capsule
- Calorie-free drink or 6 ounces tea
- 16 ounces water before bed

SNACK

- ¾ cup sugar-free low-fat chocolate pudding

EXERCISE SUGGESTION

Moderate exercise (from list on page 235) for 30 minutes.

DAY 12 NUTRITIONAL VALUES

Calories: 1,641
Fiber: 22 grams
Percent fat: 35
AA: 51 milligrams
GLA: 450 milligrams
EPA: 1,441 milligrams
DHA + DPA: 1,774 milligrams
Long-chain omega-6/omega-3 ratio: .02
Cholesterol: 213 milligrams

Day 13

BREAKFAST

- 6 ounces low-fat vanilla yogurt
- ½ medium oat bran bagel with 1 tablespoon reduced-fat cream cheese
- 1 cup cantaloupe chunks (or 1 serving other in-season high-polyphenol fruit)
- 6 ounces hot or cold brewed tea blended with ¼ cup recommended juice (see page 256)
- 1 fish oil and 1 borage oil capsule
- 6 ounces hot coffee if desired (sugar substitute and fat-free milk if needed)
- 16 ounces water between breakfast and lunch

LUNCH

SALMON PASTA SALAD WITH CRACKERS

1 tablespoon olive oil
Lemon juice, to taste
Herbs and seasonings of choice
3 ounces canned pink salmon
1 cup cooked whole-wheat macaroni
¼ cup diced red bell pepper
¼ cup diced celery
¼ cup diced red onion
6 small whole-wheat crackers

Mix together the olive oil, lemon juice, and seasonings. In a serving bowl, combine the salmon, macaroni, bell pepper, celery, and onion. Add the dressing and toss to combine. Serve the salad with crackers.

MARINATED CUCUMBERS: 1 cup sliced cucumbers tossed with vinegar, chopped fresh dill, and spices of choice

- Calorie-free drink or 6 ounces tea
- 16 ounces water between lunch and dinner

DINNER

BBQ PORK CHOP: 3 ounces lean top loin pork chop cooked in a nonstick skillet with 1 tablespoon barbecue sauce

- 1 cup cooked asparagus (or other in-season, high-polyphenol vegetable)
- ½ cup cooked yellow corn

TOMATO-MOZZARELLA SALAD: 1 ounce sliced fresh mozzarella layered with 4 large tomato slices, then drizzled with 2 teaspoons olive oil, balsamic vinegar to taste, and fresh herbs (such as parsley, chives, dill, or thyme)

- 2 fish oil capsules and 1 borage oil capsule
- Calorie-free drink or 6 ounces tea
- 16 ounces water before bed

SNACK

- 1 slice whole-wheat bread with 1 tablespoon peanut butter and 1 tablespoon reduced-sugar or sugar-free berry jam

EXERCISE SUGGESTION

Light circuit training (15/20/15) as described on page 240.

DAY 13 NUTRITIONAL VALUES

Calories: 1,617	
Fiber: 24 grams	
Percent fat: 35	
AA: 65 milligrams	
GLA: 450 milligrams	
EPA: 1,258 milligrams	
DHA + DPA: 1,086 milligrams	
Long-chain omega-6/omega-3 ratio: .03	
Cholesterol: 142 milligrams	

Day 14

BREAKFAST

- 2 slices whole-wheat toast with 1 tablespoon nut butter
- 1 medium banana
- 1 cup 1% milk
- 6 ounces hot or cold brewed tea blended with ¼ cup recommended juice (see page 256)
- 1 fish oil and 1 borage oil capsule
- 6 ounces hot coffee if desired (sugar substitute and fat-free milk if needed)
- 16 ounces water between breakfast and lunch

LUNCH

PORTOBELLO SANDWICH: 1 multigrain hamburger bun spread with 1 tablespoon cholesterol-free mayonnaise and topped with 2 dark green lettuce leaves, 3 ounces grilled portobello mushroom, and 1 ounce sliced provolone or Swiss cheese

CABBAGE-APPLE SALAD: ¼ cup shredded Chinese cabbage, ¼ cup shredded common green cabbage, ¼ cup shredded red cabbage, and ½ cup diced apple tossed with 1 teaspoon olive oil, vinegar to taste, and seasonings of choice

- 1 cup strawberries
- Calorie-free drink or 6 ounces tea
- 16 ounces water between lunch and dinner

DINNER

SOUTHERN MACKEREL

2 teaspoons olive oil
¼ cup sliced green bell pepper
¼ cup sliced red bell pepper
¼ cup sliced yellow bell pepper
¼ cup sliced red onion
6 sliced cherry tomatoes
5 ounces Atlantic mackerel (or other Category 1 fish; see page 217)

Heat the oil in a large nonstick skillet over medium-high heat. Add the bell peppers, onion, and tomatoes and cook, stirring occasionally, until softened, about 5 minutes. Push the vegetables to the side of the pan. Add the mackerel and cook, turning once, until the fish flakes easily with a fork, 6 to 8 minutes.

- 1 cup cooked brown rice with 1 tablespoon trans-free margarine
- ½ cup canned mixed tropical fruit, drained and rinsed of syrup (save remaining fruit to make Tropical Gelatin on Day 16)
- 2 fish oil capsules and 1 borage oil capsule
- Calorie-free drink or 6 ounces tea
- 16 ounces water before bed

SNACK

- 1 small dark chocolate brownie

EXERCISE SUGGESTION
Rest.

DAY 14 NUTRITIONAL VALUES

Calories: 1,580	
Fiber: 20 grams	
Percent fat: 38	
AA: 64 milligrams	
GLA: 450 milligrams	
EPA: 1,110 milligrams	
DHA + DPA: 1,272 milligrams	
Long-chain omega-6/omega-3 ratio: .03	
Cholesterol: 133 milligrams	

Day 15

SOUP FAST

Take your pick from No-Cook Cold Cucumber Soup (below), Celery Soup (page 260), and Leek and Parsley Soup (page 267). Enjoy 1 to 1 ½ cups soup every 2 to 3 hours from waking until 3 hours before bedtime. Drink 8 ounces green tea or black tea or water in between soup servings. You may use regular or decaf tea. Do not engage in vigorous exercise today.

NO-COOK COLD CUCUMBER SOUP

6 medium cucumbers, peeled, halved lengthwise, seeds scraped out, and chopped

½ cup chopped fresh parsley

Juice of 1 lemon

1 ½ cups low-sodium chicken broth

1 ½ cups fat-free half-and-half

1 cup fat-free plain yogurt

Salt and freshly ground black pepper, to taste

Chopped fresh dill

In a food processor or blender, combine the cucumbers, parsley, and lemon juice and process until pureed. Remove half of the puree and set aside.

In a medium bowl, combine the broth, half-and-half, and yogurt. Add half of the broth mixture to the puree in the blender. Puree again to mix completely. Season with salt and pepper and transfer to a container and refrigerate. Repeat with the remaining puree and broth mixture.

Stir the soup before serving, garnished with fresh dill.

Makes 4-6 servings (enough for one person)

EXERCISE SUGGESTION

Light exercise (such as walking, stretching, housework, or yardwork) for 30 minutes early in the day.

DAY 15 NUTRITIONAL VALUES

Calories: 572
Fiber: 11 grams
Percent fat: 15
AA: 0 milligrams
EPA: 0 milligrams
GLA: 0 milligrams
DHA + DPA: 0 milligrams
Long-chain omega-6/omega-3 ratio: .01
Cholesterol: 22 milligrams

Day 16

BREAKFAST

- 2 (6") buckwheat pancakes (make extra for toasting later)

BUCKWHEAT PANCAKES

½ cup buckwheat flour (available at natural foods stores)

½ cup all-purpose flour

2 teaspoons double-acting baking powder

2 teaspoons sugar

1 teaspoon salt

½ stick (¼ cup) cold unsalted butter, cut into bits

2 large eggs

1 cup milk

1 ½ cups blueberries, preferably wild, picked over and, if large, halved

Vegetable oil for brushing the griddle

Pure maple syrup as an accompaniment

In a food processor blend together the flours, the baking powder, the sugar, and the salt, add the butter, and blend the mixture until it resembles fine meal. In a large bowl whisk together the eggs and the milk, add the flour mixture, and whisk the batter until it is combined well. Let the batter stand for 5 minutes and stir in the blueberries.

Preheat the oven to 200°F. Heat a griddle over moderate heat until it is hot enough to make drops of water scatter over its surface and brush it with the oil. Spoon the batter onto the griddle to form 3-inch rounds and cook the pancakes for 1 to 2 minutes on each side, or until they are golden. Transfer the pancakes as they are cooked to a heatproof platter and keep them warm in the oven. Serve the pancakes with the syrup.

- ½ cup liquid egg substitute, cooked in a nonstick pan coated with 1 teaspoon trans-free margarine
- 1 cup blueberries
- ⅓ cup low-fat granola cereal
- 6 ounces hot or cold brewed tea blended with ¼ cup recommended juice (see page 256)
- 1 fish oil and 1 borage oil capsule
- 6 ounces hot coffee if desired (sugar substitute and fat-free milk if needed)
- 16 ounces water between breakfast and lunch

Makes about twenty-four 3-inch pancakes

LUNCH

CLASSIC CAESAR SALAD

2 cups dark green lettuce

6 cherry tomatoes

⅓ cup sliced mushrooms

5 canned anchovy fillets, chopped

2 tablespoons reduced-fat Caesar dressing

In a large bowl, toss together the lettuce, tomatoes, and mushrooms. In a small bowl, whisk together the anchovies and dressing. Drizzle over the salad and serve.

TROPICAL GELATIN: 1 cup sugar-free gelatin made with leftover ¾ cup drained tropical mix fruit (from Day 14 dinner) with 1 tablespoon chopped pecans sprinkled on top

- 6 small whole-wheat crackers
- Calorie-free drink or 6 ounces tea
- 16 ounces water between lunch and dinner

DINNER

- 4 ounces cooked lean eye of round beef, thinly sliced and served au jus (make extra for roast beef sandwich tomorrow)
- 1 medium baked sweet potato with 1 teaspoon trans-free margarine

ROASTED VEGETABLES

½ cup sliced summer squash or parsnips

4 asparagus spears or ¼ cup green beans

¼ cup sliced red onion

¼ cup cubed peeled eggplant

6 cherry tomatoes

1 tablespoon olive oil

In a small roasting pan, combine the squash or parsnips, asparagus or beans, onion, eggplant, and tomatoes. Drizzle with the olive oil and toss to mix. Roast in a 400°F oven for about 15 minutes, or until the vegetables are browned and tender.

- 1 small whole-wheat dinner roll with 1 teaspoon trans-free margarine
- 2 fish oil capsules and 1 borage oil capsule
- Calorie-free drink or 6 ounces tea
- 16 ounces water before bed

SNACK

BAKED PEACH: 1 medium peach, peeled, cubed, and sprinkled with 2 tablespoons oats, 1 tablespoon slivered almonds, and 1 tablespoon trans-free margarine, then baked in 350°F oven for about 15 minutes.

EXERCISE SUGGESTION

Moderate circuit training (15/35/15) as described on page 241.

DAY 16 NUTRITIONAL VALUES

Calories: 1,528
Fiber: 22 grams
Percent fat: 37
AA: 25 milligrams
GLA: 450 milligrams
EPA: 693 milligrams
DHA + DPA: 626 milligrams
Long-chain omega-6/omega-3 ratio: .02
Cholesterol: 174 milligrams

Day 17

BREAKFAST

BAGEL AND LOX: 1 medium oat bran bagel with 1 tablespoon reduced-fat cream cheese and 3 ounces lox (smoked Chinook salmon)

- 6 ounces hot or cold brewed tea blended with ¼ cup recommended juice (see page 256)
- 1 fish oil and 1 borage oil capsule
- 6 ounces hot coffee if desired (sugar substitute and fat-free milk if needed)
- 16 ounces water between breakfast and lunch

LUNCH

OPEN-FACED ROAST BEEF SANDWICH: 1 slice whole-grain bread spread with 2 teaspoons Dijon mustard and 1 tablespoon cholesterol-free mayonnaise, then topped with 2 dark green lettuce leaves, 2 tomato slices, 2 ounces cooked lean eye of round beef (sliced as thinly as possible), and 1 ounce reduced-fat Swiss cheese

CORN AND BLACK BEAN SALAD: ⅓ cup canned yellow corn, ⅓ cup canned black beans (rinsed and drained), ¼ cup chopped red bell pepper, 1 ½ teaspoons canola oil, and lemon juice, vinegar, cilantro, and seasonings to taste (make extra salad for quesadilla tomorrow)

- 1 purple plum (or 1 serving other in-season high-polyphenol fruit)
- Calorie-free drink or 6 ounces tea
- 16 ounces water between lunch and dinner

DINNER

SEAFOOD PASTA ITALIANO

1 ½ teaspoons olive oil

3 sliced cherry tomatoes

½ cup chopped green bell pepper

2 ounces cooked shrimp

2 ounces cooked scallops

2 ounces cooked clams

½ cup cooked whole-wheat spaghetti

½ ounce Parmesan cheese, grated

Heat the oil in a medium nonstick skillet over medium heat. Add the tomatoes and bell pepper and cook, stirring, until softened. Add the shrimp, scallops, and clams and heat through. Add the pasta and toss to combine. Sprinkle with the Parmesan and broil until just crunchy before serving.

TOSSED SALAD: 1 cup romaine lettuce or baby spinach and 3 cherry tomatoes tossed with 1 tablespoon reduced-fat Italian dressing

- 2 fish oil capsules and 1 borage oil capsule
- Calorie-free drink or 6 ounces tea
- 16 ounces water before bed

SNACK

- ⅓ cup dry-roasted mixed nuts

EXERCISE SUGGESTION

Moderate exercise (from list on page 235) for 30 minutes.

DAY 17 NUTRITIONAL VALUES

Calories: 1,589	
Fiber: 25 grams	
Percent fat: 42	
AA: 124 milligrams	
GLA: 450 milligrams	
EPA: 976 milligrams	
DHA + DPA: 1,030 milligrams	
Long-chain omega-6/omega-3 ratio: .06	
Cholesterol: 248 milligrams	

Day 18

BREAKFAST

- 2 (6") buckwheat pancakes with 1 tablespoon reduced-fat cream cheese and 1 tablespoon sugar-free berry jam
- 8 ounces low-fat yogurt (any flavor)
- 6 ounces hot or cold brewed tea blended with ¼ cup recommended juice (see page 256)
- 1 fish oil and 1 borage oil capsule
- 6 ounces hot coffee if desired (sugar substitute and fat-free milk if needed)
- 16 ounces water between breakfast and lunch

LUNCH

CHICKEN QUESADILLA

2 ounces diced cooked skinless chicken breast

¼ sliced red onion

⅓ cup Corn and Black Bean Salad (from Day 17 lunch)

1 (10") whole-wheat flour tortilla

1 tablespoon reduced-fat sour cream

Mix together the chicken, onion, and salad. Spoon on half of the tortilla and top with the sour cream. Fold the tortilla over and serve.

TOMATO SALAD: 6 halved cherry tomatoes tossed with ½ tablespoon reduced-fat Italian salad dressing

- Calorie-free drink or 6 ounces tea
- 16 ounces water between lunch and dinner

DINNER

SHRIMP COCKTAIL: 6 ounces cooked shrimp (or other Category 1 or 2 fish; see page 217) served with 2 tablespoons cocktail sauce

- 1 medium baked sweet potato

ZUCCHINI BROIL: ½ cup shredded zucchini, cooked until soft in the microwave and then topped with 1 tablespoon plain bread crumbs and 1 ounce reduced-fat shredded mozzarella cheese and broiled

- 1 medium pear (or other in-season high-polyphenol fruit)
- 2 fish oil capsules and 1 borage oil capsule
- Calorie-free drink or 6 ounces tea
- 16 ounces water before bed

SNACK

- 2 pitted Medjool dates, split open and stuffed with 2 teaspoons peanut butter

EXERCISE SUGGESTION

Rest.

DAY 18 NUTRITIONAL VALUES

Calories: 1,597
Fiber: 27 grams
Percent fat: 17
AA: 121 milligrams
GLA: 450 milligrams
EPA: 831 milligrams
DHA + DPA: 639 milligrams
Long-chain omega-6/omega-3 ratio: .09
Cholesterol: 480 milligrams

Day 19

BREAKFAST

- 1 multigrain English muffin with 2 teaspoons trans-free margarine
- ½ cup 1% cottage cheese
- 1 cup blueberries
- 6 ounces hot or cold brewed tea blended with ¼ cup recommended juice (see page 256)
- 1 fish oil and 1 borage oil capsule
- 6 ounces hot coffee if desired (sugar substitute and fat-free milk if needed)
- 16 ounces water between breakfast and lunch

LUNCH

STEAK AND SWISS SANDWICH:

1 multigrain hamburger bun spread with 1½ teaspoons cholesterol-free mayonnaise and topped with 2 ounces cooked beef flank steak (thinly sliced against the grain) and 1 ounce reduced-fat Swiss cheese

- 1 cup red or purple seedless grapes
- Calorie-free drink or 6 ounces tea
- 16 ounces water between lunch and dinner

DINNER

SALMON WITH LENTILS AU GRATIN

4 ounces broiled or grilled sockeye salmon (or other Category 1 fish; see page 217) (cook extra for the Salmon Salad tomorrow)

1 cup cooked lentils

1 tablespoon plain bread crumbs

½ ounce Parmesan cheese, grated

Combine the salmon and lentils in a shallow oven-proof dish. Top with the bread crumbs and Parmesan and broil until lightly browned.

CAESAR SALAD: 1 cup romaine lettuce tossed with 1 tablespoon reduced-fat Caesar salad dressing and topped with 2 tablespoons plain croutons and ½ ounce grated Parmesan cheese

- 2 fish oil capsules and 1 borage oil capsule
- Calorie-free drink or 6 ounces tea
- 16 ounces water before bed

SNACK

- 1 cup sugar-free, fat-free frozen yogurt
- 2 tablespoons chopped pecans

EXERCISE SUGGESTION

Vigorous exercise (from list on page 236) for 30 minutes.

DAY 19 NUTRITIONAL VALUES

Calories: 1,670
Fiber: 34 grams
Percent fat: 28
AA: 68 milligrams
GLA: 450 milligrams
EPA: 1,139 milligrams
DHA + DPA: 1,300 milligrams
Long-chain omega-6/omega-3 ratio: .03
Cholesterol: 208 milligrams

Day 20

BREAKFAST

- ¾ cup Multigrain Cheerios with ½ cup 1% milk
- 1 small banana with 1 tablespoon peanut butter
- 6 ounces hot or cold brewed tea blended with ¼ cup recommended juice (see page 256)
- 1 fish oil and 1 borage oil capsule
- 6 ounces hot coffee if desired (sugar substitute and fat-free milk if needed)
- 16 ounces water

LUNCH

SALMON SALAD

2 cups romaine lettuce or baby spinach

3 ounces cooked sockeye salmon (or other Category 1 fish; see page 217)

6 chopped cherry tomatoes

¼ cup cubed unpeeled cucumber

2 tablespoons chopped green onion

1 ½ teaspoons olive oil

Vinegar, to taste

Herbs of choice

1 ounce feta cheese or soft goat cheese, crumbled

3 Greek olives or 15 pine nuts

In a medium bowl, toss together the lettuce, salmon, tomatoes, cucumber, and green onion. Mix together the olive oil, vinegar, and herbs. Drizzle over the salad and toss. Top with the cheese and olives or pine nuts and serve.

- 1 (4") whole-wheat pita

STRAWBERRY PARFAIT: 1 cup strawberries layered with 8 ounces low-fat vanilla yogurt

- Calorie-free drink or 6 ounces tea
- 16 ounces water

DINNER

CRANBERRIED ACORN SQUASH

2 tablespoons chopped cranberries

2 tablespoons crushed walnuts or pecans

½ medium acorn squash, seeds and tough fibers discarded

Mix together the cranberries and nuts and spoon the mixture into the cavity of the squash. Place the squash in a shallow baking dish and add ½" water to the bottom of the dish. Cover the squash loosely with foil and bake in a 400°F oven until tender, about 45 minutes.

- 3 ounces lean baked ham
- 1 cup cooked broccoli with 1 teaspoon trans-free margarine
- 1 cup sugar-free chocolate pudding
- 2 fish oil capsules and 1 borage oil capsule
- Calorie-free drink or 6 ounces tea
- 16 ounces water before bed

SNACK

- 4 (5") celery sticks with 1 tablespoon reduced-fat cream cheese

EXERCISE SUGGESTION

Light circuit training (15/20/15) as described on page 240.

DAY 20 NUTRITIONAL VALUES

Calories: 1,685
Fiber: 25 grams
Percent fat: 37
AA: 25 milligrams
GLA: 450 milligrams
EPA: 990 milligrams
DHA + DPA: 1,067 milligrams
Long-chain omega-6/omega-3 ratio: .01
Cholesterol: 202 milligrams

Day 21

BREAKFAST

- 2 (6") whole-grain frozen waffles with 2 teaspoons trans-free margarine and 1 tablespoon reduced-calorie pancake syrup
- ½ cup 1% cottage cheese
- 6 ounces hot or cold brewed tea blended with ¼ cup recommended juice (see page 256)
- 1 fish oil and 1 borage oil capsule
- 6 ounces hot coffee if desired (sugar substitute and fat-free milk if needed)
- 16 ounces water between breakfast and lunch

LUNCH

CHEESE TOAST: 1 slice whole-wheat toast topped with 2 ounces reduced-fat cheese and broiled until the cheese melts

- 1 cup canned, low-sodium tomato soup
- 8 ounces low-fat sugar-free fruit yogurt
- Calorie-free drink or 6 ounces tea
- 16 ounces water between lunch and dinner

DINNER

LEMON-CAPER TROUT

1 tablespoon all-purpose flour

Salt and freshly ground pepper, to taste

3 ounces trout fillet (or other Category 1 fish; see page 217)

1 teaspoon olive oil

Juice of 1 lemon

1 tablespoon capers, drained

2 teaspoons butter

In a shallow bowl, combine the flour and salt and pepper. Dredge the trout in the flour mixture and shake off excess. Heat the oil in a small skillet over medium heat. Add the fish and cook, turning once, until it flakes easily with a fork, about 6 minutes. Transfer the fish to a plate. To the skillet, add the lemon juice, capers, and butter and cook until slightly reduced, about 2 minutes. Pour the sauce over the fish and serve.

VEGETABLE SAUTÉ

2 teaspoons olive oil

12 (4") sweet potato sticks

3 baby carrots, cut into sticks

12 (4") zucchini sticks

½ small green onion, thinly sliced

Heat the oil in a small skillet over medium-high heat. Add the sweet potato and cook, stirring, until slightly softened. Add the carrots and cook for 2 minutes. Add the zucchini and green onion and cook, stirring, until the zucchini is crisp-tender and the sweet potato is cooked through.

- ½ cup cooked brown rice
- ½ cup tropical fruit (or 1 serving in-season high-polyphenol fruit)
- 2 fish oil capsules and 1 borage oil capsule
- Calorie-free drink or 6 ounces tea
- 16 ounces water before bed

SNACK

BAKED APPLE: ½ cup apple slices topped with 2 tablespoons oats, 2 tablespoons sliced almonds, and 1 teaspoon trans-free margarine, then baked in a 350°F oven until softened, 15 to 30 minutes.

EXERCISE SUGGESTION

Rest.

DAY 21 NUTRITIONAL VALUES

Calories: 1,637
Fiber: 18 grams
Percent fat: 34
AA: 102 milligrams
GLA: 450 milligrams
EPA: 938 milligrams
DHA + DPA: 802 milligrams
Long-chain omega-6/omega-3 ratio: .06
Cholesterol: 186 milligrams

Day 22

BREAKFAST

- ⅔ cup muesli cereal with ½ cup 1% milk
- 1 small peach (or 1 serving other in-season high-polyphenol fruit)
- 1 ounce reduced-fat mozzarella cheese
- 6 ounces hot or cold brewed tea blended with ¼ cup recommended juice (see page 256)
- 1 fish oil and 1 borage oil capsule
- 6 ounces hot coffee if desired (sugar substitute and fat-free milk if needed)
- 16 ounces water between breakfast and lunch

LUNCH

EASY CHILI

4 ounces ground beef (95% lean)

½ cup canned kidney beans, rinsed and drained

½ cup canned diced tomatoes

Chili seasoning, to taste

2 ounces reduced-fat Cheddar cheese, grated

Coat a nonstick skillet with cooking spray and heat over medium heat. Add the beef and cook, breaking up the meat with a wooden spoon, until browned, about 5 minutes. Add the beans, tomatoes, and chili seasoning and cook, stirring occasionally, until thickened slightly, about 10 minutes. Serve with the cheese sprinkled on top.

- 6 small whole-wheat crackers
- 1 medium apple (with skin)
- Calorie-free drink or 6 ounces tea
- 16 ounces water between lunch and dinner

DINNER

CHICKEN PARMESAN WITH PASTA

1 tablespoon olive oil

4 ounces skinless chicken breast

¼ cup prepared marinara sauce

1 ounce reduced-fat mozzarella cheese, grated

2 tablespoons seasoned dry bread crumbs

½ cup cooked whole-wheat spaghetti

Heat the oil in a medium ovenproof skillet over medium-high heat. Add the chicken and cook, turning once, until cooked through. Add the marinara sauce and cook until heated through. Sprinkle the mozzarella over the chicken, and sprinkle the bread crumbs on top. Place the skillet under the broiler and broil until the mozzarella is melted and the bread crumbs are golden brown. Place the spaghetti on a serving plate and top with the chicken and sauce.

GREEN BEANS VINAIGRETTE: 1 cup cooked green beans mixed with 1 tablespoon diced red bell pepper, then topped with 1 tablespoon reduced-sugar or sugar-free berry jam mixed with 2 teaspoons fruit-based vinegar

- 1 fish oil and 1 borage oil capsule
- Calorie-free drink or 6 ounces tea
- 16 ounces water before bed

SNACK

CRAB SPREAD: 3 ounces imitation crabmeat (surimi) mixed with 2 tablespoons diced celery, 1 tablespoon cholesterol-free mayonnaise, and 1 teaspoon chopped fresh parsley

- 6 small whole-wheat crackers

EXERCISE SUGGESTION

Light exercise (such as walking, stretching, housework, or yardwork) for 30 minutes.

DAY 22 NUTRITIONAL VALUES

Calories: 1,731
Fiber: 25 grams
Percent fat: 28
AA: 59 milligrams
EPA: 567 milligrams
DHA + DPA: 562 milligrams
Long-chain omega 6/omega-3 ratio: .05
Cholesterol: 244 milligrams

Day 23

BREAKFAST

- 2 bran muffins (made from scratch) with 1 tablespoon reduced-fat cream cheese

ALL-BRAN MUFFINS

Kellogg's All-Bran Bran Buds Muffins

1 ½ cups All-Bran Bran Buds

1 ¼ cups all-purpose flour

½ cup sugar

1 tablespoon baking powder

¼ teaspoon salt

1 ¼ cups fat-free milk

2 egg whites

¼ cup vegetable oil

In electric blender or food processor, crush Kellogg's All-Bran Bran Buds cereal to fine crumbs.

In mixing bowl, stir together crushed cereal, flour, sugar, baking powder, and salt. Set aside.

In large mixing bowl, combine milk, egg whites, and oil; mix well. Add cereal mixture, stirring only until combined. Portion batter evenly into twelve 2½-inch muffin-pan cups coated with cooking spray.

Bake at 400°F for 20 minutes or until lightly browned. Serve warm.

Makes 12 servings

- 1 medium peach (or 1 serving of other in-season high-polyphenol fruit)
- 6 ounces hot or cold brewed tea blended with ¼ cup recommended juice (see page 256)
- 1 fish oil and 1 borage oil capsule
- 6 ounces hot coffee if desired (sugar substitute and fat-free milk if needed)
- 16 ounces water between breakfast and lunch

LUNCH

BLUE CHEESE–STEAK SALAD

2 cups dark green lettuce

¼ cup sliced carrot

¼ cup sliced red onion

2 tablespoons bottled Champagne salad dressing

1 ounce blue cheese, crumbled

3 ounces cooked beef flank steak, thinly sliced against the grain

In a bowl, toss together the lettuce, carrot, and onion. Drizzle with the dressing and toss. Sprinkle the cheese over the salad and top with the steak.

- 1 small whole-wheat roll with 1 teaspoon trans-free margarine
- 2 kiwifruit (or 1 serving other in-season high-polyphenol fruit)
- Calorie-free drink or 6 ounces tea
- 16 ounces water between lunch and dinner

DINNER

- 3 ounces cooked lean top loin pork roast
- 1 medium baked sweet potato with 1 tablespoon trans-free margarine
- 1 cup cooked brussels sprouts or broccoli with 1 ½ teaspoons trans-free margarine
- ½ cup fat-free, sugar-free vanilla yogurt with ½ cup raspberries
- 1 fish oil and 1 borage oil capsule
- Calorie-free drink or 6 ounces tea
- 16 ounces water before bed

SNACK

SALMON SPREAD: 2 ounces canned pink salmon mixed with 2 tablespoons reduced-fat cream cheese and herbs and seasonings of choice

- 4 small whole-wheat crackers

EXERCISE SUGGESTION

Moderate circuit training (15/35/15) as described on page 241.

DAY 23 NUTRITIONAL VALUES

Calories: 1,781
Fiber: 26 grams
Percent fat: 39
AA: 58 milligrams
EPA: 834 milligrams
DHA + DPA: 723 milligrams
Long-chain omega-6/omega-3 ratio: .04
Cholesterol: 188 milligrams

Day 24

BREAKFAST

- 1 multigrain English muffin with 2 teaspoons trans-free margarine
- ½ cup grapefruit sections and ½ cup orange sections (or 1 serving other in-season high-polyphenol fruit)
- 6 ounces hot or cold brewed tea blended with ¼ cup recommended juice (see page 256)
- 1 fish oil and 1 borage oil capsule
- 6 ounces hot coffee if desired (sugar substitute and fat-free milk if needed)
- 16 ounces water between breakfast and lunch

LUNCH

TUNA SALAD: 2 cups red leaf lettuce, ¼ cup chopped red onion, and ¼ cup grated carrots tossed with 2 tablespoons reduced-fat ranch dressing, then topped with 5 ounces grilled or broiled bluefin tuna

THREE-BEAN SALAD: ¼ cup canned green beans (rinsed and drained), ¼ cup canned chickpeas (rinsed and drained), and ¼ cup canned wax beans (rinsed and drained) tossed with 1 tablespoon canola oil, vinegar to taste, and herbs and seasonings of choice

- 4 small whole-wheat crackers
- Calorie-free drink or 6 ounces tea
- 16 ounces water between lunch and dinner

DINNER

- 3 ounces baked skinless chicken breast (make extra for the chicken pita tomorrow)
- ¾ cup cooked brown rice mixed with ½ cup cooked green peas and pearl onions and ½ cup cooked carrots
- 1 whole-wheat dinner roll with 1 teaspoon trans-free margarine
- 12 Bing cherries
- 1 fish oil and 1 borage oil capsule
- Calorie-free drink or 6 ounces tea
- 16 ounces water before bed

SNACK

- 8 ounces low-fat vanilla yogurt
- ¼ cup Fiber One cereal

EXERCISE SUGGESTION

Moderate exercise (as listed on page 235) for 30 minutes.

DAY 24 NUTRITIONAL VALUES

Calories: 1,759
Fiber: 33 grams
Percent fat: 27
AA: 78 milligrams
EPA: 872 milligrams
DHA + DPA: 2,076 milligrams
Long-chain omega-6/omega-3 ratio: .03
Cholesterol: 202 milligrams

Day 25

BREAKFAST

- 2 bran muffins (made from scratch) with 1 tablespoon reduced-fat cream cheese
- 1 small peach (or 1 serving other in-season high-polyphenol fruit)
- 6 ounces hot or cold brewed tea blended with 1/4 cup recommended juice (see page 256)
- 1 fish oil and 1 borage oil capsule
- 6 ounces hot coffee if desired (sugar substitute and fat-free milk if needed)
- 16 ounces water between breakfast and lunch

LUNCH

GREEK CHICKEN PITA: 2 ounces diced baked skinless chicken, 1/2 cup diced cucumber, 1 ounce feta cheese, and 2 tablespoons vinaigrette stuffed into 1 (4") whole-wheat pita

TOMATO-BULGUR SALAD: 1/2 cup tabbouleh (bulgur wheat salad) tossed with 1/4 cup chopped tomato, 1 tablespoon olive oil, and lemon juice and vinegar to taste

- Calorie-free drink or 6 ounces tea
- 16 ounces water between lunch and dinner

DINNER

GRILLED DIJON SALMON: 6 ounces sockeye salmon (or other Category 1 fish; see page 217) brushed with 1 teaspoon canola oil and 1 tablespoon Dijon mustard and grilled or broiled

- 3/4 cup cooked wild rice

PEAS AND CARROTS: 1/2 cup cooked green peas and 3/4 cup diced cooked carrots tossed with 1 1/2 teaspoons trans-free margarine

FRUIT GELATIN: 1 cup sugar-free gelatin made with 8.5 ounces canned fruit (drained)

- 1 fish oil and 1 borage oil capsule
- Calorie-free drink or 6 ounces tea
- 16 ounces water before bed

SNACK

- 4 (4") celery stalks with 1 tablespoon peanut butter

EXERCISE SUGGESTION

Rest.

DAY 25 NUTRITIONAL VALUES

Calories: 1,868
Fiber: 24 grams
Percent fat: 40
AA: 54 milligrams
EPA: 1,108 milligrams
DHA + DPA: 1,417 milligrams
Long-chain omega-6/omega-3 ratio: .02
Cholesterol: 219 milligrams

Day 26

BREAKFAST

- 1 medium whole-wheat bagel with 1 ounce reduced-fat cream cheese flavored with chives, scallions, or walnuts
- 1 cup mixed fresh berries (or ½ cup frozen mixed berries) blended with 8 ounces low-fat vanilla yogurt
- 6 ounces hot or cold brewed tea blended with ¼ cup recommended juice (see page 256)
- 1 fish oil and 1 borage oil capsule
- 6 ounces hot coffee if desired (sugar substitute and fat-free milk if needed)
- 16 ounces water between breakfast and lunch

LUNCH

SALMON PASTA SALAD WITH CRACKERS

3 ounces canned pink salmon
½ cup cooked whole-wheat macaroni
¼ cup diced red bell pepper
¼ cup diced celery
¼ cup diced red onion
1 tablespoon olive oil
Lemon juice, to taste
Herbs and seasonings of choice
6 whole-wheat crackers

In a medium bowl, combine the salmon, macaroni, bell pepper, celery, and onion. Mix together the olive oil, lemon juice, and herbs and seasonings. Drizzle the dressing over the salad and toss. Serve with the crackers.

MARINATED CUCUMBERS: 1 cup sliced cucumbers tossed with 1 teaspoon canola oil, vinegar to taste, fresh dill, and seasonings of choice

- Calorie-free drink or 6 ounces tea
- 16 ounces water between lunch and dinner

DINNER

SPICY MAPLE PORK MEDALLIONS

5 ounces pork tenderloin medallions

1 cup dark beer

1 tablespoon real maple syrup

Cayenne pepper, to taste

Place the pork in a shallow dish and pour the beer over it. Cover and marinate in the refrigerator for 4 to 12 hours. Drain the pork and pat dry. Brush the pork with the maple syrup and season with cayenne. Grill or broil the pork, turning once, until just cooked through, 4 to 6 minutes.

- 1 cup mashed rutabaga and russet potatoes with 1 teaspoon trans-free margarine
- 1 cup cooked broccoli with 1 tablespoon Parmesan cheese
- 1 small whole-wheat roll with 1 teaspoon margarine
- 1 fish oil and 1 borage oil capsule
- Calorie-free drink or 6 ounces tea
- 16 ounces water before bed

SNACK

- 1 (4") whole-wheat pita with 1 ounce reduced-fat Cheddar cheese and ¼ cup chopped red bell pepper

EXERCISE SUGGESTION

Vigorous exercise (as listed on page 236) for 30 minutes.

DAY 26 NUTRITIONAL VALUES

Calories: 1,755
Fiber: 36 grams
Percent fat: 29
AA: 65 milligrams
EPA: 1,078 milligrams
DHA + DPA: 966 milligrams
Long-chain omega-6/omega-3 ratio: .03
Cholesterol: 147 milligrams

Day 27

BREAKFAST

- 1 cup muesli cereal with ¾ cup 1% milk
- 1 small peach (or 1 serving other in-season high-polyphenol fruit)
- 1 ounce reduced-fat mozzarella cheese
- 6 ounces hot or cold brewed tea blended with ¼ cup recommended juice (see page 256)
- 1 fish oil and 1 borage oil capsule
- 6 ounces hot coffee if desired (sugar substitute and fat-free milk if needed)
- 16 ounces water between breakfast and lunch

LUNCH

HAM AND CHEESE SANDWICH: 2 slices whole-wheat bread spread with 2 teaspoons cholesterol-free mayonnaise and topped with 3 ounces extra-lean sliced ham, 1 ounce reduced-fat cheese, 1 leaf dark green lettuce, and 2 slices tomato

- 1 medium apple (with skin) or 1 serving other in-season high-polyphenol fruit
- Calorie-free drink or 6 ounces tea
- 16 ounces water between lunch and dinner

DINNER

BEEF AND VEGETABLE TERIYAKI OVER PASTA

5 ounces beef flank steak

2 tablespoons teriyaki sauce

1 tablespoon peanut oil

½ cup snow peas

½ cup sliced red bell pepper

½ cup sliced carrots

½ cup cooked whole-wheat pasta

2 tablespoons sesame seeds, toasted

Place the steak in a shallow bowl and drizzle with the teriyaki sauce. Cover and marinate in the refrigerator for 6 to 10 hours.

Heat the oil in a medium nonstick skillet over medium-high heat. Add the steak and cook, turning once, to desired doneness. Transfer the steak to a plate and keep warm. Add the snow peas, bell pepper, and carrots to the skillet and cook, stirring, until crisp-tender, about 5 minutes.

Thinly slice the steak against the grain. In a bowl, toss together the pasta, steak strips, and sautéed vegetables. Sprinkle with the sesame seeds and serve.

- ½ cup raspberries with ¾ cup sugar-free dark chocolate mousse
- 1 fish oil and 1 borage oil capsule
- Calorie-free drink or 6 ounces tea
- 16 ounces water before bed

SNACK

TUNA SPREAD: 3 ounces drained canned white tuna mixed with 2 tablespoons diced celery and 2 teaspoons cholesterol-free mayonnaise

- 6 small whole-wheat crackers

EXERCISE SUGGESTION

Moderate circuit training (15/35/15) as described on page 241.

DAY 27 NUTRITIONAL VALUES

Calories: 1,789
Fiber: 31 grams
Percent fat: 34
AA: 43 milligrams
EPA: 558 milligrams
DHA + DPA: 790 milligrams
Long-chain omega-6/omega-3 ratio: .03
Cholesterol: 207 milligrams

Day 28

BREAKFAST

- 2 slices whole-wheat toast with 1 tablespoon nut butter
- 1 medium banana, sliced
- ¾ cup 1% milk
- 6 ounces hot or cold brewed tea blended with ¼ cup recommended juice (see page 256)
- 1 fish oil and 1 borage oil capsule
- 6 ounces hot coffee if desired (sugar substitute and fat-free milk if needed)
- 16 ounces water between breakfast and lunch

LUNCH

LENTIL SOUP

¼ cup chopped red onion
¼ cup diced carrot
¼ cup diced celery
½ cup cooked lentils
1 cup fat-free chicken broth

Coat a nonstick saucepan with cooking spray and place over medium heat. Add the onion, carrot, and celery and cook, stirring, until softened, about 5 minutes. Add the lentils and stir well. Add the broth, cover, and bring just to a simmer before serving.

ANTIPASTO SALAD

2 teaspoons olive oil
Vinegar, to taste
Seasonings of choice
2 cups romaine lettuce
2 ounces reduced-fat mozzarella cheese, grated
2 ounces sliced beef salami
5 cherry tomatoes
5 large black olives

Mix together the olive oil, vinegar, and seasonings. Place the lettuce in a large bowl and toss with the dressing. Top the salad with the mozzarella, salami, tomatoes, and olives and serve.

- 4 small whole-wheat crackers
- Calorie-free drink or 6 ounces tea
- 16 ounces water between lunch and dinner

DINNER

CRAB OMELET

1 teaspoon canola oil

¼ cup diced green bell pepper

¼ cup diced red bell pepper

1 cup liquid egg substitute

3 ounces cooked Alaskan king
crabmeat, flaked

Heat the oil in a medium nonstick skillet over medium-high heat. Add the bell peppers and cook, stirring, until softened. Add the egg substitute, reduce the heat, and cook without stirring until the bottom sets, about 3 minutes. Add the crab and carefully fold the egg over to cover the crab. Cook for 2 minutes. Turn the omelet and cook until set throughout, 3 to 5 minutes longer.

- 1 slice whole-wheat bread with 1 teaspoon trans-free margarine
- 1 medium orange (or 1 serving other in-season high-polyphenol fruit)
- 1 fish oil and 1 borage oil capsule
- Calorie-free drink or 6 ounces tea
- 16 ounces water before bed

SNACK

- ⅓ cup dry-roasted mixed nuts

EXERCISE SUGGESTION

Rest.

DAY 28 NUTRITIONAL VALUES

Calories: 1,825
Fiber: 33 grams
Percent fat: 42
AA: 37 milligrams
EPA: 611 milligrams
DHA + DPA: 366 milligrams
Long-chain omega 6/omega-3 ratio: .04
Cholesterol: 126 milligrams

Day 29

BREAKFAST

- ½ cup Kellogg's All-Bran cereal with ¾ cup strawberries and ½ cup 1% milk
- 1 multigrain English muffin with 1 ounce reduced-fat cheese
- 6 ounces hot or cold brewed tea blended with ¼ cup recommended juice (see page 256)
- 1 fish oil and 1 borage oil capsule
- 6 ounces hot coffee if desired (sugar substitute and fat-free milk if needed)
- 16 ounces water between breakfast and lunch

LUNCH

CURRIED CHICKEN SALAD

2 tablespoons cholesterol-free mayonnaise

2 teaspoons curry powder

Lemon juice, to taste

Seasonings of choice

3 ounces diced cooked skinless chicken breast

½ cup cooked brown rice

¼ cup diced celery

Mix together the mayonnaise, curry powder, lemon juice, and seasonings. In a medium bowl, combine the chicken, rice, and celery. Add the dressing and toss to coat.

FRUIT SALAD: ¼ cup sliced peach, ¼ cup sliced seedless red grapes, ¼ cup blueberries, and ¼ cup kiwi slices or cubed mango

- Calorie-free drink or 6 ounces tea
- 16 ounces water between lunch and dinner

DINNER

BLUE CHEESEBURGER: 1 whole-wheat hamburger bun with 3 ounces cooked ground beef (95% lean), 1 tablespoon crumbled blue cheese, and 1 slice red onion

THREE-BEAN SALAD: ¼ cup canned green beans (rinsed and drained), ¼ cup canned chickpeas (rinsed and drained), and ¼ cup canned wax beans (rinsed and drained) tossed with 1 tablespoon canola oil, vinegar to taste, and seasonings of choice

- 1 fish oil and 1 borage oil capsule
- Calorie-free drink or 6 ounces tea
- 16 ounces water before bed

SNACK

SALMON SPREAD: 3 ounces canned pink salmon mixed with 2 tablespoons cholesterol-free reduced-fat mayonnaise and herbs and seasonings of choice

- 4 small whole-wheat crackers

EXERCISE SUGGESTION

Light exercise (such as walking, stretching, housework, or yardwork) for 30 minutes.

DAY 29 NUTRITIONAL VALUES

Calories: 1,765
Fiber: 30 grams
Percent fat: 33
AA: 109 milligrams
EPA: 1,078 milligrams
DHA + DPA: 966 milligrams
Long-chain omega-6/omega-3 ratio: .05
Cholesterol: 256 milligrams

Day 30

BREAKFAST

VEGETABLE SCRAMBLE WRAP

2 tablespoons chopped green bell pepper

2 tablespoons chopped red onion

¾ cup liquid egg substitute

1 (10") whole-wheat flour tortilla

Coat a small nonstick skillet with cooking spray and place over medium heat. Add the bell pepper and onion and cook, stirring, until softened. Add the egg substitute and cook, stirring occasionally, until cooked to your liking. Spoon the egg mixture onto the tortilla, roll up, and serve.

- ½ medium grapefruit (or 1 serving other in-season high-polyphenol fruit)
- 6 ounces hot or cold brewed tea blended with ¼ cup recommended juice (see page 256)
- 1 fish oil and 1 borage oil capsule
- 6 ounces hot coffee if desired (sugar substitute and fat-free milk if needed)
- 16 ounces water between breakfast and lunch

LUNCH

HAM AND PLUM SALAD

2 cups dark green lettuce or baby spinach

¼ cup bite-size chunks fresh or canned plums (rinsed and drained if canned)

2 ounces reduced-fat mozzarella cheese, grated

2 ounces cubed lean ham

4 cherry tomatoes, sliced

1 tablespoon vinaigrette

In a large bowl, combine the lettuce, plums, mozzarella, ham, and tomatoes. Drizzle with the vinaigrette and toss.

- 6 small whole-wheat crackers
- 1 ½ cups red seedless grapes
- Calorie-free drink or 6 ounces tea
- 16 ounces water between lunch and dinner

DINNER

OYSTER PO' BOY: 1 medium whole-grain hoagie with 4 ounces (8 medium) breaded and fried oysters, ¼ cup sliced red onion, and 1 tablespoon reduced-fat ranch salad dressing

- 1 medium pear (or 1 serving other high-polyphenol fruit of choice)
- 1 fish oil and 1 borage oil capsule
- Calorie-free drink or 6 ounces tea
- 16 ounces water before bed

SNACK

- 4 Medjool dates, split open and stuffed with 2 tablespoons peanut butter

EXERCISE SUGGESTION

Vigorous circuit training (15/45/15) as described on page 242.

DAY 30 NUTRITIONAL VALUES

Calories: 1,899
Fiber: 27 grams
Percent fat: 28
AA: 82 milligrams
EPA: 597 milligrams
DHA + DPA: 552 milligrams
Long-chain omega-6/omega-3 ratio: .07
Cholesterol: 165 milligrams

Day 31

BREAKFAST

- 2 (7") whole-grain frozen waffles or pancakes with 2 teaspoons trans-free margarine, and apple topping (below)

WARM APPLE TOPPING: 1 medium apple, peeled, sliced, and cooked in a nonstick pan until soft

- 6 ounces hot or cold brewed tea blended with ¼ cup recommended juice (see page 256)
- 1 fish oil and 1 borage oil capsule
- 6 ounces hot coffee if desired (sugar substitute and fat-free milk if needed)
- 16 ounces water between breakfast and lunch

LUNCH

TUNA MELT

3 ounces drained canned white tuna
1 tablespoon reduced-fat mayonnaise
1 tablespoon pickle relish
1 slice whole-wheat bread, toasted
1 ounce reduced-fat cheese

Mix together the tuna, mayonnaise, and relish. Spread on the toast and top with the cheese. Broil until the cheese melts.

- 8 ounces low-fat sugar-free fruited yogurt blended with ½ cup frozen berries
- Calorie-free drink or 6 ounces tea
- 16 ounces water between lunch and dinner

DINNER

SPAGHETTI WITH RED MEAT SAUCE

4 ounces ground beef (95% lean)
½ cup prepared marinara sauce
½ cup cooked whole-wheat spaghetti
1 tablespoon grated Parmesan cheese

Coat a medium nonstick pan with cooking spray and place over medium heat. Add the beef and cook, breaking up the meat with a wooden spoon, until browned. Add the marinara sauce and cook until heated through. Add the pasta and toss to coat. Sprinkle with the Parmesan and serve.

TOSSED SALAD: 1 cup romaine lettuce, ½ cup sliced fresh mushrooms, and 6 cherry tomatoes tossed with 1 tablespoon reduced-fat Italian dressing

STRAWBERRY PARFAIT: ½ cup reduced-fat ricotta cheese layered with ½ cup strawberries

- 1 fish oil and 1 borage oil capsule
- Calorie-free drink or 6 ounces tea
- 16 ounces water before bed

SNACK

1 large carrot, peeled and cut into sticks, with 1 tablespoon reduced-fat ranch dressing

EXERCISE SUGGESTION

Moderate exercise (as listed on page 235) for 30 minutes.

DAY 31 NUTRITIONAL VALUES

Calories: 1,853
Fiber: 23 grams
Percent fat: 29
AA: 72 milligrams
EPA: 558 milligrams
DHA + DPA: 790 milligrams
Long-chain omega-6/omega-3 ratio: .05
Cholesterol: 243 milligrams

Day 32

BREAKFAST

- 2 slices whole-wheat toast with 1 tablespoon nut butter
- 1 medium banana, sliced
- 1 cup 1% milk
- 6 ounces hot or cold brewed tea blended with ¼ cup recommended juice (see page 256)
- 1 fish oil and 1 borage oil capsule
- 6 ounces hot coffee if desired (sugar substitute and fat-free milk if needed)
- 16 ounces water between breakfast and lunch

LUNCH

CHEESEBURGER: 1 multigrain hamburger bun with 3 ounces cooked ground beef (95% lean) and 1 ounce reduced-fat cheese

SPINACH SALAD: 1 cup baby spinach, ¼ cup unpeeled cucumber slices, 6 cherry tomatoes, and 4–6 thin slices red onion tossed with 1 tablespoon vinaigrette

- Calorie-free drink or 6 ounces tea
- 16 ounces water between lunch and dinner

DINNER

- 3 ounces cooked lean pork loin chop

ROASTED VEGETABLES: ¾ cup green beans and ¾ cup cubed root vegetables (red potatoes, parsnips, rutabagas, turnips) tossed with 1 tablespoon melted trans-free margarine and roasted in a 400°F oven until browned and softened

- 1 cup cooked carrots topped with 1½ teaspoons trans-free margarine and 2 teaspoons light brown sugar

- 1 medium apple (with skin)
- 1 fish oil and 1 borage oil capsule
- Calorie-free drink or 6 ounces tea
- 16 ounces water before bed

SNACK

- ⅓ cup dry-roasted mixed nuts

EXERCISE SUGGESTION

Rest.

DAY 32 NUTRITIONAL VALUES

Calories: 1,794
Fiber: 30 grams
Percent fat: 37
AA: 78 milligrams
EPA: 360 milligrams
DHA + DPA: 240 milligrams
Long-chain omega-6/omega-3 ratio: .13
Cholesterol: 154 milligrams

Day 33

BREAKFAST

- 1 multigrain English muffin
- 1 slice reduced-fat cheese melted on top

CITRUS SALAD: ½ cup grapefruit sections and ½ cup orange sections sprinkled with 3 chopped dried plums (prunes), or 1 serving other in-season high-polyphenol fruit

- 6 ounces hot or cold brewed tea blended with ¼ cup recommended juice (see page 256)
- 1 fish oil and 1 borage oil capsule
- 6 ounces hot coffee if desired (sugar substitute and fat-free milk if needed)
- 16 ounces water between breakfast and lunch

LUNCH

CHICKEN SALAD WITH CRACKERS

3 ounces chopped cooked skinless chicken breast

¼ cup chopped red onion

¼ cup chopped celery

¼ cup chopped fresh parsley

1 tablespoon cholesterol-free mayonnaise

8 small whole-wheat crackers

Mix together the chicken, onion, celery, parsley, and mayonnaise. Serve with the crackers.

MARINATED CUCUMBERS: ½ cup sliced cucumbers tossed with 1 teaspoon canola oil, vinegar to taste, and seasonings of choice

- 1 medium apple (with skin)
- Calorie-free drink or 6 ounces tea
- 16 ounces water between lunch and dinner

DINNER

SHRIMP CREOLE

1 tablespoon olive oil

¼ cup diced celery

¼ cup diced red or green bell pepper

¼ cup diced shallots

6 cherry tomatoes, diced

5 ounces cooked shrimp

Heat the oil in a medium skillet over medium heat. Add the celery, bell pepper, shallots, and tomatoes and cook, stirring, until softened. Add the cooked shrimp and heat through. (Make extra for the soup tomorrow.)

- 1 cup cooked brown rice
- ½ cup cooked okra mixed with ½ cup stewed tomatoes
- 1 fish oil and 1 borage oil capsule
- Calorie-free drink or 6 ounces tea
- 16 ounces water before bed

SNACK

BERRIES AND YOGURT: 8 ounces low-fat vanilla yogurt mixed with ¼ cup strawberries, ¼ cup raspberries, and ¼ cup blueberries

EXERCISE SUGGESTION

Vigorous exercise (as listed on page 236) for 20 minutes.

DAY 33 NUTRITIONAL VALUES

Calories: 1,834	
Fiber: 25 grams	
Percent fat: 26	
AA: 123 milligrams	
EPA: 724 milligrams	
DHA + DPA: 618 milligrams	
Long-chain omega-6/omega-3 ratio: .09	
Cholesterol: 365 milligrams	

Day 34

BREAKFAST

YOGURT SUNDAE: 8 ounces low-fat vanilla yogurt mixed with ¾ cup frozen mixed berries and topped with ⅓ cup low-fat granola

- 6 ounces hot or cold brewed tea blended with ¼ cup recommended juice (see page 256)
- 1 fish oil and 1 borage oil capsule
- 6 ounces hot coffee if desired (sugar substitute and fat-free milk if needed)
- 16 ounces water between breakfast and lunch

LUNCH

CREOLE SHRIMP SOUP: ¾ cup leftover Shrimp Creole (from Day 33) mixed with 1 cup canned, low-sodium tomato soup

- 1 ounce whole-wheat pretzels
- 1 cup sugar-free chocolate pudding
- Calorie-free drink or 6 ounces tea
- 16 ounces water between lunch and dinner

DINNER

OPEN-FACED REUBEN

1 tablespoon reduced-fat Thousand Island dressing

1 slice pumpernickel bread, toasted

¼ cup sauerkraut

4 ounces cooked lean eye of round beef, thinly sliced

1 slice reduced-fat Swiss cheese

Spread the dressing on the bread and top with the sauerkraut. Layer the beef and then the cheese on top. Broil until the cheese melts.

CORN AND BLACK BEAN SALAD: ⅓ cup cooked yellow corn, ⅓ cup canned black beans (rinsed and drained), and ¼ cup chopped red bell pepper mixed with 1 tablespoon canola oil, lemon juice to taste, vinegar to taste, chopped fresh cilantro, and seasonings of choice

- 1 serving in-season high-polyphenol fruit
- 1 fish oil and 1 borage oil capsule
- Calorie-free drink or 6 ounces tea
- 16 ounces water before bed

SNACK

- ½ medium banana with 1 tablespoon chocolate-flavored hazelnut spread

EXERCISE SUGGESTION

Moderate circuit training (15/35/15) as described on page 241.

DAY 34 NUTRITIONAL VALUES

Calories: 1,876
Fiber: 26 grams
Percent fat: 22
AA: 23 milligrams
EPA: 451 milligrams
DHA + DPA: 333 milligrams
Long-chain omega-6/omega-3 ratio: .05
Cholesterol: 243 milligrams

Day 35

BREAKFAST

BAGEL AND LOX: 1 medium oat bran bagel with 2 tablespoons reduced-fat cream cheese, 3 ounces lox (smoked Chinook salmon), and 2 teaspoons drained capers

- 6 ounces hot or cold brewed tea blended with ¼ cup recommended juice (see page 256)
- 1 fish oil and 1 borage oil capsule
- 6 ounces hot coffee if desired (sugar substitute and fat-free milk if needed)
- 16 ounces water between breakfast and lunch

LUNCH

PITA PIZZA

1 (4") whole-wheat pita

¼ cup marinara sauce

2 ounces diced cooked Canadian bacon

¼ cup chopped red onion

¼ cup sliced mushrooms

2 ounces reduced-fat mozzarella cheese, shredded

Top the pita with the marinara sauce, bacon, onion, mushrooms, and mozzarella. Place on a baking sheet and bake in a 350°F oven for 15 minutes, or until the pita is heated through and the cheese is melted.

- 1 ½ cups red or purple seedless grapes
- Calorie-free drink or 6 ounces tea
- 16 ounces water between lunch and dinner

DINNER

LEMON-HERB HALIBUT

1 tablespoon trans-free margarine

6 ounces Greenland halibut (or other Category 1 fish; see page 217)

2 tablespoons lemon juice

2 tablespoons chopped fresh parsley

¼ teaspoon chopped fresh dill

Melt the margarine in a nonstick skillet over medium-high heat. Add the fish and cook, turning once, until it flakes easily with a fork, 6 to 8 minutes. Transfer the fish to a plate and keep warm. To the skillet, add the lemon juice, parsley, and dill and cook, stirring, until slightly reduced, about 2 minutes. Pour the sauce over the fish and serve.

- ¾ cup cooked brown rice mixed with 1 cup cooked carrots and 1 cup cooked green beans
- ⅓ cup yogurt cheese (to make, drain plain or vanilla yogurt in a strainer over cheesecloth for 24 hours) mixed with ½ cup fresh or canned pineapple chunks
- 1 fish oil and 1 borage oil capsule
- Calorie-free drink or 6 ounces tea
- 16 ounces water before bed

SNACK

PITA CRISPS: 1 (4″) whole-wheat pita, cut into 4 sections and baked in a 350°F oven until crisp

- 2 tablespoons roasted red pepper hummus

EXERCISE SUGGESTION
Rest.

DAY 35 NUTRITIONAL VALUES

Calories: 1,792	
Fiber: 24 grams	
Percent fat: 35	
AA: 134 milligrams	
EPA: 1,661 milligrams	
DHA: 1,580 milligrams	
Long-chain omega-6/omega-3 ratio: .04	
Cholesterol: 203 milligrams	

Optimal Maintenance Phase Menus

You can enter the Optimal Maintenance Phase whenever you are ready. You often hit a plateau while losing weight, and sometimes moving up in calories for a week and then backing down to a caloric reduction level works best to move your body back into a weight-loss phase. The biggest challenge is to not get so frustrated that a binge occurs or that you just give up altogether and slide back into old habits. Rely on the principles of the Gene Smart Diet Pyramid and eat sensibly in accordance with your appetite, hunger, and satiety cues. It is a fine idea to rotate through the whole plan (3 weeks of Adaptive Response, 2 weeks of Preconditioning, and 1 week of Optimal Maintenance) over and over until the desired amount of weight loss is achieved.

A person in the Optimal Maintenance Phase can eat any of the meals laid out in the Adaptive Response or Preconditioning Phases and just increase some of the portion sizes accordingly. (Note that all of the menu plans are for one serving, but all of the recipes below make two servings.) Maintenance is easy because all of the menu ideas are interchangeable.

The Optimal Maintenance Phase is based on a 2,000-calorie diet. If you want to think about the plan in a fairly structured manner, then the following meal pattern will help guide your food choices.

Breakfast: 2 servings whole-grain bread or cereal, 2 servings fruit, 1 serving low-fat milk , 2 servings low-fat protein, and 2 servings fat

Lunch: 2 servings whole-grain bread, 2 servings colorful high-polyphenol vegetable, 1 serving starchy vegetable, 1 serving high-polyphenol fruit, 3 servings (ounces) low-fat protein, and 2 servings fat

Dinner: 2 servings whole-grain bread, 2 servings colorful high-polyphenol vegetable, 1 serving starchy vegetable, 1 serving high-polyphenol fruit, 4 servings (ounces) low-fat protein, and 2 servings fat

Snacks: 2 servings whole-grain bread or cereal or 2 servings fruit, or 1 serving low-fat milk

Supplements: As in the Preconditioning Phase, I want you to take one gel capsule of fish oil and one capsule of borage oil at breakfast and the same (one and one) at dinner.

Remember to eat the suggested types of seafood at least three to six times a week. Choose lean cuts of beef and pork as alternatives. Occasional vegetarian dishes that are based on legumes (beans) for lunch or dinner are another great way to build fiber and polyphenols into your diet.

If you find yourself on a binge or have days where you are constantly hungry, eat fiber to achieve a feeling of fullness. A large bowl of Kashi is my personal favorite, but you can chose any high-fiber source that you want.

And don't forget, the Optimal Maintenance Phase is where you get to include the dark chocolate and red wine as a regular part of your diet. Both should be taken in with the keys of balance and moderation in mind. There are dozens of great chocolate cookbooks on the market today: Make sure you buy at least one. Remember to use cocoa powder or dark cooking chocolate in the recipes—experiment and create desserts and entrées that appeal to you. And remember that the spiciness of some chiles pairs beautifully with chocolate.

And although it's a reiteration, it is important to remember that if you have a problem with alcohol consumption, sulfites consumption, or if drinking alcohol causes you to overeat, then you should forgo the red wine recommendations. A problem handling alcohol outstrips by far any plant chemical (phytochemical) boost you would get from drinking red wine. Know thyself, be judicious in your consumption, and never drink and drive.

There are a fair number of seafood recipes in this section and you can try all of them, but I would strongly suggest that you also buy a few great cookbooks devoted to seafood. On a personal note I want to tell you that cooking seafood is like anything else—it will take some time and patience to get it right, but you will get it. I struggled when I was learning to cook fish—I had to really learn what pans and temperatures work best with which fish. I have undercooked a lot of fish—only to turn around and overcook it. But I find that if I cook it in a delicious marinade or with lots of fruits and vegetables in a steam packet (*en papillote*, pronounced en pah-pee-YOHT), the fish is fine despite being a little overcooked. So, don't give up and keep at it. All good things are worth the effort!

Please remember to use the categories of fish listed on page 217 as an index of what you can consume. On days where it is not possible to prepare a nice fillet of salmon, you can open a can of albacore tuna or other listed fish on page 217. Put it on a whole-grain roll with some reduced-fat mayonnaise and *voilá!*—you have achieved the same bioactive profile as that large salmon meal. Remember, you are developing a lifestyle that must be flexible to be successful.

OPTIMAL MAINTENANCE BREAKFAST RECIPES
ALL RECIPES MAKE 2 SERVINGS.

First, remember that all the breakfast recipes listed in the Adaptive Response and Preconditioning menus can be utilized at any time in the Optimal Maintenance Phase. In addition, the following recipes may be used:

Egg Muffin Sandwiches

½ tablespoon trans-free margarine

1 cup liquid egg substitute

3 ounces cooked Canadian bacon, chopped

2 whole-wheat English muffins, split

3 ounces reduced-fat cheese slices

Melt the margarine in a medium skillet over medium heat. Add the egg substitute and cook, stirring, until beginning to set. Add the bacon and cook, stirring, until the eggs are cooked to your liking. Divide the eggs between the 2 muffin bottoms, top with the cheese, and cover with the muffin tops.

Covered and Studded Scrambled Eggs and Toast

2 ounces diced Canadian bacon

2 tablespoons diced red onion

1 cup liquid egg substitute

2 ounces reduced-fat cheese, grated

2 teaspoons trans-free margarine

2 tablespoons reduced-sugar or sugar-free berry jam

4 slices oat bran bread, toasted

Coat a medium nonstick skillet with cooking spray and place over medium heat. Add the bacon and cook, stirring occasionally, until crisp. Add the onion and cook, stirring, until softened. Add the egg substitute and cook, stirring occasionally, until the eggs are cooked to your liking. Divide the eggs among 2 plates and top with the cheese. Spread the margarine and jam on the toast slices and serve with the eggs.

Veggie Frittata with Toast

½ cup diced summer squash or zucchini

¼ cup chopped red bell pepper

1 ½ cups liquid egg substitute

¼ cup reduced-fat ricotta cheese

2 teaspoons trans-free margarine

2 tablespoons reduced-sugar or sugar-free berry jam

4 slices multigrain bread, toasted

Preheat the broiler. Coat an ovenproof nonstick skillet with cooking spray. (If the skillet's handle is not ovenproof, wrap it in aluminum foil.)

Place the prepared skillet over medium heat. Add the squash and bell pepper and cook, stirring, until softened. Add the egg substitute and cook, without stirring, until the egg begins to set on the bottom, about 4 minutes. Drop the ricotta in small spoonfuls over the eggs. Place the skillet under the broiler and cook until the frittata is set and cooked through, 6 to 8 minutes.

Spread the margarine and jam on the toast slices and serve with the frittata.

Oatmeal and Berries

1 cup strawberries, hulled and chopped

2 cups cooked old-fashioned oatmeal (not instant)

2 tablespoons crushed walnuts or pecans

¼ cup organic real maple syrup

2 cups 1% milk

Stir the strawberries into the oatmeal and divide between 2 bowls. Top with the nuts and maple syrup. Serve with the milk.

Loaded Bagels

4 teaspoons trans-free margarine

1 cup liquid egg substitute

4 slices cooked lean bacon

2 medium oat bran bagels, each cut in half

2 ounces reduced-fat cheese, grated

Melt the margarine in a medium skillet over medium heat. Add the egg substitute and cook, stirring occasionally, until it begins to set. Add the bacon and cook, stirring, until the eggs are cooked to your liking. Spoon the eggs on the bagel halves and top with the cheese.

Cereal Delight

1 cup fiber-enriched cereal (at least 6 grams fiber per ½ cup)

1 cup 1% milk

1 cup blueberries (fresh or frozen)

MAINTENANCE SEAFOOD RECIPES
ALL RECIPES MAKE 2 SERVINGS.

Remember, the single-serving seafood suggestions and recipes in the Adaptive Response and Preconditioning menus can be utilized at any time in the Optimal Maintenance Phase. In addition, the following recipes, all serving two, can also be used:

Grilled Salmon Teriyaki

- 2 (8-ounce) salmon fillets
- 2 tablespoons teriyaki sauce
- ½ teaspoon coarsely ground black pepper

Place the salmon in a bowl or shallow dish. Pour the teriyaki sauce over fillets; cover and let stand at room temperature for 10 minutes.

Spray a grill with cooking spray and heat to 450°F. Remove the salmon from the marinade. Rub the pepper into skinless side of each fillet. Place the salmon on the grill, skin side up, and cook over medium-high (400°F) heat for 3 to 4 minutes. Turn and cook until the salmon flakes easily with a fork, 2 minutes longer. Serve immediately.

Tuna Pasta Salad

- 2 cups cooked whole-wheat pasta
- 1 (6-ounce) can albacore tuna in water, drained
- ½ cup diced celery
- ½ cup diced red bell pepper
- ¼ cup cholesterol-free mayonnaise
- Salt and freshly ground black pepper, to taste

In a bowl, combine the pasta, tuna, celery, bell pepper, mayonnaise, and salt and pepper. Cover and refrigerate at least 6 hours.

Shrimp and Vegetable Stir-Fry I

4 tablespoons olive oil, divided

12 ounces fresh or frozen shrimp, peeled and deveined

1 tablespoon minced fresh garlic

1 cup diced celery

1 cup diced green bell pepper

1 cup diced tomatoes

2 cups cooked whole-wheat spaghetti

In a large skillet, heat 2 tablespoons of the oil over medium-high heat. Add the shrimp and garlic and cook, turning occasionally, until the shrimp are cooked through, 5 minutes. Transfer the shrimp to a plate.

In the same skillet, heat the remaining oil. Add the celery and bell pepper and cook, stirring constantly, until crisp-tender, 2 minutes. Stir in the shrimp and tomatoes and cook until heated through. Serve over the spaghetti.

Salmon Cakes

1 (6-ounce) can pink salmon

¼ cup liquid egg substitute

¼ cup dry bread crumbs

1½ teaspoons Dijon mustard

3 tablespoons finely chopped onion

¼ teaspoon garlic salt

¼ cup canola oil

Remove any large bones from the salmon and flake into a bowl. Add the egg substitute, bread crumbs, and mustard and mix well. Stir in the onion and garlic salt.

Heat the oil in a large skillet over medium-high heat. Drop the salmon mixture into the skillet by ¼-cup portions and flatten with a spatula. Cook until browned on the bottoms, 3 to 4 minutes. Turn the cakes and cook on the other side until brown, about 4 minutes longer.

Shrimp Chowder

¼ cup trans-free margarine

¼ cup chopped onion

¼ cup all-purpose flour

2 cups 1% milk

½–¾ cup fat-free chicken broth

1 cup canned, fresh, or frozen corn

8 ounces cooked shrimp

1 teaspoon dried basil

Salt and freshly ground black pepper, to taste

In a saucepan, heat the margarine over medium heat until melted. Add the onion and cook, stirring, until golden. Add the flour and stir continuously until smooth and bubbly. Slowly add the milk, stirring constantly. Cook, stirring, until thickened. Add the broth, corn, shrimp, basil, and salt and pepper. Cook over low heat just until heated through.

Crab Salad

4–6 ounces artificial crabmeat (surimi)

2–4 tablespoons minced celery

2 tablespoons cholesterol-free mayonnaise

1 tablespoon lemon juice

Whole-wheat crackers

In a medium bowl, combine the crabmeat, celery, mayonnaise, and lemon juice. Cover and chill 2 hours. Serve with crackers.

Lemon-Herb Fish

12 ounces fresh or frozen wild mackerel, halibut, or salmon fillets

2 tablespoons lemon juice

2 tablespoons chopped fresh parsley

$\frac{1}{4}$ teaspoon dill weed

$\frac{1}{4}$ teaspoon salt

$\frac{1}{8}$ teaspoon coarsely ground black pepper

Line a broiler pan with aluminum foil and spray rack with cooking spray. Place the fish on the rack.

In a small bowl, combine the lemon juice, parsley, dill, salt, and pepper. Baste the fish with the lemon mixture. Broil the fish 4" from the heat until it flakes easily with a fork, about 10 minutes per inch of thickness measured at thickest point. Do not turn the fillets. Baste several times during cooking time. Serve immediately.

Crab Lasagna Rolls

4 whole-wheat lasagna noodles

1 (8-ounce) can blue crabmeat

$\frac{1}{2}$ cup 1% cottage cheese

1 tablespoon dried parsley

$\frac{1}{4}$ teaspoon onion powder

$\frac{1}{4}$ teaspoon freshly ground black pepper

1 cup tomato sauce

$\frac{1}{4}$ cup grated Parmesan cheese

Preheat the oven to 375°F. Spray a baking dish with cooking spray.

Cook the noodles in a large pot of boiling water according to package directions. Rinse under cold water and drain well.

In a small bowl, combine the crabmeat, cottage cheese, parsley, onion powder, and pepper. Lay the cooked noodles flat on a work surface and spread one-fourth of filling over each. Roll up as tightly as possible.

Place the rolls seam-side down in the prepared baking dish and pour the tomato sauce on top. Cover the dish and bake for 30 minutes. Sprinkle with the Parmesan cheese and bake, uncovered, until the cheese is melted, about 5 minutes.

Mackerel and Crab Jambalaya

½ cup chopped green and/or yellow onion

½ cup chopped green bell pepper

½ cup chopped yellow bell pepper

2 stalks celery with leaves, chopped

½ teaspoon minced garlic

8 ounces fresh or frozen Atlantic or canned mackerel, chopped

4 ounces fresh, frozen, or canned crabmeat, flaked

1 (14.5-ounce) can diced tomatoes

2 cups fat-free chicken broth

1 cup uncooked brown rice

½ teaspoon salt

¼ teaspoon cayenne pepper

Coat a large skillet with cooking spray and place over medium-high heat. Add the onion, bell peppers, celery, and garlic and cook, stirring, until tender but not brown. Stir in the mackerel and crabmeat and cook 5 minutes longer. Add the tomatoes, broth, rice, salt, and cayenne. Stir, cover, and cook over low heat until the rice is tender, 30 to 40 minutes. If mixture becomes too dry, add tomato juice or water.

Seafood Pasta Salad

4 ounces canned crabmeat, drained and flaked

4 ounces chopped cooked shrimp

2 cups cooked small shell pasta

1 cup chopped asparagus, blanched

½ cup cholesterol-free mayonnaise

2 tablespoons chopped fresh dill

1 teaspoon lemon zest

Salt and freshly ground black pepper, to taste

Juice of 1 lemon

In a bowl, combine the crab, shrimp, pasta, asparagus, mayonnaise, dill, lemon zest, and salt and pepper and toss to combine well. Cover and refrigerate for 2 hours. Before serving, add the lemon juice and adjust seasonings.

Shrimp and Scallop Scampi

2 tablespoons olive oil

2 cloves garlic, minced

½ cup fat-free chicken broth

½ teaspoon dried oregano

½ teaspoon dried basil

¼ teaspoon crushed red pepper flakes

6 ounces fresh or frozen scallops (sea or bay)

6 ounces shrimp, peeled and deveined

½ lemon

In a large skillet, heat the oil over medium-high heat. Add the garlic and cook until just browned, about 3 minutes. Stir in the broth, oregano, basil, and red pepper flakes and bring to a simmer. Cook 3 minutes. Add the scallops and shrimp and cook just until the shrimp are cooked through, 3 to 5 minutes. Squeeze lemon juice over the top and serve immediately.

Tuna Melts

1 (6-ounce) can albacore tuna in water, drained and flaked

1/4 cup chopped green onions

1 tablespoon cholesterol-free mayonnaise

1/4 teaspoon ground cumin

1/8 teaspoon freshly ground black pepper

2 English muffins, split and lightly toasted

4 (1-ounce) slices reduced-fat Swiss cheese

Preheat the broiler.

In a medium bowl, combine the tuna, green onions, mayonnaise, cumin, and pepper. Top each muffin half with one-fourth of the tuna mixture. Place on a baking sheet and broil for 1 minute. Top each muffin half with 1 slice cheese and broil until the cheese begins to melt and brown, 1 to 2 minutes longer.

Crab Cakes

12 ounces cooked or canned crabmeat, flaked

1/2 cup dry bread crumbs

1/4 cup liquid egg substitute

1 tablespoon prepared mustard

1 teaspoon Worcestershire sauce

Garlic powder, to taste

Salt and freshly ground black pepper, to taste

1/4 cup canola oil

In a medium bowl, combine the crab, 1/4 cup of the bread crumbs, the egg substitute, mustard, Worcestershire, garlic powder, and salt and pepper.

Place the remaining 1/4 cup bread crumbs in a shallow bowl. Form the crab mixture into 4 cakes and dredge each one in the bread crumbs.

In a medium skillet, heat the oil over medium-high heat. Add the cakes and cook, turning once, just until well-browned, about 10 minutes.

Scalloped Oysters

½ cup dry bread crumbs

¼ cup trans-free margarine, melted

10 ounces oysters (about 30 medium), drained with ¼ cup liquid reserved

Salt and freshly ground black pepper, to taste

Preheat the oven to 450°F. Coat a shallow baking dish with cooking spray.

In a small bowl, combine ¼ cup of the bread crumbs and the melted margarine. Spread in the prepared dish. Place half of the oysters on top of the bread crumb mixture and season with salt and pepper. Sprinkle with half of the reserved oyster liquid. Repeat with remaining oysters and liquid. Top with the remaining bread crumbs.

Bake for 30 minutes, or until the oysters are cooked through.

Curried Shrimp Salad

1 ⅓ cups water

⅔ cup uncooked long-grain brown rice

½ teaspoon salt

10 ounces chopped cooked shrimp

½ cup cholesterol-free mayonnaise

⅔ cup frozen peas, thawed

2 tablespoons grated onion

1 tablespoon lemon juice

2 teaspoons curry powder

In a small saucepan, bring the water to a boil over high heat. Stir in the rice and salt. Reduce the heat, cover, and simmer until the rice is tender, 30 to 40 minutes. Fluff lightly with a fork and cool to room temperature.

In a medium bowl, combine the shrimp, mayonnaise, peas, onion, lemon juice, and curry powder. Stir in the rice. Refrigerate until ready to serve.

Salmon in Sun-Dried Tomato-Cream Sauce

½ cup sun-dried tomatoes (not oil-packed)

2 tablespoons trans-free margarine

2 cloves garlic, minced

2 tablespoons all-purpose flour

¼ teaspoon salt

¼ teaspoon freshly ground black pepper

1 cup fat-free half-and-half

8 ounces cooked wild sockeye or canned pink salmon, flaked

½ cup chopped fresh basil

2 cups cooked whole-wheat pasta

2 ounces (¾ cup) grated fresh Parmesan cheese

Place the sun-dried tomatoes in a small bowl and add boiling water to cover. Let soak while making the sauce.

Coat a skillet with cooking spray and place over medium heat. Add the margarine and cook until melted, being careful to not let it burn. Add the garlic and cook, stirring, until just browned. Stir in the flour, salt, and pepper. Cook over low heat, stirring constantly, until smooth and bubbly. Stir in the half-and-half and heat to boiling, stirring constantly.

Drain the sun-dried tomatoes and chop; stir into the sauce. Add the salmon and basil and heat gently for 2 minutes. Serve the salmon mixture over the pasta, topped with the Parmesan.

Grilled Foil-Wrapped Shrimp

2 tablespoons chopped fresh parsley

4 teaspoons canola oil

2 cloves garlic, minced

12 ounces fresh or frozen shrimp, peeled and deveined

Heat a grill to medium.

In a small bowl, whisk the parsley, oil, and garlic vigorously to blend well. Evenly divide the shrimp between 2 pieces of heavy-duty aluminum foil and top with the sauce. Fold and seal foil securely.

Grill the packets over medium heat for 10 to 12 minutes, or until the shrimp are cooked through.

Waldorf Tuna Salad

6 ounces canned white albacore tuna in water, drained

½ small red apple, cored and chopped

½ cup chopped celery

¼ cup cholesterol-free mayonnaise

¼ cup English walnut pieces

In a medium bowl, combine the tuna, apple, celery, mayonnaise, and walnuts. Cover and refrigerate 2 hours before serving.

Broiled Salmon

1 pound wild sockeye salmon

Freshly ground black pepper, to taste

1/4 cup lemon juice

1/4 cup white vinegar

1 teaspoon minced fresh ginger

1 teaspoon minced garlic

1/4 teaspoon white pepper

Salt, to taste

Preheat the broiler. Season the salmon with black pepper and refrigerate.

In a small saucepan over high heat, combine the lemon juice, vinegar, ginger, garlic, white pepper, and salt. Bring to a boil and cook for 2 to 3 minutes. Let cool.

Brush the salmon with the vinegar mixture and place on a broiler pan. Place the pan under the broiler and broil, turning once, until the salmon flakes easily with a fork, about 10 minutes.

Grilled Tuna Salad

6 ounces fresh or thawed frozen wild bluefin tuna or sockeye salmon steaks

2 tablespoons lemon juice

2 cloves garlic, minced

2 cups salad greens

1 cup chopped vegetables of choice

2 tablespoons vinaigrette

Heat a grill to medium-hot.

Place the fish in a shallow bowl. In a small bowl, combine the lemon juice and garlic; pour over fish. Refrigerate 1 hour, turning once.

Remove the fish from marinade and place on the grill rack. Cook, turning once, until it flakes easily with a fork, 10 to 12 minutes, depending on thickness.

In a large serving bowl, toss the greens with the vegetables. Add the vinaigrette and toss again. Place the warm fish steaks on top and serve.

Greek Salmon Salad

2 tablespoons olive oil

2 tablespoons lemon juice

1/4 teaspoon garlic salt

Pinch of coarsely ground black pepper

Pinch of crushed oregano leaves

4 cups torn romaine lettuce or other salad greens

1 cup chopped fresh Roma tomatoes

1/2 cup sliced cucumbers

1/4 cup chopped green onions

8 large black olives, sliced (1/4 cup)

8 ounces grilled or baked wild sockeye or canned pink salmon

2 ounces feta cheese

To make the dressing, in a small bowl, whisk together the oil, lemon juice, garlic salt, black pepper, and oregano until well blended. Refrigerate until ready to serve.

Place the lettuce in a bowl or on serving platter. Top with the tomatoes, cucumbers, green onions, and olives. Flake the salmon (removing large bones if using canned salmon) over the vegetables. Crumble the feta cheese over the top. Drizzle the dressing over the salad and serve.

Shrimp and Vegetable Stir-Fry II

1 cup thinly sliced red onion

Zest and juice of 1 lemon

1 tablespoon Dijon mustard

1 clove garlic, crushed

2 tablespoons olive oil

Salt and freshly ground black pepper, to taste

8 ounces fresh or thawed frozen shrimp, peeled and deveined

1 cup sliced red bell pepper

1 cup snow peas

2 cups cherry tomatoes, each halved

2 cups cooked whole-wheat spaghetti

In a medium bowl, combine the onion, lemon zest and juice, mustard, and garlic. Add 1 tablespoon of the olive oil and whisk until thoroughly blended. Season with salt and pepper. Add the shrimp and toss. Cover and marinate in the refrigerator for 6 to 8 hours.

Coat a large skillet with cooking spray. Add the remaining 1 tablespoon oil and heat over medium-high heat. Add the red pepper and snow peas and cook, stirring, until crisp-tender. Remove the shrimp from the marinade (reserving the marinade) and add to the skillet. Cook, stirring frequently, until the shrimp are just cooked through, 3 to 5 minutes. Add the tomatoes and reserved marinade and bring to a boil. Serve over the spaghetti.

Albacore Tuna Salad

1 (6-ounce) can white albacore tuna in water, drained

¼ cup finely chopped celery

4 teaspoons cholesterol-free mayonnaise

Salt and freshly ground black pepper, to taste

In a medium bowl, combine the tuna, celery, mayonnaise, and salt and pepper. Cover and refrigerate for 2 hours before serving.

Grilled Salmon Dijon

2 tablespoons Dijon mustard

2 tablespoons canola oil

1 tablespoon lemon juice

2 (6-ounce) wild sockeye salmon fillets

Heat a grill to medium-hot. Cut 2 large pieces of heavy-duty aluminum foil. Coat 1 piece of foil with cooking spray.

In a small bowl, combine the mustard, oil, and lemon juice. Place the salmon skin-side down on the greased piece of foil. Brush the mustard sauce over the salmon. Form a tent over salmon with the second piece of foil and seal edges.

Place the packet on the grill rack and cook until the salmon flakes easily with a fork, 8 to 15 minutes, depending on thickness of the fish (total cooking time will be about 10 minutes per inch of thickness at the thickest point.)

Salmon Spread

1 (4-ounce) can pink salmon

¼ cup reduced-fat cream cheese

1 tablespoon chopped fresh parsley

1 teaspoon Dijon mustard

⅛ teaspoon freshly ground black pepper

⅛ teaspoon cayenne pepper

Whole-wheat crackers

In a medium bowl, combine the salmon, cream cheese, parsley, mustard, black pepper, and cayenne pepper. Cover and refrigerate at least 2 hours before serving. Serve with the crackers.

Shrimp, Scallops (Bay or Sea), and Clams Italiano

6 ounces shrimp, peeled and deveined

4 ounces fresh or thawed frozen bay or sea scallops

4 ounces fresh, thawed frozen, or canned clams

¼ cup olive oil

1 cup chopped green bell pepper

4 cloves garlic, minced

1 cup canned or fresh diced tomatoes

2 tablespoons chopped fresh parsley

Salt and freshly ground black pepper, to taste

2 cups cooked whole-wheat spaghetti

2 ounces grated fresh Parmesan cheese

Fill a medium saucepan with water and bring to a boil. Add the shrimp, scallops, and uncooked clams (if using cooked canned or frozen clams, add them later). Reduce the heat and poach until the seafood is cooked through, 3 to 5 minutes. Drain, reserving ½ cup of the cooking liquid. Keep the shellfish warm.

Heat the oil in a large skillet over medium heat. Add the bell pepper and garlic and cook, stirring, until softened. Add the reserved cooking liquid, tomatoes, parsley, and salt and pepper; simmer gently for 5 minutes. Add the poached shellfish (including canned or frozen clams, if using) to the tomato sauce. Reduce the heat to low and simmer gently for 5 minutes.

Place the pasta in a hot serving dish, add the sauce, and toss to mix well. Top with the Parmesan.

Salmon Pasta Salad

1 (6-ounce) can pink salmon
2 cups cooked whole-wheat macaroni
½ cup chopped green bell pepper
¼ cup chopped celery
¼ cup chopped red onion
¼ cup lemon juice
2 tablespoons olive oil
2 tablespoons chopped fresh basil or 2 teaspoons dried
⅛ teaspoon salt
¼ teaspoon freshly ground black pepper
Garlic powder, to taste

In a medium bowl, combine the salmon, macaroni, bell pepper, celery, onion, lemon juice, olive oil, basil, salt, black pepper, and garlic powder. Gently stir until well mixed. Cover and refrigerate at least 8 hours before serving.

Baked Salmon

2 (6-ounce) sockeye salmon steaks
¼ cup dry white wine
¼ cup sliced green onions (white and green parts)
1 teaspoon fresh dill
¼ teaspoon freshly ground black pepper

Place the salmon in a baking dish. Drizzle with the wine and sprinkle with the green onions, dill, and black pepper. Cover and refrigerate for 30 minutes, turning once.

Preheat the oven to 350°F.

Remove the salmon from refrigerator and let stand at room temperature for 20 minutes. Bake the salmon, uncovered, occasionally basting with the marinade, for 30 to 35 minutes, or until it flakes easily with a fork.

Fried Oyster Salad

¼ cup yellow cornmeal or fine dry bread crumbs

Salt and freshly ground black pepper, to taste

Cayenne pepper, to taste

18 shucked oysters (about 10 ounces), drained

¼ cup canola oil

4 cups torn green leaf lettuce or other salad greens

½ cup sliced red onion

½ cup reduced-fat ranch dressing

In a ziptop bag, combine the cornmeal, salt, black pepper, and cayenne pepper and mix well. Place the oysters, 6 at a time, in the bag and shake to coat completely. Tap oysters to remove excess coating.

In a heavy skillet, heat the oil over medium-high heat to 375°F. Add the oysters, 6 at a time, and fry, turning occasionally, until golden brown. With a slotted spoon, transfer to paper towels to drain.

Divide the greens between two salad bowls. Add the onion (and other salad vegetables if you like). Drizzle with the dressing and top each salad with 9 fried oysters.

Scallop and Asparagus Sauté

1 cup whole-wheat pasta

16 medium asparagus stalks, cut into 3"–4" lengths (about 2 cups)

2 tablespoons canola oil

1 pound bay or sea scallops

1 cup fish stock, divided

1 tablespoon cornstarch

Juice of 2 lemons

Salt and freshly ground black pepper, to taste

In a large pot of boiling water, cook the pasta according to package directions. Drain and keep warm.

Meanwhile, place the asparagus in a steamer basket and place over boiling water. Cover and steam until crisp-tender; drain and set aside.

In a large skillet, heat the oil over medium-high heat. Add the scallops and cook until just cooked through, 2 to 3 minutes. (Scallops are a delicate seafood and require very little cooking time. Be careful not to overcook.)

In a small saucepan, whisk together ¼ cup of the fish stock and the cornstarch, removing all lumps. Whisk in the remaining stock and bring to a boil over medium-high heat, whisking continuously. Cook, whisking, until slightly thickened. Reduce the heat, add the lemon juice and salt and pepper, and simmer for 1 to 2 minutes.

Divide the cooked pasta between 2 plates. Top with the asparagus and scallops and drizzle with the sauce. Serve immediately.

Shrimp Creole

2 tablespoons olive oil

½ cup chopped celery

½ cup chopped green bell pepper

½ cup chopped onion

2 cloves garlic, chopped

1 cup chopped peeled tomatoes

¾ cup water

2 tablespoons chopped fresh parsley

1 packet sugar substitute

2 teaspoons Worcestershire sauce

½ teaspoon crushed dried thyme

¼ teaspoon hot pepper sauce

⅛ teaspoon cayenne pepper

1 bay leaf

¼ teaspoon salt

¼ teaspoon freshly ground black pepper

12 ounces shrimp, peeled and deveined

1 cup cooked brown rice

In a large skillet, heat the oil over medium heat. Add the celery, bell pepper, onion, and garlic and cook, stirring, until softened. Add the tomatoes, water, parsley, sugar substitute, Worcestershire, thyme, pepper sauce, cayenne, bay leaf, salt, and black pepper. Cook slowly, stirring occasionally, until slightly thickened, 20 to 30 minutes. (The sauce may be prepared a day in advance.)

Coat a medium skillet with cooking spray and heat over medium-high heat. Add the shrimp and cook, turning occasionally, until cooked through. Add the shrimp to the sauce and heat through. Discard the bay leaf. Serve over brown rice.

Some of My Favorite High-Fiber Foods

Below is a list of some of my favorite high-fiber foods. These foods have proven invaluable for me and for the participants in the Hillsdale Study. Why? They're low-calorie ways to keep yourself full—and your mouth busy when you're about to lose control and blow your diet.

Major food companies recognize the benefit of high-fiber foods and are introducing more and more new products. I will continue to update my list of favorite high-fiber foods at www.genesmart.com.

High-Fiber Cereals

Fiber One Cereal: Honey Clusters—
13 grams of fiber (per serving)

Bran—14 grams of fiber (per serving)

Kashi Cereal: different varieties—
8-10 grams of fiber (per serving)

All-Bran: different varieties—
10-13 grams of fiber

Raisin Bran: 7 grams of fiber
(per serving)

Frosted Mini Wheats: 6 grams of fiber
(per serving)

High-Fiber Bars

Fiber One Bars: different varieties—
9 grams of fiber

Kashi Bars: different varieties—
4 grams of fiber

MAINTENANCE EXERCISE SUGGESTIONS

Congratulations! You have gotten yourself in shape for the Maintenance Exercise Program. Please remember the program suggested below is only one of an infinite number of possibilities. The most important aspect of any program is that it incorporates an aerobic component, a strength resistance component, and a stretching component. My 7-day program begins with moderate exercise for 30 minutes on Day 1. Day 2 incorporates vigorous circuit training, 15/45/15. On Day 3, I suggest moderate exercise for 30 minutes. You will rest on Day 4. On Day 5, you will exercise vigorously for 20–30 minutes. Day 6 utilizes vigorous circuit training, 15/45/15, and on Day 7, you rest again.

CONCLUSION

THE NOTION OF A NOSTRUM—a magical potion to cure all ills—might be pure fantasy, but the discovery of the master gene regulators amounts to something very similar. We may not be aware of this lightning-fast switching system, or of the busy whir of signals that trigger or still the expression of thousands of genes every day. Indeed, until now, these master health regulators have been operating below your doctor's radar, too! But, even without our awareness, these gatekeepers determine our fate, for good or for ill.

My research for this book enabled me to begin to understand, for the first time, why our nation is suffering from an epidemic of inflammatory disease. Clearly, the standard American diet and lifestyle are making us very sick indeed. It also helped me to understand that science has provided the beginning of a strategy to reverse that epidemic—one that utilizes the most elegant solution possible: the body's own survival system.

We now know some of the ways that we can control the master health regulators that control wide swaths of genes determining whether we stay well or get ill, whether we grow old before our time or defy the clock. The levers we use to control the master regulators of our genes—the bioactives in our foods and exercise—*are* things that we control, and must, if we want to reverse this destructive trend.

These are early days for this science; we're right on the edge of an extremely personalized era in nutrition and medicine. I'll be first in line to know precisely which foods I should choose and avoid, given the specific information encoded in my personal genome. But we don't have to wait for the science to advance in order to have a dramatic, life-changing, and life-extending impact on our health.

These master regulators give us access right now to a built-in, genetically programmed system that can protect us from obesity and chronic disease at a level much more precise than we'd even dared to imagine possible. Currently, changes in what and how we eat have turned these regulators against us, so that we've had to rely on medications to drag us back toward the light.

Gene Smart not only gets us back on track, but it goes one step further by asking, "What happens if we give these regulators precisely what they need?" Gene Smart provides our miraculous bodies with the positive "stress" they are genetically programmed to read as a signal to protect themselves. In so doing, we not only recruit these powerful switches, helping to make us healthy and whole, but catapult ourselves into a world of much better health, rigor, greater fitness, and perhaps unimaginable longevity.

ABOUT GENE SMART COMPASSION

DURING THE TIME I WAS WRITING THIS BOOK, my wife, Briana, and I had the opportunity to go to Africa to work with orphans affected by HIV/AIDS. We washed their feet, gave them shoes, and prayed with them. My group directly interacted with almost 2,000 orphans during our stay there.

On the third day of our trip, we traveled to a banana plantation. It was the saddest place I'd ever been, and I immediately knew my life would be changed by it. When we arrived, hundreds of children were playing in a big field surrounded by a fence. The older ones stuck their heads through the fence, like trapped livestock, to get a better look at us. About 50 infants, all under 2 years old, were sitting in the mud crying. When we asked one of the caretakers the name of one infant, she couldn't answer. The baby was one of hundreds of children without names, looked after by a few "grannies."

I was immediately drawn to one of the infants. His eyes were deep yellow from liver failure as a result of AIDS and hepatitis, his face badly distorted from a birth defect and the ravages of malnutrition. He was crying, too, but only half-heartedly. As I looked at him, I thought, "I can't pick him up; it's too much of a risk for me and my family." Then, with great clarity, I heard God's voice asking me: "Who are you? *Whose* are you?" I immediately picked up the child, washed his face, and sang the lullaby that my mom had sung to me when I was a baby. The little boy stopped crying and looked me right in the eyes. And in his eyes, I saw what I believed to be the face of God for the first time in my life.

On a more recent trip, I visited Jach, an area on the border between southern Sudan and Darfur. When it became known that I was a researcher in the field of nutrition, I was introduced to a 4-year-old girl named Abuk, who was left an orphan by the surrounding genocide. Abuk was so severely malnourished that she weighed just 12 pounds; she clearly was just days from death. Over the next 10 days, I was blessed to be able to love that child, and to help bring her back to life by providing basic nutrition.

There are more than 140 million orphans worldwide, and 16 million in southern Africa who have lost their parents to AIDS. That number is expected to exceed 25 million in the next 2 years; that's two and a half times the population of North Carolina, my home state. Millions more have been orphaned as a result of genocide. When we talk about malnutrition, we are talking about millions of beautiful, loving children like Abuk. And I know that we must do something now to help children like her.

These children are malnourished by the amount and the type of food they eat. When it doesn't kill, malnutrition:

- Is responsible for hundreds of thousands of serious birth defects each year
- Impairs mental development and stunts physical growth
- Weakens immune function and renders children susceptible to infectious diseases, including malaria, tuberculosis, and HIV.
- Diminishes their capacity to work when they grow up, which undermines an entire nation's prospects for economic stability

I have decided to devote the rest of my life to using the latest, most sophisticated first-world technology to help alleviate the suffering of African children. I have founded a nonprofit organization called Gene Smart Compassion, which is setting up feeding stations and developing a therapeutic food designed to provide malnourished orphans with the micro- and macro-nutrients that they will need to survive and prosper given their current food supply.

The Gene Smart Diet is devoted to using food to alter the expression of inflammatory genes, which are constantly switched on thanks to the over-abundant environment in which we find ourselves. Gene Smart Compassion will use the same approach to address the other end of the malnutrition spectrum: in this case, to *increase* the expression of inflammatory genes in children who desperately need to build their immune systems.

We must do this now. Millions of children are missing their "window of opportunity" for normal growth and development; thousands are dying every day. As the late Nobel laureate Gabriela Mistral wrote:

> *We are guilty of many errors and many faults, but our worst crime is abandoning the children, neglecting the foundation of life. Many of the things we need can wait. The child cannot. Right now is the time his bones are being formed, his blood is being made and his senses are being developed. To him we cannot answer "Tomorrow." His name is "Today."*

Ten percent of all royalties that I receive from this book will be tithed to enriching the lives of orphans and other vulnerable children in Africa. If you are interested in helping with this effort, please visit www.genesmartcompassion.org.

ACKNOWLEDGMENTS

MY THANKS TO GOD for unconditional love, and for giving my life hope and meaning. To my wife, Briana, for opening my mind to new approaches to helping others and for her continued support. To my children, Candice, Josh, Shane, and Sarah, and my stepchildren, Jarret, Gianna, and Jordan, and my beautiful granddaughter, Grace, for providing me constant joy and purpose. To my mom, Ruby, and to my sisters Tammy and Tanya for being my biggest fans.

I'm grateful to my friend and agent, Laurie Bernstein, for continuing to guide my publishing career; to Laura Tucker, for taking what I believe are very helpful and at times very complex ideas and helping me articulate them; to Anne-Marie Scott, PhD, RD, assistant professor and director of the Undergraduate Dietetics Program at the University of North Carolina at Greensboro, for her assistance in creating the diets; and to Susan Berg and the staff at Rodale for helping me to reach a wide audience.

I owe thanks to mentors too numerous to mention individually at Western Carolina University, Wake Forest University School of Medicine, National Jewish Medical and Research Center, and Johns Hopkins University School of Medicine. And I would like to thank the National Institutes of Health and, in particular, the National Center for Complementary and Alternative Medicine and the Office of Dietary Supplements for their generous support of my research.

Finally, my thanks goes to the members and study participants from Hillsdale United Methodist Church and the surrounding community for helping me to understand the deep connection between physical and spiritual wellness.

REFERENCE LIST

Abramson, J.L., Williams, S.A., Krumholz, H.M., and Vaccarino, V. 2001. Moderate alcohol consumption and risk of heart failure among older persons. *JAMA* **285**:1971-1977.

Adams, K.F., Schatzkin, A., Harris, T.B., Kipnis, V., Mouw, T., Ballard-Barbash, R., Hollenbeck, A., and Leitzman, M.F. 2006. Overweight, obesity, and mortality in a large prospective cohort of persons 50 to 71 years old. *N. Engl. J. Med.* **355**:763-778.

Adams, P.B., Lawson, S., Sanigorski, A., and Sinclair, A.J. 1996. Arachidonic acid to eicosapentaenoic acid ratio in blood correlates positively with clinical symptoms of depression. *Lipids* **31 Suppl**:S157-S161.

Ahima, R.S. 2008. Revisiting leptin's role in obesity and weight loss. *J. Clin. Invest* **118**:2380-2383.

Ajani, U.A., Gaziano, J.M., Lotufo, P.A., Liu, S., Hennekens, C.H., Buring, J.E., and Manson, J.E. 2000. Alcohol consumption and risk of coronary heart disease by diabetes status. *Circulation* **102**:500-505.

Albert, C.M., Hennekens, C.H., O'Donnell, C.J., Ajani, U.A., Carey, V.J., Willett, W.C., Ruskin, J.N., and Manson, J.E. 1998. Fish consumption and risk of sudden cardiac death. *JAMA* **279**:23-28.

Albert, C.M., Manson, J.E., Cook, N.R., Ajani, U.A., Gaziano, J.M., and Hennekens, C.H. 1999. Moderate alcohol consumption and the risk of sudden cardiac death among US male physicians. *Circulation* **100**:944-950.

Albert, C.M., Campos, H., Stampfer, M.J., Ridker, P.M., Manson, J.E., Willett, W.C., and Ma, J. 2002. Blood levels of long-chain n-3 fatty acids and the risk of sudden death. *N. Engl. J. Med.* **346**:1113-1118.

Alfieri, M.A., Pomerleau, J., Grace, D.M., and Anderson, L. 1995. Fiber intake of normal weight, moderately obese and severely obese subjects. *Obes. Res.* **3**:541-547.

Antebi, A. 2007. Ageing: when less is more. *Nature* **447**:536-537.

Appleby, P.N., Thorogood, M., Mann, J.I., and Key, T.J. 1998. Low body mass index in non-meat eaters: the possible roles of animal fat, dietary fibre and alcohol. *Int. J. Obes. Relat Metab Disord.* **22**:454-460.

Aronson, D., Sheikh-Ahmad, M., Avizohar, O., Kerner, A., Sella, R., Bartha, P., Markiewicz, W., Levy, Y., and Brook, G.J. 2004. C-Reactive protein is inversely related to physical fitness in middle-aged subjects. *Atherosclerosis* **176**:173-179.

Aronson, D., Avizohar, O., Levy, Y., Bartha, P., Jacob, G., and Markiewicz, W. 2008. Factor analysis of risk variables associated with low-grade inflammation. *Atherosclerosis*.

Auger, C., Teissedre, P.L., Gerain, P., Lequeux, N., Bornet, A., Serisier, S., Besancon, P., Caporiccio, B., Cristol, J.P., and Rouanet, J.M. 2005. Dietary wine phenolics catechin, quercetin, and resveratrol efficiently protect hypercholesterolemic hamsters against aortic fatty streak accumulation. *J. Agric. Food Chem.* **53**:2015-2021.

Austin, M.A., Hokanson, J.E., and Edwards, K.L. 1998. Hypertriglyceridemia as a cardiovascular risk factor. *Am. J. Cardiol.* **81**:7B-12B.

Bagga, D., Wang, L., Farias-Eisner, R., Glaspy, J.A., and Reddy, S.T. 2003. Differential effects of prostaglandin derived from omega-6 and omega-3 polyunsaturated fatty acids on COX-2 expression and IL-6 secretion. *Proc. Natl. Acad. Sci. U. S. A.*. **100**:1751-1756.

Bang, H.O., Dyerberg, J., and Nielsen, A.B. 1971. Plasma lipid and lipoprotein pattern in Greenlandic West-coast Eskimos. *Lancet* 1:1143-1145.

Bang, H.O., and Dyerberg, J. 1972. Plasma lipids and lipoproteins in Greenlandic west coast Eskimos. *Acta Med. Scand.* **192**:85-94.

Bang, H.O., Dyerberg, J., and Hjoorne, N. 1976. The composition of food consumed by Greenland Eskimos. *Acta Med. Scand.* **200**:69-73.

Banz, W.J., Maher, M.A., Thompson, W.G., Bassett, D.R., Moore, W., Ashraf, M., Keefer, D.J., and Zemel, M.B. 2003. Effects of resistance versus aerobic training on coronary artery disease risk factors. *Exp. Biol. Med. (Maywood.)* **228**:434-440.

Barrett-Connor, E.L., Cohn, B.A., Wingard, D.L., and Edelstein, S.L. 1991. Why is diabetes mellitus a stronger risk factor for fatal ischemic heart disease in women than in men? The Rancho Bernardo Study. *JAMA* **265**:627-631.

Baur, J.A., Pearson, K.J., Price, N.L., Jamieson, H.A., Lerin, C., Kalra, A., Prabhu, V.V., Allard, J.S., Lopez-Lluch, G., Lewis, K. et al 2006. Resveratrol improves health and survival of mice on a high-calorie diet. *Nature* **444**:337-342.

Beilin, L. 2005. Alcohol and hypertension: balancing the risks and benefits. *J. Hypertens.* **23**:1953-1955.

Berger, K., Ajani, U.A., Kase, C.S., Gaziano, J.M., Buring, J.E., Glynn, R.J., and Hennekens, C.H. 1999. Light-to-moderate alcohol consumption and risk of stroke among U.S. male physicians. *N. Engl. J. Med.* **341**:1557-1564.

Bergman, B.C., and Brooks, G.A. 1999. Respiratory gas-exchange ratios during graded exercise in fed and fasted trained and untrained men. *J. Appl. Physiol* **86**:479-487.

Bes-Rastrollo, M., Martinez-Gonzalez, M.A., Sanchez-Villegas, A., de la Fuente, A.C., and Martinez, J.A. 2006. Association of fiber intake and fruit/vegetable consumption with weight gain in a Mediterranean population. *Nutrition* **22**:504-511.

Beulens, J.W., Rimm, E.B., Ascherio, A., Spiegelman, D., Hendriks, H.F., and Mukamal, K.J. 2007. Alcohol consumption and risk for coronary heart disease among men with hypertension. *Ann. Intern. Med.* **146**:10-19.

Bjelakovic, G., Nikolova, D., Simonetti, R.G., and Gluud, C. 2004. Antioxidant supplements for prevention of gastrointestinal cancers: a systematic review and meta-analysis. *Lancet* **364**:1219-1228.

Bjelakovic, G., Nikolova, D., Gluud, L.L., Simonetti, R.G., and Gluud, C. 2007. Mortality in randomized trials of antioxidant supplements for primary and secondary prevention: systematic review and meta-analysis. *JAMA* **297**:842-857.

Bordone, L., and Guarente, L. 2005. Calorie restriction, SIRT1 and metabolism: understanding longevity. *Nat. Rev. Mol. Cell Biol.* **6**:298-305.

Bouzan, C., Cohen, J.T., Connor, W.E., Kris-Etherton, P.M., Gray, G.M., Konig, A., Lawrence, R.S., Savitz, D.A., and Teutsch, S.M. 2005. A quantitative analysis of fish consumption and stroke risk. *Am. J. Prev. Med.* **29**:347-352.

Braith, R.W., and Stewart, K.J. 2006. Resistance exercise training: its role in the prevention of cardiovascular disease. *Circulation* **113**:2642-2650.

Broeder, C.E., Burrhus, K.A., Svanevik, L.S., and Wilmore, J.H. 1992. The effects of either high-intensity resistance or endurance training on resting metabolic rate. *Am. J. Clin. Nutr.* **55**:802-810.

Brooks, N., Layne, J.E., Gordon, P.L., Roubenoff, R., Nelson, M.E., and Castaneda-Sceppa, C. 2007. Strength training improves muscle quality and insulin sensitivity in Hispanic older adults with type 2 diabetes. *Int. J. Med. Sci.* **4**:19-27.

Bruunsgaard, H. 2005. Physical activity and modulation of systemic low-level inflammation. *J. Leukoc. Biol.* **78**:819-835.

Bryson, C.L., Mukamal, K.J., Mittleman, M.A., Fried, L.P., Hirsch, C.H., Kitzman, D.W., and Siscovick, D.S. 2006. The association of alcohol consumption and incident heart failure: the Cardiovascular Health Study. *J. Am. Coll. Cardiol.* **48**:305-311.

Bulpitt, C.J. 2005. How many alcoholic drinks might benefit an older person with hypertension? *J. Hypertens.* **23**:1947-1951.

Burr, M.L., Fehily, A.M., Gilbert, J.F., Rogers, S., Holliday, R.M., Sweetnam, P.M., Elwood, P.C., and Deadman, N.M. 1989. Effects of changes in fat, fish, and fibre intakes on death and myocardial reinfarction: diet and reinfarction trial (DART). *Lancet* **2**:757-761.

Calabro, P., Willerson, J.T., and Yeh, E.T. 2003. Inflammatory cytokines stimulated C-reactive protein production by human coronary artery smooth muscle cells. *Circulation* **108**: 1930-1932.

Calder, P.C. 2002. Dietary modification of inflammation with lipids. *Proc. Nutr. Soc.* **61**:345-358.

Calder, P.C., and Grimble, R.F. 2002. Polyunsaturated fatty acids, inflammation and immunity. *Eur. J. Clin. Nutr.* **56 Suppl 3**:S14-S19.

Canto, J.G., and Iskandrian, A.E. 2003. Major risk factors for cardiovascular disease: debunking the "only 50%" myth. *JAMA* **290**:947-949.

Castaneda, C., Layne, J.E., Munoz-Orians, L., Gordon, P.L., Walsmith, J., Foldvari, M., Roubenoff, R., Tucker, K.L., and Nelson, M.E. 2002. A randomized controlled trial of resistance exercise training to improve glycemic control in older adults with type 2 diabetes. *Diabetes Care* **25**:2335-2341.

Cawthorne, M.A. 2007. Opportunities and challenges for the development of pharmacological therapies for obesity treatment. *Obes. Rev.* **8 Suppl 1**:131-136.

Chen, D., Steele, A.D., Lindquist, S., and Guarente, L. 2005. Increase in activity during calorie restriction requires Sirt1. *Science* **310**: 1641.

Chen, F., Castranova, V., Shi, X., and Demers, L.M. 1999. New insights into the role of nuclear factor-kappaB, a ubiquitous transcription factor in the initiation of diseases. *Clin. Chem.* **45**:7-17.

Christensen, J.H. 2003. n-3 fatty acids and the risk of sudden cardiac death. Emphasis on heart rate variability. *Dan. Med. Bull.* **50**:347-367.

Christman, J.W., Lancaster, L.H., and Blackwell, T.S. 1998. Nuclear factor kappa B: a pivotal role in the systemic inflammatory response syndrome and new target for therapy. *Intensive Care Med.* **24**:1131-1138.

Cohen, J.T., Bellinger, D.C., Connor, W.E., and Shaywitz, B.A. 2005. A quantitative analysis of prenatal intake of n-3 polyunsaturated fatty acids and cognitive development. *Am. J. Prev. Med.* **29**:366-374.

Cohen, J.T., Bellinger, D.C., and Shaywitz, B.A. 2005. A quantitative analysis of prenatal methyl mercury exposure and cognitive development. *Am. J. Prev. Med.* **29**:353-365.

Cohen, J.T., Bellinger, D.C., Connor, W.E., Kris-Etherton, P.M., Lawrence, R.S., Savitz, D.A., Shaywitz, B.A., Teutsch, S.M., and Gray, G.M. 2005. A quantitative risk-benefit analysis of changes in population fish consumption. *Am. J. Prev. Med.* **29**:325-334.

Colliander, E.B., and Tesch, P.A. 1988. Blood pressure in resistance-trained athletes. *Can. J. Sport Sci.* **13**:31-34.

Cordain, L., Eaton, S.B., Sebastian, A., Mann, N., Lindeberg, S., Watkins, B.A., O'Keefe, J.H., and Brand-Miller, J. 2005. Origins and evolution of the Western diet: health implications for the 21st century. *Am. J. Clin. Nutr.* **81**: 341-354.

Cordain, L., Eaton, S.B., Sebastian, A., Mann, N., Lindeberg, S., Watkins, B.A., O'Keefe, J.H., and Brand-Miller, J. 2005. Origins and evolution of the Western diet: health implications for the 21st century. *Am. J. Clin. Nutr.* **81**: 341-354.

Cornelissen, V.A., and Fagard, R.H. 2005. Effect of resistance training on resting blood pressure: a meta-analysis of randomized controlled trials. *J. Hypertens.* **23**:251-259.

Curtis, C.L., Hughes, C.E., Flannery, C.R., Little, C.B., Harwood, J.L., and Caterson, B. 2000. n-3 fatty acids specifically modulate catabolic factors involved in articular cartilage degradation. *J. Biol. Chem.* **275**:721-724.

Cushman, W.C., Cutler, J.A., Hanna, E., Bingham, S.F., Follmann, D., Harford, T., Dubbert, P., Allender, P.S., Dufour, M., Collins, J.F. et al 1998. Prevention and Treatment of Hypertension Study (PATHS): effects of an alcohol treatment program on blood pressure. *Arch. Intern. Med.* **158**:1197-1207.

Dallongeville, J., Yarnell, J., Ducimetiere, P., Arveiler, D., Ferrieres, J., Montaye, M., Luc, G., Evans, A., Bingham, A., Hass, B. et al 2003. Fish consumption is associated with lower heart rates. *Circulation* **108**:820-825.

Daviglus, M.L., Stamler, J., Orencia, A.J., Dyer, A.R., Liu, K., Greenland, P., Walsh, M.K., Morris, D., and Shekelle, R.B. 1997. Fish consumption and the 30-year risk of fatal myocardial infarction. *N. Engl. J. Med.* **336**:1046-1053.

De, L.M., and Salen, P. 1999. Wine ethanol, platelets, and Mediterranean diet. *Lancet* **353**:1067.

De, M.M., Franceschi, C., Monti, D., and Ginaldi, L. 2006. Inflammation markers predicting frailty and mortality in the elderly. *Exp. Mol. Pathol.* **80**:219-227.

De, R., V, Procaccini, C., Cali, G., Pirozzi, G., Fontana, S., Zappacosta, S., La, C.A., and Matarese, G. 2007. A key role of leptin in the control of regulatory T cell proliferation. *Immunity.* **26**:241-255.

Denu, J.M. 2005. The Sir 2 family of protein deacetylases. *Curr. Opin. Chem. Biol.* **9**:431-440.

Di, C.A., Costanzo, S., Bagnardi, V., Donati, M.B., Iacoviello, L., and de, G.G. 2006. Alcohol dosing and total mortality in men and women: an updated meta-analysis of 34 prospective studies. *Arch. Intern. Med.* **166**:2437-2445.

Dolecek, T.A., and Granditis, G. 1991. Dietary polyunsaturated fatty acids and mortality in the Multiple Risk Factor Intervention Trial (MRFIT). *World Rev. Nutr. Diet.* **66**:205-216.

Donahue, R.P., Abbott, R.D., Reed, D.M., and Yano, K. 1986. Alcohol and hemorrhagic stroke. The Honolulu Heart Program. *JAMA* **255**:2311-2314.

Dunstan, D.W., Puddey, I.B., Beilin, L.J., Burke, V., Morton, A.R., and Stanton, K.G. 1998. Effects of a short-term circuit weight training program on glycaemic control in NIDDM. *Diabetes Res. Clin. Pract.* **40**:53-61.

Dunstan, D.W., Daly, R.M., Owen, N., Jolley, D., de Court, Shaw, J., and Zimmet, P. 2002. High-intensity resistance training improves glycemic control in older patients with type 2 diabetes. *Diabetes Care* **25**:1729-1736.

Dvorakova-Lorenzova, A., Suchanek, P., Havel, P.J., Stavek, P., Karasova, L., Valenta, Z., Tintera, J., and Poledne, R. 2006. The decrease in C-reactive protein concentration after diet and physical activity induced weight reduction is associated with changes in plasma lipids, but not interleukin-6 or adiponectin. *Metabolism* **55**:359-365.

Dwyer, J.H., Allayee, H., Dwyer, K.M., Fan, J., Wu, H., Mar, R., Lusis, A.J., and Mehrabian, M. 2004. Arachidonate 5-lipoxygenase promoter genotype, dietary arachidonic acid, and atherosclerosis. *N. Engl. J. Med.* **350**:29-37.

Dyer, A.R., Stamler, J., Paul, O., Berkson, D.M., Lepper, M.H., McKean, H., Shekelle, R.B., Lindberg, H.A., and Garside, D. 1977. Alcohol consumption, cardiovascular risk factors, and mortality in two Chicago epidemiologic studies. *Circulation* **56**:1067-1074.

Dyerberg, J., Bang, H.O., and Hjorne, N. 1975. Fatty acid composition of the plasma lipids in Greenland Eskimos. *Am. J. Clin. Nutr.* **28**:958-966.

Dyerberg, J., Bang, H.O., and Hjorne, N. 1977. Plasma cholesterol concentration in Caucasian Danes and Greenland West-coast Eskimos. *Dan. Med. Bull.* **24**:52-55.

Elkind, M.S., Sciacca, R., Boden-Albala, B., Rundek, T., Paik, M.C., and Sacco, R.L. 2006. Moderate alcohol consumption reduces risk of ischemic stroke: the Northern Manhattan Study. *Stroke* **37**:13-19.

Eriksson, J., Taimela, S., Eriksson, K., Parviainen, S., Peltonen, J., and Kujala, U. 1997. Resistance training in the treatment of non-insulin-dependent diabetes mellitus. *Int. J. Sports Med.* **18**:242-246.

Eriksson, J., Tuominen, J., Valle, T., Sundberg, S., Sovijarvi, A., Lindholm, H., Tuomilehto, J., and Koivisto, V. 1998. Aerobic endurance exercise or circuit-type resistance training for individuals with impaired glucose tolerance? *Horm. Metab Res.* **30**:37-41.

Estruch, R., Sacanella, E., Badia, E., Antunez, E., Nicolas, J.M., Fernandez-Sola, J., Rotilio, D., de, G.G., Rubin, E., and Urbano-Marquez, A. 2004. Different effects of red wine and gin consumption on inflammatory biomarkers of atherosclerosis: a prospective randomized crossover trial. Effects of wine on inflammatory markers. *Atherosclerosis* **175**:117-123.

Ettinger, W.H., Jr., Burns, R., Messier, S.P., Applegate, W., Rejeski, W.J., Morgan, T., Shumaker, S., Berry, M.J., O'Toole, M., Monu, J. et al 1997. A randomized trial comparing aerobic exercise and resistance exercise with a health education program in older adults with knee osteoarthritis. The Fitness Arthritis and Seniors Trial (FAST). *JAMA* **277**:25-31.

Fenicchia, L.M., Kanaley, J.A., Azevedo, J.L., Jr., Miller, C.S., Weinstock, R.S., Carhart, R.L., and Ploutz-Snyder, L.L. 2004. Influence of resistance exercise training on glucose control in women with type 2 diabetes. *Metabolism* **53**:284-289.

Ferretti, A., Nelson, G.J., Schmidt, P.C., Kelley, D.S., Bartolini, G., and Flanagan, V.P. 1997. Increased dietary arachidonic acid enhances the synthesis of vasoactive eicosanoids in humans. *Lipids* **32**:435-439.

Flight, I., and Clifton, P. 2006. Cereal grains and legumes in the prevention of coronary heart disease and stroke: a review of the literature. *Eur. J. Clin. Nutr.* **60**:1145-1159.

Flowers, M.T., Miyazaki, M., Liu, X., and Ntambi, J.M. 2006. Probing the role of stearoyl-CoA desaturase-1 in hepatic insulin resistance. *J. Clin. Invest* **116**:1478-1481.

Folsom, A.R., and Demissie, Z. 2004. Fish intake, marine omega-3 fatty acids, and mortality in a cohort of postmenopausal women. *Am. J. Epidemiol.* **160**:1005-1010.

Fontana, L., Meyer, T.E., Klein, S., and Holloszy, J.O. 2004. Long-term calorie restriction is highly effective in reducing the risk for atherosclerosis in humans. *Proc. Natl. Acad. Sci. U. S. A.* **101**:6659-6663.

Fontana, L., and Klein, S. 2007. Aging, adiposity, and calorie restriction. *JAMA* **297**:986-994.

Gaziano, J.M., Buring, J.E., Breslow, J.L., Goldhaber, S.Z., Rosner, B., VanDenburgh, M., Willett, W., and Hennekens, C.H. 1993. Moderate alcohol intake, increased levels of high-density lipoprotein and its subfractions, and decreased risk of myocardial infarction. *N. Engl. J. Med.* **329**:1829-1834.

Gaziano, J.M., Gaziano, T.A., Glynn, R.J., Sesso, H.D., Ajani, U.A., Stampfer, M.J., Manson, J.E., Hennekens, C.H., and Buring, J.E. 2000. Light-to-moderate alcohol consumption and mortality in the Physicians' Health Study enrollment cohort. *J. Am. Coll. Cardiol.* **35**:96-105.

Geleijnse, J.M., Giltay, E.J., Grobbee, D.E., Donders, A.R., and Kok, F.J. 2002. Blood pressure response to fish oil supplementation: metaregression analysis of randomized trials. *J. Hypertens.* **20**:1493-1499.

Goldberg, R.J., Burchfiel, C.M., Reed, D.M., Wergowske, G., and Chiu, D. 1994. A prospective study of the health effects of alcohol consumption in middle-aged and elderly men. The Honolulu Heart Program. *Circulation* **89**:651-659.

Goldhammer, E., Tanchilevitch, A., Maor, I., Beniamini, Y., Rosenschein, U., and Sagiv, M. 2005. Exercise training modulates cytokines activity in coronary heart disease patients. *Int. J. Cardiol.* **100**:93-99.

Gronbaek, M., Becker, U., Johansen, D., Gottschau, A., Schnohr, P., Hein, H.O., Jensen, G., and Sorensen, T.I. 2000. Type of alcohol consumed and mortality from all causes, coronary heart disease, and cancer. *Ann. Intern. Med.* **133**:411-419.

Gronbaek, M., Johansen, D., Becker, U., Hein, H.O., Schnohr, P., Jensen, G., Vestbo, J., and Sorensen, T.I. 2004. Changes in alcohol intake and mortality: a longitudinal population-based study. *Epidemiology* **15**:222-228.

Guarente, L., and Picard, F. 2005. Calorie restriction—the SIR2 connection. *Cell* **120**:473-482.

Guiraud, A., de, L.M., Boucher, F., Berthonneche, C., Rakotovao, A., and de, L.J. 2004. Cardioprotective effect of chronic low dose ethanol drinking: insights into the concept of ethanol preconditioning. *J. Mol. Cell Cardiol.* **36**:561-566.

Gutierrez-Juarez, R., Pocai, A., Mulas, C., Ono, H., Bhanot, S., Monia, B.P., and Rossetti, L. 2006. Critical role of stearoyl-CoA desaturase-1 (SCD1) in the onset of diet-induced hepatic insulin resistance. *J. Clin. Invest* **116**:1686-1695.

Hale, S.L., and Kloner, R.A. 2001. Effects of resveratrol, a flavinoid found in red wine, on infarct size in an experimental model of ischemia/reperfusion. *J. Stud. Alcohol* **62**:730-735.

Hamilton, M.C., Hites, R.A., Schwager, S.J., Foran, J.A., Knuth, B.A., and Carpenter, D.O. 2005. Lipid composition and contaminants in farmed and wild salmon. *Environ. Sci. Technol.* **39**:8622-8629.

Hammett, C.J., Oxenham, H.C., Baldi, J.C., Doughty, R.N., Ameratunga, R., French, J.K., White, H.D., and Stewart, R.A. 2004. Effect of six months' exercise training on C-reactive protein levels in healthy elderly subjects. *J. Am. Coll. Cardiol.* **44**:2411-2413.

Hannah, V.C., Ou, J., Luong, A., Goldstein, J.L., and Brown, M.S. 2001. Unsaturated fatty acids down-regulate srebp isoforms 1a and 1c by two mechanisms in HEK-293 cells. *J. Biol. Chem.* **276**:4365-4372.

Hansagi, H., Romelsjo, A., Gerhardsson, d., V, Andreasson, S., and Leifman, A. 1995. Alcohol consumption and stroke mortality. 20-year follow-up of 15,077 men and women. *Stroke* **26**:1768-1773.

Harris, W.S. 1997. n-3 fatty acids and serum lipoproteins: human studies. *Am. J. Clin. Nutr.* **65**:1645S-1654S.

Harris, W.S. 2007. Omega-3 fatty acids and cardiovascular disease: a case for omega-3 index as a new risk factor. *Pharmacol. Res.* **55**:217-223.

Harris, W.S., Poston, W.C., and Haddock, C.K. 2007. Tissue n-3 and n-6 fatty acids and risk for coronary heart disease events. *Atherosclerosis* **193**:1-10.

Harris, W.S., DiRienzo, M.A., Sands, S.A., George, C., Jones, P.G., and Eapen, A.K. 2007. Stearidonic acid increases the red blood cell and heart eicosapentaenoic acid content in dogs. *Lipids* **42**:325-333.

Haskell, W.L., Lee, I.M., Pate, R.R., Powell, K.E., Blair, S.N., Franklin, B.A., Macera, C.A., Heath, G.W., Thompson, P.D., and Bauman, A. 2007. Physical activity and public health: updated recommendation for adults from the American College of Sports Medicine and the American Heart Association. *Circulation* **116**:1081-1093.

He, K., Song, Y., Daviglus, M.L., Liu, K., Van, H.L., Dyer, A.R., and Greenland, P. 2004. Accumulated evidence on fish consumption and coronary heart disease mortality: a meta-analysis of cohort studies. *Circulation* **109**:2705-2711.

He, K., Song, Y., Daviglus, M.L., Liu, K., Van, H.L., Dyer, A.R., Goldbourt, U., and Greenland, P. 2006. Risks and benefits of seafood consumption. *Am. J. Prev. Med.* **30**:440-441.

Heilbronn, L.K., de, J.L., Frisard, M.I., DeLany, J.P., Larson-Meyer, D.E., Rood, J., Nguyen, T., Martin, C.K., Volaufova, J., Most, M.M. et al 2006. Effect of 6-month calorie restriction on biomarkers of longevity, metabolic adaptation, and oxidative stress in overweight individuals: a randomized controlled trial. *JAMA* **295**: 1539-1548.

Hibbeln, J.R., Ferguson, T.A., and Blasbalg, T.L. 2006. Omega-3 fatty acid deficiencies in neurodevelopment, aggression and autonomic dysregulation: opportunities for intervention. *Int. Rev. Psychiatry* **18**:107-118.

Hites, R.A., Foran, J.A., Carpenter, D.O., Hamilton, M.C., Knuth, B.A., and Schwager, S.J. 2004. Global assessment of organic contaminants in farmed salmon. *Science* **303**:226-229.

Hites, R.A., Foran, J.A., Schwager, S.J., Knuth, B.A., Hamilton, M.C., and Carpenter, D.O. 2004. Global assessment of polybrominated diphenyl ethers in farmed and wild salmon. *Environ. Sci. Technol.* **38**:4945-4949.

Hites, R.A., Foran, J.A., Carpenter, D.O., Hamilton, M.C., Knuth, B.A., and Schwager, S.J. 2004. Global assessment of organic contaminants in farmed salmon. *Science* **303**:226-229.

Holliday, R. 1989. Food, reproduction and longevity: is the extended lifespan of calorie-restricted animals an evolutionary adaptation? *Bioessays* **10**:125-127.

Holliday, R. 2006. Aging is no longer an unsolved problem in biology. *Ann. N. Y. Acad. Sci.* **1067**:1-9.

Honkola, A., Forsen, T., and Eriksson, J. 1997. Resistance training improves the metabolic profile in individuals with type 2 diabetes. *Acta Diabetol.* **34**:245-248.

Howarth, N.C., Saltzman, E., and Roberts, S.B. 2001. Dietary fiber and weight regulation. *Nutr. Rev.* **59**:129-139.

Hu, F.B., Bronner, L., Willett, W.C., Stampfer, M.J., Rexrode, K.M., Albert, C.M., Hunter, D., and Manson, J.E. 2002. Fish and omega-3 fatty acid intake and risk of coronary heart disease in women. *JAMA* **287**:1815-1821.

Hung, J., Knuiman, M.W., Divitini, M.L., Davis, T., and Beilby, J.P. 2008. Prevalence and risk factor correlates of elevated C-reactive protein in an adult Australian population. *Am. J. Cardiol.* **101**:193-198.

Hurley, B.F., and Roth, S.M. 2000. Strength training in the elderly: effects on risk factors for age-related diseases. *Sports Med.* **30**:249-268.

Ibanez, J., Izquierdo, M., Arguelles, I., Forga, L., Larrion, J.L., Garcia-Unciti, M., Idoate, F., and Gorostiaga, E.M. 2005. Twice-weekly progressive resistance training decreases abdominal fat and improves insulin sensitivity in older men with type 2 diabetes. *Diabetes Care* **28**:662-667.

Imhof, A., Woodward, M., Doering, A., Helbecque, N., Loewel, H., Amouyel, P., Lowe, G.D., and Koenig, W. 2004. Overall alcohol intake, beer, wine, and systemic markers of inflammation in western Europe: results from three MONICA samples (Augsburg, Glasgow, Lille). *Eur. Heart J.* **25**:2092-2100.

Ingram, D.K., Zhu, M., Mamczarz, J., Zou, S., Lane, M.A., Roth, G.S., and deCabo, R. 2006. Calorie restriction mimetics: an emerging research field. *Aging Cell* **5**:97-108.

Ishii, T., Yamakita, T., Sato, T., Tanaka, S., and Fujii, S. 1998. Resistance training improves insulin sensitivity in NIDDM subjects without altering maximal oxygen uptake. *Diabetes Care* **21**:1353-1355.

Iso, H., Kobayashi, M., Ishihara, J., Sasaki, S., Okada, K., Kita, Y., Kokubo, Y., and Tsugane, S. 2006. Intake of fish and n3 fatty acids and risk of coronary heart disease among Japanese: the Japan Public Health Center-Based (JPHC) Study Cohort I. *Circulation* **113**:195-202.

Janszky, I., Mukamal, K.J., Orth-Gomer, K., Romelsjo, A., Schenck-Gustafsson, K., Svane, B., Kirkeeide, R.L., and Mittleman, M.A. 2004. Alcohol consumption and coronary atherosclerosis progression—the Stockholm Female Coronary Risk Angiographic Study. *Atherosclerosis* **176**:311-319.

Jee, S.H., Sull, J.W., Park, J., Lee, S.Y., Ohrr, H., Guallar, E., and Samet, J.M. 2006. Body-mass index and mortality in Korean men and women. *N. Engl. J. Med.* **355**:779-787.

Jeffcoat, R. 2007. Obesity—a perspective based on the biochemical interrelationship of lipids and carbohydrates. *Med. Hypotheses* **68**:1159-1171.

Jensen, T., Retterstol, L.J., Sandset, P.M., Godal, H.C., and Skjonsberg, O.H. 2006. A daily glass of red wine induces a prolonged reduction in plasma viscosity: a randomized controlled trial. *Blood Coagul. Fibrinolysis* **17**:471-476.

Jolly, C.A. 2005. Diet manipulation and prevention of aging, cancer and autoimmune disease. *Curr. Opin. Clin. Nutr. Metab Care* **8**:382-387.

Jouven, X., Zureik, M., Desnos, M., Guerot, C., and Ducimetiere, P. 2001. Resting heart rate as a predictive risk factor for sudden death in middle-aged men. *Cardiovasc. Res.* **50**:373-378.

Jump, D.B. 2002. Dietary polyunsaturated fatty acids and regulation of gene transcription. *Curr. Opin. Lipidol.* **13**:155-164.

Jurca, R., Lamonte, M.J., Church, T.S., Earnest, C.P., Fitzgerald, S.J., Barlow, C.E., Jordan, A.N., Kampert, J.B., and Blair, S.N. 2004. Associations of muscle strength and fitness with metabolic syndrome in men. *Med. Sci. Sports Exerc.* **36**:1301-1307.

Kalra, S.P. 2008. Central leptin insufficiency syndrome: an interactive etiology for obesity, metabolic and neural diseases and for designing new therapeutic interventions. *Peptides* **29**:127-138.

Kannel, W.B., Kannel, C., Paffenbarger, R.S., Jr., and Cupples, L.A. 1987. Heart rate and cardiovascular mortality: the Framingham Study. *Am. Heart J.* **113**:1489-1494.

Karapanagiotidis, I.T., Bell, M.V., Little, D.C., Yakupitiyage, A., and Rakshit, S.K. 2006. Polyunsaturated fatty acid content of wild and farmed tilapias in Thailand: effect of aquaculture practices and implications for human nutrition. *J. Agric. Food Chem.* **54**:4304-4310.

Karatzi, K., Papamichael, C., Aznaouridis, K., Karatzis, E., Lekakis, J., Matsouka, C., Boskou, G., Chiou, A., Sitara, M., Feliou, G. et al 2004. Constituents of red wine other than alcohol improve endothelial function in patients with coronary artery disease. *Coron. Artery Dis.* **15**:485-490.

Kelley, D.S., Nelson, G.J., Love, J.E., Branch, L.B., Taylor, P.C., Schmidt, P.C., Mackey, B.E., and Iacono, J.M. 1993. Dietary alpha-linolenic acid alters tissue fatty acid composition, but not blood lipids, lipoproteins or coagulation status in humans. *Lipids* **28**:533-537.

Kelley, D.S., Taylor, P.C., Nelson, G.J., and Mackey, B.E. 1998. Dietary docosahexaenoic acid and immunocompetence in young healthy men. *Lipids* **33**:559-566.

Kelley, G.A., and Kelley, K.S. 2006. Effects of aerobic exercise on C-reactive protein, body composition, and maximum oxygen consumption in adults: a meta-analysis of randomized controlled trials. *Metabolism* **55**:1500-1507.

Khaodhiar, L., Ling, P.R., Blackburn, G.L., and Bistrian, B.R. 2004. Serum levels of interleukin-6 and C-reactive protein correlate with body mass index across the broad range of obesity. *JPEN J. Parenter. Enteral Nutr.* **28**:410-415.

Kimm, S.Y. 1995. The role of dietary fiber in the development and treatment of childhood obesity. *Pediatrics* **96**:1010-1014.

Kiyohara, Y., Kato, I., Iwamoto, H., Nakayama, K., and Fujishima, M. 1995. The impact of alcohol and hypertension on stroke incidence in a general Japanese population. The Hisayama Study. *Stroke* **26**:368-372.

Klatsky, A.L., Friedman, G.D., and Armstrong, M.A. 1986. The relationships between alcoholic beverage use and other traits to blood pressure: a new Kaiser Permanente study. *Circulation* **73**:628-636.

Klatsky, A.L., Armstrong, M.A., and Friedman, G.D. 1992. Alcohol and mortality. *Ann. Intern. Med.* **117**:646-654.

Kloner, R.A., and Rezkalla, S.H. 2007. To drink or not to drink? That is the question. *Circulation* **116**:1306-1317.

Konig, A., Bouzan, C., Cohen, J.T., Connor, W.E., Kris-Etherton, P.M., Gray, G.M., Lawrence, R.S., Savitz, D.A., and Teutsch, S.M. 2005. A quantitative analysis of fish consumption and coronary heart disease mortality. *Am. J. Prev. Med.* **29**:335-346.

Kris-Etherton, P.M., Taylor, D.S., Yu-Poth, S., Huth, P., Moriarty, K., Fishell, V., Hargrove, R.L., Zhao, G., and Etherton, T.D. 2000. Polyunsaturated fatty acids in the food chain in the

United States. *Am. J. Clin. Nutr.* **71**:179S-188S.

Kris-Etherton, P.M., Lefevre, M., Beecher, G.R., Gross, M.D., Keen, C.L., and Etherton, T.D. 2004. Bioactive compounds in nutrition and health-research methodologies for establishing biological function: the antioxidant and anti-inflammatory effects of flavonoids on athero-sclerosis. *Annu. Rev. Nutr.* **24**:511-538.

Kristensen, S.D., Iversen, A.M., and Schmidt, E.B. 2001. n-3 polyunsaturated fatty acids and coronary thrombosis. *Lipids* **36 Suppl**:S79-S82.

Kromhout, D., Bosschieter, E.B., and de Lezenne, C.C. 1985. The inverse relation between fish con-sumption and 20-year mortality from coronary heart disease. *N. Engl. J. Med.* **312**:1205-1209.

Kromhout, D., Feskens, E.J., and Bowles, C.H. 1995. The protective effect of a small amount of fish on coronary heart disease mortality in an elderly population. *Int. J. Epidemiol.* **24**:340-345.

Kromhout, D., Bloemberg, B., Seidell, J.C., Nis-sinen, A., and Menotti, A. 2001. Physical activ-ity and dietary fiber determine population body fat levels: the Seven Countries Study. *Int. J. Obes. Relat Metab Disord.* **25**:301-306.

Kunesova, M., Braunerova, R., Hlavaty, P., Tvrzicka, E., Stankova, B., Skrha, J., Hilgertova, J., Hill, M., Kopecky, J., Wagenknecht, M. et al 2006. The influence of n-3 polyunsaturated fatty acids and very low calorie diet during a short-term weight reducing regimen on weight loss and serum fatty acid composition in severely obese women. *Physiol Res.* **55**:63-72.

Lairon, D. 1996. Dietary fibres: effects on lipid metabolism and mechanisms of action. *Eur. J. Clin. Nutr.* **50**:125-133.

Lairon, D., Arnault, N., Bertrais, S., Planells, R., Clero, E., Hercberg, S., and Boutron-Ruault, M.C. 2005. Dietary fiber intake and risk factors for cardiovascular disease in French adults. *Am. J. Clin. Nutr.* **82**:1185-1194.

Lairon, D. 2007. Dietary fiber and control of body weight. *Nutr. Metab Cardiovasc. Dis.* **17**:1-5.

Lazarevic, A.M., Nakatani, S., Neskovic, A.N., Marinkovic, J., Yasumura, Y., Stojicic, D., Miyatake, K., Bojic, M., and Popovic, A.D. 2000. Early changes in left ventricular function in chronic asymptomatic alcoholics: relation to the duration of heavy drinking. *J. Am. Coll. Cardiol.* **35**:1599-1606.

Leaf, A., Kang, J.X., Xiao, Y.F., and Billman, G.E. 2003. Clinical prevention of sudden car-diac death by n-3 polyunsaturated fatty acids and mechanism of prevention of arrhythmias by n-3 fish oils. *Circulation* **107**:2646-2652.

Leaf, A., Albert, C.M., Josephson, M., Stein-haus, D., Kluger, J., Kang, J.X., Cox, B., Zhang, H., and Schoenfeld, D. 2005. Prevention of fatal arrhythmias in high-risk subjects by fish oil n-3 fatty acid intake. *Circulation* **112**:2762-2768.

Leikert, J.F., Rathel, T.R., Wohlfart, P., Cheynier, V., Vollmar, A.M., and Dirsch, V.M. 2002. Red wine polyphenols enhance endothe-lial nitric oxide synthase expression and subse-quent nitric oxide release from endothelial cells. *Circulation* **106**:1614-1617.

Lemaitre, R.N., King, I.B., Mozaffarian, D., Kuller, L.H., Tracy, R.P., and Siscovick, D.S. 2003. n-3 Polyunsaturated fatty acids, fatal ischemic heart disease, and nonfatal myocardial infarction in older adults: the Cardiovascular Health Study. *Am. J. Clin. Nutr.* **77**:319-325.

Lichtenstein, A.H., Appel, L.J., Brands, M., Carnethon, M., Daniels, S., Franch, H.A., Franklin, B., Kris-Etherton, P., Harris, W.S., Howard, B. et al 2006. Diet and lifestyle recom-mendations revision 2006: a scientific state-ment from the American Heart Association Nutrition Committee. *Circulation* **114**:82-96.

Liu, S. 2002. Intake of refined carbohydrates and whole grain foods in relation to risk of type 2 diabetes mellitus and coronary heart disease. *J. Am. Coll. Nutr.* **21**:298-306.

Liu, S., Willett, W.C., Manson, J.E., Hu, F.B., Rosner, B., and Colditz, G. 2003. Relation between changes in intakes of dietary fiber and grain products and changes in weight and development of obesity among middle-aged women. *Am. J. Clin. Nutr.* **78**:920-927.

Loeser, R.F. 2003. Systemic and local regula-tion of articular cartilage metabolism: where does leptin fit in the puzzle? *Arthritis Rheum.* **48**:3009-3012.

Lord, G.M., Matarese, G., Howard, J.K., Baker, R.J., Bloom, S.R., and Lechler, R.I. 1998. Leptin modulates the T-cell immune response and reverses starvation-induced immunosuppression. *Nature* **394**:897-901.

Lucas, M., and Harris, W.S. 2007. Risks and benefits of fish intake. *JAMA* **297**:585.

Ludwig, D.S., Pereira, M.A., Kroenke, C.H., Hilner, J.E., Van, H.L., Slattery, M.L., and Jacobs, D.R., Jr. 1999. Dietary fiber, weight gain, and cardiovascular disease risk factors in young adults. *JAMA* **282**:1539-1546.

Maclure, M. 1993. Demonstration of deductive meta-analysis: ethanol intake and risk of myocardial infarction. *Epidemiol. Rev.* **15**:328-351.

Macmahon, S., Peto, R., Cutler, J., Collins, R., Sorlie, P., Neaton, J., Abbott, R., Godwin, J., Dyer, A., and Stamler, J. 1990. Blood pressure, stroke, and coronary heart disease. Part 1, Prolonged differences in blood pressure: prospective observational studies corrected for the regression dilution bias. *Lancet* **335**:765-774.

Maiorana, A., O'Driscoll, G., Goodman, C., Taylor, R., and Green, D. 2002. Combined aerobic and resistance exercise improves glycemic control and fitness in type 2 diabetes. *Diabetes Res. Clin. Pract.* **56**:115-123.

Malinski, M.K., Sesso, H.D., Lopez-Jimenez, F., Buring, J.E., and Gaziano, J.M. 2004. Alcohol consumption and cardiovascular disease mortality in hypertensive men. *Arch. Intern. Med.* **164**:623-628.

Manley, S. 2003. Haemoglobin A1c—a marker for complications of type 2 diabetes: the experience from the UK Prospective Diabetes Study (UKPDS). *Clin. Chem. Lab Med.* **41**:1182-1190.

Mann, J.I., De, L., I, Hermansen, K., Karamanos, B., Karlstrom, B., Katsilambros, N., Riccardi, G., Rivellese, A.A., Rizkalla, S., Slama, G. et al 2004. Evidence-based nutritional approaches to the treatment and prevention of diabetes mellitus. *Nutr. Metab Cardiovasc. Dis.* **14**:373-394.

Manning, J.M., Dooly-Manning, C.R., White, K., Kampa, I., Silas, S., Kesselhaut, M., and Ruoff, M. 1991. Effects of a resistive training program on lipoprotein—lipid levels in obese women. *Med. Sci. Sports Exerc.* **23**:1222-1226.

Maraldi, C., Volpato, S., Kritchevsky, S.B., Cesari, M., Andresen, E., Leeuwenburgh, C., Harris, T.B., Newman, A.B., Kanaya, A., Johnson, K.C. et al 2006. Impact of inflammation on the relationship among alcohol consumption, mortality, and cardiac events: the health, aging, and body composition study. *Arch. Intern. Med.* **166**:1490-1497.

Marlett, J.A., McBurney, M.I., and Slavin, J.L. 2002. Position of the American Dietetic Association: health implications of dietary fiber. *J. Am. Diet. Assoc.* **102**:993-1000.

Matarese, G., Leiter, E.H., and La, C.A. 2007. Leptin in autoimmunity: many questions, some answers. *Tissue Antigens* **70**:87-95.

Mattson, M.P., and Cheng, A. 2006. Neurohormetic phytochemicals: Low-dose toxins that induce adaptive neuronal stress responses. *Trends Neurosci.* **29**:632-639.

Mattusch, F., Dufaux, B., Heine, O., Mertens, I., and Rost, R. 2000. Reduction of the plasma concentration of C-reactive protein following nine months of endurance training. *Int. J. Sports Med.* **21**:21-24.

McCartney, N. 1998. Role of resistance training in heart disease. *Med. Sci. Sports Exerc.* **30**: S396-S402.

McFarlin, B.K., Flynn, M.G., Campbell, W.W., Craig, B.A., Robinson, J.P., Stewart, L.K., Timmerman, K.L., and Coen, P.M. 2006. Physical activity status, but not age, influences inflammatory biomarkers and toll-like receptor 4. *J. Gerontol. A Biol. Sci. Med. Sci.* **61**:388-393.

Metoyer, C.F., and Pruitt, K. 2008. The role of sirtuin proteins in obesity. *Pathophysiology* **15**:103-108.

Mickleborough, T.D., Lindley, M.R., Ionescu, A.A., and Fly, A.D. 2006. Protective effect of fish oil supplementation on exercise-induced bronchoconstriction in asthma. *Chest* **129**:39-49.

Miech, R.A., Kumanyika, S.K., Stettler, N., Link, B.G., Phelan, J.C., and Chang, V.W. 2006.

Trends in the association of poverty with overweight among US adolescents, 1971-2004. *JAMA* **295**:2385-2393.

Miller, E.R., III, Pastor-Barriuso, R., Dalal, D., Riemersma, R.A., Appel, L.J., and Guallar, E. 2005. Meta-analysis: high-dosage vitamin E supplementation may increase all-cause mortality. *Ann. Intern. Med.* **142**:37-46.

Miller, W.C., Niederpruem, M.G., Wallace, J.P., and Lindeman, A.K. 1994. Dietary fat, sugar, and fiber predict body fat content. *J. Am. Diet. Assoc.* **94**:612-615.

Montecucco, F., Steffens, S., and Mach, F. 2008. Insulin resistance: a proinflammatory state mediated by lipid-induced signaling dysfunction and involved in atherosclerotic plaque instability. *Mediators. Inflamm.* **2008**:767623.

Montonen, J., Knekt, P., Jarvinen, R., Aromaa, A., and Reunanen, A. 2003. Whole-grain and fiber intake and the incidence of type 2 diabetes. *Am. J. Clin. Nutr.* **77**:622-629.

Mozaffarian, D., Lemaitre, R.N., Kuller, L.H., Burke, G.L., Tracy, R.P., and Siscovick, D.S. 2003. Cardiac benefits of fish consumption may depend on the type of fish meal consumed: the Cardiovascular Health Study. *Circulation* **107**:1372-1377.

Mozaffarian, D., Ascherio, A., Hu, F.B., Stampfer, M.J., Willett, W.C., Siscovick, D.S., and Rimm, E.B. 2005. Interplay between different polyunsaturated fatty acids and risk of coronary heart disease in men. *Circulation* **111**:157-164.

Mozaffarian, D., Geelen, A., Brouwer, I.A., Geleijnse, J.M., Zock, P.L., and Katan, M.B. 2005. Effect of fish oil on heart rate in humans: a meta-analysis of randomized controlled trials. *Circulation* **112**:1945-1952.

Mozaffarian, D., and Rimm, E.B. 2006. Fish intake, contaminants, and human health: evaluating the risks and the benefits. *JAMA* **296**:1885-1899.

Mozaffarian, D., Gottdiener, J.S., and Siscovick, D.S. 2006. Intake of tuna or other broiled or baked fish versus fried fish and cardiac structure, function, and hemodynamics. *Am. J. Cardiol.* **97**:216-222.

Mozaffarian, D., and Rimm, E.B. 2006. Fish intake, contaminants, and human health: evaluating the risks and the benefits. *JAMA* **296**:1885-1899.

Mukamal, K.J., Maclure, M., Muller, J.E., Sherwood, J.B., and Mittleman, M.A. 2001. Prior alcohol consumption and mortality following acute myocardial infarction. *JAMA* **285**:1965-1970.

Mukamal, K.J., Chiuve, S.E., and Rimm, E.B. 2006. Alcohol consumption and risk for coronary heart disease in men with healthy lifestyles. *Arch. Intern. Med.* **166**:2145-2150.

Nakamura, Y., Ueshima, H., Okamura, T., Kadowaki, T., Hayakawa, T., Kita, Y., Tamaki, S., and Okayama, A. 2005. Association between fish consumption and all-cause and cause-specific mortality in Japan: NIPPON DATA 80, 1980-99. *Am. J. Med.* **118**:239-245.

Narkar, V.A., Downes, M., Yu, R.T., Embler, E., Wang, Y.X., Banayo, E., Mihaylova, M.M., Nelson, M.C., Zou, Y., Juguilon, H. et al 2008. AMPK and PPARdelta agonists are exercise mimetics. *Cell* **134**:405-415.

Nassis, G.P., Papantakou, K., Skenderi, K., Triandafillopoulou, M., Kavouras, S.A., Yannakoulia, M., Chrousos, G.P., and Sidossis, L.S. 2005. Aerobic exercise training improves insulin sensitivity without changes in body weight, body fat, adiponectin, and inflammatory markers in overweight and obese girls. *Metabolism* **54**:1472-1479.

Needleman, P., Raz, A., Minkes, M.S., Ferrendelli, J.A., and Sprecher, H. 1979. Triene prostaglandins: prostacyclin and thromboxane biosynthesis and unique biological properties. *Proc. Natl. Acad. Sci. U. S. A.* **76**:944-948.

Needleman, P., Whitaker, M.O., Wyche, A., Watters, K., Sprecher, H., and Raz, A. 1980. Manipulation of platelet aggregation by prostaglandins and their fatty acid precursors: pharmacological basis for a therapeutic approach. *Prostaglandins* **19**:165-181.

Nelson, M.E., Fiatarone, M.A., Morganti, C.M., Trice, I., Greenberg, R.A., and Evans, W.J.

1994. Effects of high-intensity strength training on multiple risk factors for osteoporotic fractures. A randomized controlled trial. *JAMA* **272**:1909-1914.

Nestel, P.J. 2000. Fish oil and cardiovascular disease: lipids and arterial function. *Am. J. Clin. Nutr.* **71**:228S-231S.

Nicklas, B.J., You, T., and Pahor, M. 2005. Behavioural treatments for chronic systemic inflammation: effects of dietary weight loss and exercise training. *CMAJ.* **172**:1199-1209.

Okita, K., Nishijima, H., Murakami, T., Nagai, T., Morita, N., Yonezawa, K., Iizuka, K., Kawaguchi, H., and Kitabatake, A. 2004. Can exercise training with weight loss lower serum C-reactive protein levels? *Arterioscler. Thromb. Vasc. Biol.* **24**:1868-1873.

Oomen, C.M., Feskens, E.J., Rasanen, L., Fidanza, F., Nissinen, A.M., Menotti, A., Kok, F.J., and Kromhout, D. 2000. Fish consumption and coronary heart disease mortality in Finland, Italy, and The Netherlands. *Am. J. Epidemiol.* **151**:999-1006.

Otero, M., Lago, R., Lago, F., Casanueva, F.F., Dieguez, C., Gomez-Reino, J.J., and Gualillo, O. 2005. Leptin, from fat to inflammation: old questions and new insights. *FEBS Lett.* **579**:295-301.

Ounpuu, S., Negassa, A., and Yusuf, S. 2001. INTER-HEART: A global study of risk factors for acute myocardial infarction. *Am. Heart J.* **141**:711-721.

Pais, P., Pogue, J., Gerstein, H., Zachariah, E., Savitha, D., Jayprakash, S., Nayak, P.R., and Yusuf, S. 1996. Risk factors for acute myocardial infarction in Indians: a case-control study. *Lancet* **348**:358-363.

Parks, J.S., Kaduck-Sawyer, J., Bullock, B.C., and Rudel, L.L. 1990. Effect of dietary fish oil on coronary artery and aortic atherosclerosis in African green monkeys. *Arteriosclerosis* **10**:1102-1112.

Pawlosky, R.J., Hibbeln, J.R., Novotny, J.A., and Salem, N., Jr. 2001. Physiological compartmental analysis of alpha-linolenic acid metabolism in adult humans. *J. Lipid Res.* **42**:1257-1265.

Pereira, M.A., and Ludwig, D.S. 2001. Dietary fiber and body-weight regulation. Observations and mechanisms. *Pediatr. Clin. North Am.* **48**:969-980.

Phelan, S., Wyatt, H.R., Hill, J.O., and Wing, R.R. 2006. Are the eating and exercise habits of successful weight losers changing? *Obesity. (Silver. Spring)* **14**:710-716.

Picard, F., Kurtev, M., Chung, N., Topark-Ngarm, A., Senawong, T., hado De, O.R., Leid, M., McBurney, M.W., and Guarente, L. 2004. Sirt1 promotes fat mobilization in white adipocytes by repressing PPAR-gamma. *Nature* **429**:771-776.

Pischon, T., Hankinson, S.E., Hotamisligil, G.S., Rifai, N., and Rimm, E.B. 2003. Leisure-time physical activity and reduced plasma levels of obesity-related inflammatory markers. *Obes. Res.* **11**:1055-1064.

Pittler, M.H., and Ernst, E. 2001. Guar gum for body weight reduction: meta-analysis of randomized trials. *Am. J. Med.* **110**:724-730.

Poehlman, E.T., Dvorak, R.V., Denino, W.F., Brochu, M., and Ades, P.A. 2000. Effects of resistance training and endurance training on insulin sensitivity in nonobese, young women: a controlled randomized trial. *J. Clin. Endocrinol. Metab* **85**:2463-2468.

Popkin, B.M. 2004. The nutrition transition: an overview of world patterns of change. *Nutr. Rev.* **62**:S140-S143.

Prabhakaran, B., Dowling, E.A., Branch, J.D., Swain, D.P., and Leutholtz, B.C. 1999. Effect of 14 weeks of resistance training on lipid profile and body fat percentage in premenopausal women. *Br. J. Sports Med.* **33**:190-195.

Pratley, R., Nicklas, B., Rubin, M., Miller, J., Smith, A., Smith, M., Hurley, B., and Goldberg, A. 1994. Strength training increases resting metabolic rate and norepinephrine levels in healthy 50- to 65-yr-old men. *J. Appl. Physiol* **76**:133-137.

Rana, J.S., Nieuwdorp, M., Jukema, J.W., and Kastelein, J.J. 2007. Cardiovascular metabolic syndrome—an interplay of, obesity, inflammation, diabetes and coronary heart disease. *Diabetes Obes. Metab* **9**:218-232.

Renaud, S., and de, L.M. 1992. Wine, alcohol, platelets, and the French paradox for coronary heart disease. *Lancet* **339**:1523-1526.

Reuben, D.B., Judd-Hamilton, L., Harris, T.B., and Seeman, T.E. 2003. The associations between physical activity and inflammatory markers in high-functioning older persons: MacArthur Studies of Successful Aging. *J. Am. Geriatr. Soc.* **51**:1125-1130.

Reynolds, T.H., Supiano, M.A., and Dengel, D.R. 2004. Resistance training enhances insulin-mediated glucose disposal with minimal effect on the tumor necrosis factor-alpha system in older hypertensives. *Metabolism* **53**:397-402.

Richter, E.A., Kiens, B., and Wojtaszewski, J.F. 2008. Can exercise mimetics substitute for exercise? *Cell Metab* **8**:96-98.

Rigaud, D., Ryttig, K.R., Angel, L.A., and Apfelbaum, M. 1990. Overweight treated with energy restriction and a dietary fibre supplement: a 6-month randomized, double-blind, placebo-controlled trial. *Int. J. Obes.* **14**:763-769.

Rimm, E.B., Williams, P., Fosher, K., Criqui, M., and Stampfer, M.J. 1999. Moderate alcohol intake and lower risk of coronary heart disease: meta-analysis of effects on lipids and haemostatic factors. *BMJ* **319**:1523-1528.

Rist, M.J., Wenzel, U., and Daniel, H. 2006. Nutrition and food science go genomic. *Trends Biotechnol.* **24**:172-178.

Rosengren, A., Hawken, S., Ounpuu, S., Sliwa, K., Zubaid, M., Almahmeed, W.A., Blackett, K.N., Sitthi-amorn, C., Sato, H., and Yusuf, S. 2004. Association of psychosocial risk factors with risk of acute myocardial infarction in 11119 cases and 13648 controls from 52 countries (the INTERHEART study): case-control study. *Lancet* **364**:953-962.

Ryan, A.S., Pratley, R.E., Goldberg, A.P., and Elahi, D. 1996. Resistive training increases insulin action in postmenopausal women. *J. Gerontol. A Biol. Sci. Med. Sci.* **51** :M199-M205.

Ryttig, K.R., Tellnes, G., Haegh, L., Boe, E., and Fagerthun, H. 1989. A dietary fibre supplement and weight maintenance after weight reduction: a randomized, double-blind, placebo-controlled long-term trial. *Int. J. Obes.* **13**:165-171.

Sanchez-Villegas, A., Bes-Rastrollo, M., Martinez-Gonzalez, M.A., and Serra-Majem, L. 2006. Adherence to a Mediterranean dietary pattern and weight gain in a follow-up study: the SUN cohort. *Int. J. Obes. (Lond)* **30**:350-358.

Sanna, V., Di, G.A., La, C.A., Lechler, R.I., Fontana, S., Zappacosta, S., and Matarese, G. 2003. Leptin surge precedes onset of autoimmune encephalomyelitis and correlates with development of pathogenic T cell responses. *J. Clin. Invest* **111**:241-250.

Sato, M., Maulik, N., and Das, D.K. 2002. Cardioprotection with alcohol: role of both alcohol and polyphenolic antioxidants. *Ann. N. Y. Acad. Sci.* **957**:122-135.

Schmidt, E.B., Rasmussen, L.H., Rasmussen, J.G., Joensen, A.M., Madsen, M.B., and Christensen, J.H. 2006. Fish, marine n-3 polyunsaturated fatty acids and coronary heart disease: a minireview with focus on clinical trial data. *Prostaglandins Leukot. Essent. Fatty Acids* **75**:191-195.

Schulz, M., Nothlings, U., Hoffmann, K., Bergmann, M.M., and Boeing, H. 2005. Identification of a food pattern characterized by high-fiber and low-fat food choices associated with low prospective weight change in the EPIC-Potsdam cohort. *J. Nutr.* **135**:1183-1189.

Schwartz, R.S., and Hirth, V.A. 1995. The effects of endurance and resistance training on blood pressure. *Int. J. Obes. Relat Metab Disord.* **19 Suppl** 4:S52-S57.

Serhan, C.N., and Savill, J. 2005. Resolution of inflammation: the beginning programs the end. *Nat. Immunol.* **6**:1191-1197.

Serhan, C.N. 2007. Resolution phase of inflammation: novel endogenous anti-inflammatory and proresolving lipid mediators and pathways. *Annu. Rev. Immunol.* **25**:101-137.

Seyberth, H.W., Oelz, O., Kennedy, T., Sweetman, B.J., Danon, A., Frolich, J.C., Heimberg, M., and Oates, J.A. 1975. Increased arachidonate in lipids after administration to man: effects on prostaglandin biosynthesis. *Clin. Pharmacol. Ther.* **18**:521-529.

Siegmund, B., Sennello, J.A., Jones-Carson, J., Gamboni-Robertson, F., Lehr, H.A., Batra, A., Fedke, I., Zeitz, M., and Fantuzzi, G. 2004. Leptin receptor expression on T lymphocytes modulates chronic intestinal inflammation in mice. *Gut* **53**:965-972.

Sigal, R.J., Kenny, G.P., Wasserman, D.H., Castaneda-Sceppa, C., and White, R.D. 2006. Physical activity/exercise and type 2 diabetes: a consensus statement from the American Diabetes Association. *Diabetes Care* **29**:1433-1438.

Simopoulos, A.P. 2001. Evolutionary aspects of diet and essential fatty acids. *World Rev. Nutr. Diet.* **88**:18-27.

Sinclair, A.J., and Mann, N.J. 1996. Short-term diets rich in arachidonic acid influence plasma phospholipid polyunsaturated fatty acid levels and prostacyclin and thromboxane production in humans. *J. Nutr.* **126**:1110S-1114S.

Singer, P., Berger, I., Wirth, M., Godicke, W., Jaeger, W., and Voigt, S. 1986. Slow desaturation and elongation of linoleic and alpha-linolenic acids as a rationale of eicosapentaenoic acid-rich diet to lower blood pressure and serum lipids in normal, hypertensive and hyperlipemic subjects. *Prostaglandins Leukot. Med.* **24**:173-193.

Singer, P., Theilla, M., Fisher, H., Gibstein, L., Grozovski, E., and Cohen, J. 2006. Benefit of an enteral diet enriched with eicosapentaenoic acid and gamma-linolenic acid in ventilated patients with acute lung injury. *Crit Care Med.* **34**:1033-1038.

Singh, N.A., Clements, K.M., and Fiatarone, M.A. 1997. A randomized controlled trial of progressive resistance training in depressed elders. *J. Gerontol. A Biol. Sci. Med. Sci.* **52**: M27-M35.

Sinn, N., and Bryan, J. 2007. Effect of supplementation with polyunsaturated fatty acids and micronutrients on learning and behavior problems associated with child ADHD. *J. Dev. Behav. Pediatr.* **28**:82-91.

Sinn, N., and Bryan, J. 2007. Effect of supplementation with polyunsaturated fatty acids and micronutrients on learning and behavior problems associated with child ADHD. *J. Dev. Behav. Pediatr.* **28**:82-91.

Siscovick, D.S., Lemaitre, R.N., and Mozaffarian, D. 2003. The fish story: a diet-heart hypothesis with clinical implications: n-3 polyunsaturated fatty acids, myocardial vulnerability, and sudden death. *Circulation* **107**:2632-2634.

Slavin, J.L. 2005. Dietary fiber and body weight. *Nutrition* **21**:411-418.

Smith, W.L. 2005. Cyclooxygenases, peroxide tone and the allure of fish oil. *Curr. Opin. Cell Biol.* **17**:174-182.

Smutok, M.A., Reece, C., Kokkinos, P.F., Farmer, C.M., Dawson, P.K., DeVane, J., Patterson, J., Goldberg, A.P., and Hurley, B.F. 1994. Effects of exercise training modality on glucose tolerance in men with abnormal glucose regulation. *Int. J. Sports Med.* **15** :283-289.

Solomon, C.G., Hu, F.B., Stampfer, M.J., Colditz, G.A., Speizer, F.E., Rimm, E.B., Willett, W.C., and Manson, J.E. 2000. Moderate alcohol consumption and risk of coronary heart disease among women with type 2 diabetes mellitus. *Circulation* **102**:494-499.

Stamler, J., Caggiula, A.W., and Grandits, G.A. 1997. Relation of body mass and alcohol, nutrient, fiber, and caffeine intakes to blood pressure in the special intervention and usual care groups in the Multiple Risk Factor Intervention Trial. *Am. J. Clin. Nutr.* **65**:338S-365S.

Stamler, J., Stamler, R., Neaton, J.D., Wentworth, D., Daviglus, M.L., Garside, D., Dyer, A.R., Liu, K., and Greenland, P. 1999. Low riskfactor profile and long-term cardiovascular and noncardiovascular mortality and life expectancy: findings for 5 large cohorts of young adult and middle-aged men and women. *JAMA* **282**:2012-2018.

Stampfer, M.J., Colditz, G.A., Willett, W.C., Speizer, F.E., and Hennekens, C.H. 1988. A prospective study of moderate alcohol consumption and the risk of coronary disease and stroke in women. *N. Engl. J. Med.* **319**:267-273.

Stampfer, M.J., Hu, F.B., Manson, J.E., Rimm, E.B., and Willett, W.C. 2000. Primary prevention of coronary heart disease in women through diet and lifestyle. *N. Engl. J. Med.* **343**:16-22.

Stewart, K.J. 1992. Weight training in coronary artery disease and hypertension. *Prog. Cardiovasc. Dis.* **35**:159-168.

Stewart, K.J., Bacher, A.C., Turner, K.L., Fleg, J.L., Hees, P.S., Shapiro, E.P., Tayback, M., and Ouyang, P. 2005. Effect of exercise on blood pressure in older persons: a randomized controlled trial. *Arch. Intern. Med.* **165**:756-762.

Stewart, L.K., Flynn, M.G., Campbell, W.W., Craig, B.A., Robinson, J.P., Timmerman, K.L., McFarlin, B.K., Coen, P.M., and Talbert, E. 2007. The influence of exercise training on inflammatory cytokines and C-reactive protein. *Med. Sci. Sports Exerc.* **39**:1714-1719.

Stone, M.H., Fleck, S.J., Triplett, N.T., and Kraemer, W.J. 1991. Health- and performance-related potential of resistance training. *Sports Med.* **11**:210-231.

Suh, I., Shaten, B.J., Cutler, J.A., and Kuller, L.H. 1992. Alcohol use and mortality from coronary heart disease: the role of high-density lipoprotein cholesterol. The Multiple Risk Factor Intervention Trial Research Group. *Ann. Intern. Med.* **116**:881-887.

Teragawa, H., Fukuda, Y., Matsuda, K., Higashi, Y., Yamagata, T., Matsuura, H., and Chayama, K. 2002. Effect of alcohol consumption on endothelial function in men with coronary artery disease. *Atherosclerosis* **165**:145-152.

Thun, M.J., Peto, R., Lopez, A.D., Monaco, J.H., Henley, S.J., Heath, C.W., Jr., and Doll, R. 1997. Alcohol consumption and mortality among middle-aged and elderly U.S. adults. *N. Engl. J. Med.* **337**:1705-1714.

Toft, A.D., Jensen, L.B., Bruunsgaard, H., Ibfelt, T., Halkjaer-Kristensen, J., Febbraio, M., and Pedersen, B.K. 2002. Cytokine response to eccentric exercise in young and elderly humans. *Am. J. Physiol Cell Physiol* **283**:C289-C295.

Tolstrup, J., Jensen, M.K., Tjonneland, A., Overvad, K., Mukamal, K.J., and Gronbaek, M. 2006. Prospective study of alcohol drinking patterns and coronary heart disease in women and men. *BMJ* **332**:1244-1248.

Tomaszewski, M., Charchar, F.J., Przybycin, M., Crawford, L., Wallace, A.M., Gosek, K., Lowe, G.D., Zukowska-Szczechowska, E., Grzeszczak, W., Sattar, N. et al 2003. Strikingly low circulating CRP concentrations in ultramarathon runners independent of markers of adiposity: how low can you go? *Arterioscler. Thromb. Vasc. Biol.* **23**:1640-1644.

Valmadrid, C.T., Klein, R., Moss, S.E., Klein, B.E., and Cruickshanks, K.J. 1999. Alcohol intake and the risk of coronary heart disease mortality in persons with older-onset diabetes mellitus. *JAMA* **282**:239-246.

Van den Brink, G.R., O'Toole, T., Hardwick, J. C., van den Boogaardt, D.E., Versteeg, H.H., van Deventer, S.J., and Peppelenbosch, M.P. 2000. Leptin signaling in human peripheral blood mononuclear cells, activation of p38 and p42/44 mitogen-activated protein (MAP) kinase and p70 S6 kinase. *Mol. Cell Biol. Res. Commun.* **4**:144-150.

Van Gelder, B.M., Tijhuis, M., Kalmijn, S., and Kromhout, D. 2007. Fish consumption, n-3 fatty acids, and subsequent 5-y cognitive decline in elderly men: the Zutphen Elderly Study. *Am. J. Clin. Nutr.* **85**:1142-1147.

Vincent, K.R., Braith, R.W., Feldman, R.A., Kallas, H.E., and Lowenthal, D.T. 2002. Improved cardiorespiratory endurance following 6 months of resistance exercise in elderly men and women. *Arch. Intern. Med.* **162**:673-678.

Vincent, K.R., Braith, R.W., Bottiglieri, T., Vincent, H.K., and Lowenthal, D.T. 2003. Homocysteine and lipoprotein levels following resistance training in older adults. *Prev. Cardiol.* **6**:197-203.

Wada, M., DeLong, C.J., Hong, Y.H., Rieke, C.J., Song, I., Sidhu, R.S., Yuan, C., Warnock, M., Schmaier, A.H., Yokoyama, C. et al 2007. Enzymes and receptors of prostaglandin pathways with arachidonic acid-derived versus eicosapentaenoic acid-derived substrates and products. *J. Biol. Chem.* **282**:22254-22266.

Wald, N.J., and Law, M.R. 2003. A strategy to reduce cardiovascular disease by more than 80%. *BMJ* **326**:1419.

Walsh, C.R., Larson, M.G., Evans, J.C., Djousse, L., Ellison, R.C., Vasan, R.S., and Levy, D. 2002. Alcohol consumption and risk for congestive heart failure in the Framingham Heart Study. *Ann. Intern. Med.* **136**:181-191.

Wang, J., Obici, S., Morgan, K., Barzilai, N., Feng, Z., and Rossetti, L. 2001. Overfeeding rapidly induces leptin and insulin resistance. *Diabetes* **50**:2786-2791.

Wang, Y.X., Lee, C.H., Tiep, S., Yu, R.T., Ham, J., Kang, H., and Evans, R.M. 2003. Peroxisome-proliferator-activated receptor delta activates fat metabolism to prevent obesity. *Cell* **113**:159-170.

Wannamethee, G., and Shaper, A.G. 1992. Alcohol and sudden cardiac death. *Br. Heart J.* **68**:443-448.

Wannamethee, S.G., and Shaper, A.G. 1996. Patterns of alcohol intake and risk of stroke in middle-aged British men. *Stroke* **27**:1033-1039.

Weed, J.L., Lane, M.A., Roth, G.S., Speer, D.L., and Ingram, D.K. 1997. Activity measures in rhesus monkeys on long-term calorie restriction. *Physiol Behav.* **62**:97-103.

Whelton, S.P., Chin, A., Xin, X., and He, J. 2002. Effect of aerobic exercise on blood pressure: a meta-analysis of randomized, controlled trials. *Ann. Intern. Med.* **136**:493-503.

White, L.J., Castellano, V., and Mc Coy, S.C. 2006. Cytokine responses to resistance training in people with multiple sclerosis. *J. Sports Sci.* **24**:911-914.

Wijchers, P.J., Burbach, J.P., and Smidt, M.P. 2006. In control of biology: of mice, men and Foxes. *Biochem. J.* **397**:233-246.

Wilhelmsen, L., Rosengren, A., Johansson, S., and Lappas, G. 1997. Coronary heart disease attack rate, incidence and mortality 1975-1994 in Goteborg, Sweden. *Eur. Heart J.* **18**:572-581.

Wing, R.R., and Phelan, S. 2005. Long-term weight loss maintenance. *Am. J. Clin. Nutr.* **82**:222S-225S.

Xu, J., Teran-Garcia, M., Park, J.H., Nakamura, M.T., and Clarke, S.D. 2001. Polyunsaturated fatty acids suppress hepatic sterol regulatory element-binding protein-1 expression by accelerating transcript decay. *J. Biol. Chem.* **276**:9800-9807.

Yano, K., Rhoads, G.G., and Kagan, A. 1977. Coffee, alcohol and risk of coronary heart disease among Japanese men living in Hawaii. *N. Engl. J. Med.* **297**:405-409.

Young, G., and Conquer, J. 2005. Omega-3 fatty acids and neuropsychiatric disorders. *Reprod. Nutr. Dev.* **45**:1-28.

Yusuf, S., Reddy, S., Ounpuu, S., and Anand, S. 2001. Global burden of cardiovascular diseases: part I: general considerations, the epidemiologic transition, risk factors, and impact of urbanization. *Circulation* **104**:2746-2753.

INDEX

Underscored page references indicate boxed text and tables.
Boldface references indicate illustrations.

A

AA. *See* Arachidonic acid
Abdominal obesity, 109
Abdominals exercise, 240
Acorn squash
    Cranberried Acorn Squash, 281
Adaptive excess response, 104, 105, 112
Adaptive Response menus, 248, 252, 253,
    254–55
    Days 1 through 21, 260–83
Adaptive Response Phase, 205–12, **207**, 215,
    216, 233, 238, 248
Adaptive stress response
    beneficial effects of, 44–45, 52–53,
        63, 104, 113
    exercise as, 120
    factors inducing
        calorie reduction, 116
        CR mimetics, 62
        Gene Smart Diet, 11, 202
        red wine, 171
    factors preventing, 91–92
    fiber and, 135
    hormetic response and, 48–49
    overeating suppressing, 14
Adenomatous polyposis, 177
Aerobic activity, 235–36, 235, 236
Africa, malnutrition in, 331–32
Aging
    biomarkers of, 38, 40, 41, 43
    cellular maintenance and, 27–29, 34
    definition of, 24–25
    effect of environment and genes on, 3, 36
    Gene Smart Diet slowing, 201
    inflammatory diseases of, 23–24, 28,
        29, 30
    telomeres and, 123–24
AIDS, in Africa, 331, 332
Alcohol consumption. *See also* Wine, red
    benefits of, 49, 171
    caution with, 224

hormetic response and, 47
    in Optimal Maintenance Phase, 305
Allergic dermatitis, statistics on, 22
Allergies
    from chronic inflammation, 7, 8
    fatty acids and, 35
    omega-3 fatty acids preventing, 157
    statistics on, 22
Almonds
    Green Beans Almandine, 264
Alzheimer's disease
    incidence of, 23
    inflammation and, 9
    omega-3 fatty acids improving, 155, 156
Antioxidants, increasing mortality, 69
Antipasto
    Antipasto Salad, 294
Apples
    Baked Apple, 264, 283
    Cabbage-Apple Salad, 274
    Tuna, Apple, and Walnut Salad with
        Crackers, 270
    Waldorf Tuna Salad, 318
    Warm Apple Topping, 298
Apricots
    Apricot Crisp, 272
Aquaculture, altering fat ratios in fish, 163–66
Arachidonic acid (AA)
    in farmed fish, 164, 165
    Gene Smart Diet reducing, 167, 190
    inflammatory messengers from, 144
Arthritis. *See also* Osteoarthritis; Rheumatoid
    arthritis
    from chronic inflammation, 3, 7, 8
    as disease of aging, 29
    fatty acids and, 35
    incidence of, 23
    medications for, 82
    polyphenols and, 176–77
Artificial sweeteners, 249
Asian paradox, 172–73

Circuit with strength training, 237–40
Clams
    Seafood Pasta Italiano, 278
    Shrimp, Scallops (Bay or Sea), and Clams
      Italiano, 323
Cocoa, for blood pressure reduction, 175
Coffee, 227
Cognitive function, omega-3 fatty acids
    improving, 156, 193
Colon cancer, 12, 130, 159
Colorectal cancer, 177
Constipation, from low fiber consumption, 130
COPD, 7, 82, 157, 194
Corn
    Corn and Black Bean Salad, 278, 301
Coronary arteries, inflammation in, 8
Coronary artery disease, from chronic inflam-
    mation, 30
Coronary heart disease (CHD), fish preventing,
    152
Cortisol, harmful effects of, 19
COX-2 inhibitors, health risks from, 81
CR. *See* Calorie restriction
Crab
    Crab Cakes, 269, 315
    Crab Lasagna Rolls, 312–13
    Crab Omelet, 295
    Crab Salad, 311
    Crab Spread, 285
    Mackerel and Crab Jambalaya, 313
    Seafood Pasta Salad, 314
Cranberries
    Cranberried Acorn Squash, 281
C-reactive protein (CRP)
    as biomarker for inflammatory diseases,
      41–42, 115
    exercise and, 119, 120, 121, 122
    high
      harmful effects of, 19–20
      with overweight and obesity, 20
    predicting heart attack risk, 153
    reducing, with
      fat loss, 115–16
      fiber, 133–34
      Gene Smart Diet, 190
      red wine, 171
      weight loss, 135, 208
    synergistic effects on, 194–95
Critical-care patients, omega-3 fatty acids for,
    154–55
CR mimetics, benefits of, 60–65

Crohn's disease, 7, 8, 82, 158, 194
CRP. *See* C-reactive protein
Crunches, 240
Cucumbers
    Marinated Cucumbers, 290, 300
    No-Cook Cold Cucumber Soup, 275
Curry powder
    Curried Chicken Salad, 296
    Curried Shrimp Salad, 316

D

Dementia, as disease of aging, 29
Depression
    exercise reducing, 124
    incidence of, 23
    inflammation and, 8
    omega-3 fatty acids reducing, 154–56,
      193
Diabetes
    from chronic inflammation, 3, 7, 8, 10
    complications of, 11–12, 31
    decreased life span from, 33
    as disease of aging, 30, 31
    exercise and, 125
    fiber preventing, 133
    Gene Smart Diet and, 192–93
    interleukin-8 and, 20
    from metabolic syndrome, 109
    omega-3 fats and, 160
    polyphenols and, 175–76
    prevalence of, 11, 23, 31
    types of, 31
Diet(s)
    diseases associated with, 12
    five factors affecting, 90–91, **90**
    lack of fiber in, 129–30, 209
    modern
      vs. diet of ancestors, 95, 96–97,
        98–99
      as incompatible with genes, 86–87
    weight-loss, reasons for failure of, 16, 196,
      202
Dietary fats
    improving ratio of, 166–67
    overview of, 143–44
    reasons for poor ratios of, 144–47
Diet sodas, 249
Dinosaurs, reason for extinction of,
    88–89

DNA damage
  as biomarker of aging, 42–43
  calorie restriction slowing, 43
Drugs. *See also specific drugs*
  alternatives to, 77, 80–81
  counterbalancing poor diet, 89
  limitations of, 81–82, 83
  safety of, 81
  side effects of, 78, 80–81, <u>204</u>

E

ED, cardiovascular disease and, 125, <u>194</u>
Egg substitute
  Covered and Studded Scrambled Eggs and
    Toast, 306–7
  Crab Omelet, 295
  Egg Muffin Sandwiches, 306
  Vegetable Scramble, 261
  Vegetable Scramble Wrap, 297
  Veggie Frittata with Toast, 307
Empty calories, in American diet, 129–30
Endothelial cell function, polyphenols
  improving, 174
Endurance, exercise, resveratrol increasing,
  70–71, 72, 170–71
Environment
  genes and, 34–38, 53, 54
  master health regulators and, 85–87
Erectile dysfunction (ED), cardiovascular
  disease and, 125, <u>194</u>
Evening-primrose oil, as GLA supplement,
  220, 221
Exercise
  adaptive stress response and, 44–45
  equipment for, <u>234</u>
  in Gene Smart Diet, 126, 212, 232–43,
    253–54
  health benefits of, 48–49, 120–25, 233
  inflammatory and anti-inflammatory
    effects of, 119, 120, 121–23
  lack of, 117, 232
  in Maintenance Exercise Program, 328
  recommended amount of, 125–26
  soreness from, <u>238</u>
  starting, 236, <u>242–43</u>, 253–54
  for weight loss, 118–19, 192
Exercise endurance, resveratrol increasing,
  70–71, 72, 170–71
Exercise-induced stress response, 120, 122

F

Fasting, 250–52. *See also* Soup Fasts
Fat, body. *See* Body fat
Fat cells
  characteristics of, 14, 15
  inflammatory messengers secreted by,
    14–15, <u>19</u>
Fats, dietary. *See* Dietary fats
Fat storage
  genes promoting, 3, 5
  for survival, 14
Fatty acids, 35. *See also* Omega-3 fatty acids;
  Omega-6 fatty acids
Fiber
  anti-inflammatory effects of, 133–35
  as bioactive, 68, 72
  definition of, <u>131</u>
  in flax seeds, <u>162–63</u>
  foods high in, <u>328</u>
  in Gene Smart Diet, 114, 116, 127, 131,
    138–39, 188, 189, 209, 213, 244
  guidelines for increasing, <u>253</u>
  health benefits of, 72, 130–39, 188
  in Optimal Maintenance Phase, 305
  popular diets lacking, 139–40, <u>140</u>, 209
  recommended intake of, 138–41
  reducing hunger, <u>111</u>, 127, 136
  soluble vs. insoluble, <u>131</u>, 209
  for weight loss, 135, 137–39, 191
15/35/15 workout, 240–243
Fish and shellfish
  Albacore Tuna Salad, 322
  alternative to eating, <u>157</u>
  aquaculture altering fat ratios in, 163–66
  Bagel and Lox, 262, 271, 278, 302
  Baked Salmon, 324
  Broiled Salmon, 319
  cooking, 305
  Crab Cakes, 269, 315
  Crab Lasagna Rolls, 312–13
  Crab Omelet, 295
  Crab Salad, 311
  Crab Spread, 285
  Creole Shrimp Soup, 301
  Curried Shrimp Salad, 316
  decreased consumption of, 161–62
  fatty acid profiles of, 217–18
  Fried Oyster Salad, 325
  Greek Salmon Salad, 320–21
  Grilled Dijon Salmon, 289

High blood pressure *(cont.)*
   reducing, with
      calorie restriction, <u>40</u>, 41
      Gene Smart Diet, 188, 190
      polyphenols, 174–75
High-fructose corn syrup (HFCS), increased
   consumption of, 98
HIV/AIDS, in Africa, 331, 332
Hillsdale Study, xv, xvii, 18–19, <u>19</u>, 20–21, 63,
   65, 72, 77, 100, 127, 131, 133, 139, 188–193,
   197, 260, <u>328</u>, 334
Honey, eaten by hunter-gatherers, 97–98
Hormesis effect, 47–49
Hunger, fiber reducing, <u>111</u>, 127, 136
Hunter-gatherer ancestors
   diet of, 95, 97, 103–4, 129, 135–37, 144–45,
      186
   exercise of, 117
   fat storage in, 4, 14, 15–16
Hypertension. *See* High blood pressure

I

IL-6, 20, 121, 122
IL-8, 20–21
Immune system, fat storage and, 3, 15
Inflammation. *See also* Inflammatory diseases
   causes of, 35
   chronic
      eliminating, for disease prevention, 33
      in younger population, 31, 32
   diseases linked to, 3, 7, 8–10, <u>10</u>
   exercise and, 119, 120, 121–23
   function of, 5–6
   as normal vs. exaggerated response, 6
   from overweight and obesity, 3, 11, 13–14,
      15, 16
   reversing damage from, 186–88
   weight loss reducing, 115–16
Inflammatory diseases. *See also specific*
   diseases
   aging and, 23–24, 28, 29, 30
   calorie restriction preventing, <u>40</u>
   causes of, 329
   chronic, 6–7
   C-reactive protein and, 41–42
   epidemics of, 22–23
      reasons for, 74–76
   genes promoting, 5
   as location-specific, 8–9

   occurring with other inflammatory
      conditions, 82
   spider web approach to, 55–56
   unexplained reasons for, 3
Inflammatory messengers
   from arachidonic acid, 144
   exercise increasing, 120, 121–22
   fat secreting, 14–15
   function of, 15
   types of, 17–21, <u>19</u>
Inflammatory response, genes controlling, 35
Insulin
   in diabetes, 175
   exercise and, 125
   fiber and, 132–33
   polyphenols and, 175, 176
   reducing, with
      calorie restriction, <u>40</u>, 41
      fat loss, 115
      Gene Smart Diet, 192–93
      omega-3 fats, 160, 191
Insulin resistance, 13, 32, 133, 160, 192
Interleukin-6 (IL-6), 20, 121, 122
Interleukin-8 (IL-8), 20–21

J

Joint disease, incidence of, 23

K

Kickbacks, 239
Kitchen inventory, <u>216</u>

L

Lateral raise, 239
Leeks
   Leek and Parsley Soup, 267
Legumes. *See also* Beans; Lentils
   with polyphenols, 231
Lemons
   Lemon-Caper Trout, 282
   Lemon-Herb Fish, 312
   Lemon-Herb Halibut, 302–3
Lentils
   Lentil Soup, 294
   Salmon with Lentils au Gratin, 280

Leptin, 17–18, 115, 178
Life span
    diabetes reducing, 33
    increasing, with
        calorie restriction, 38, 39
        exercise, 123–24
        resveratrol, 70, 72, 170
Longevity. *See* Life span
Lox
    Bagel and Lox, 262, 271, 278, 302
Lunge, 240

M

Mackerel
    Lemon-Herb Fish, 312
    Mackerel and Crab Jambalaya, 313
    Southern Mackerel, 274
Macronutrients, 66
Maintenance, cellular. *See* Cellular
    maintenance
Maintenance Exercise Program, 328
Malnutrition, effects of, 332
Master gene regulators, polyphenols and, 169
Master health regulators
    altering gene expression, 54, 55, 69
    for disease protection, 329–30
    environmental factors and, 85–87
    factors suppressing, 82–83
    five factors affecting, 90–91, **90**, 93–94
    in hunter-gatherer ancestors, 186, 187
    polyphenols and, 69
    resveratrol and, 70
    role of, 35–36
    slowing aging, 201
    types of, 51–53, 55
Meat consumption. *See also* Beef; Pork
    affecting ratio of dietary fats, 145–47
    from grass- vs. corn-fed cows, 147, 203
    overconsumption of calories from, 110
Medical science, as spider web, 56
Medications. *See* Drugs
Mental health, omega-3s and, 155–56
Menus, 248, 249, 252–55, 260–305
Metabolic syndrome, 109, 192
Metastases, inflammation and, 9
Milk, reducing fat from, 250
Monounsaturated fats, 143
Muffins
    All Bran Muffins, 286

Muscle
    as anti-inflammatory organ, 48–49
    functions of, 120–22
Mushrooms
    Portobello Sandwich, 274
Myokines, exercise and, 120–21

N

NF-KB, as master health regulator, 52, 55, 169
Nrf2, as master health regulator, 55
Nuts. *See also specific nuts*
    with polyphenols, 231

O

Oats
    Oatmeal and Berries, 308
Obesity. *See* Overweight and obesity
Omega fats, 142–43. *See also* Omega-3 fatty
    acids; Omega-6 fatty acids
Omega-3 fatty acids
    added to foods, 220
    as bioactives, 72–73, 73, 142
    fed to grass-fed cows, 147
    in fish, 217–18
        aquaculture altering ratios of, 163–66
    in Gene Smart Diet, 114, 116, 167, 211–12,
        213, 245
    health benefits of, 142, 143, 147, 149–60
    safety of, 210
    for weight loss, 159–60, 191, 192, 245
Omega-6 fatty acids
    fed to cows, 147
    in fish, 217–18
        aquaculture altering ratios of, 163–66
    Gene Smart Diet reducing, 166–67
    harmful effects of, 143–44, 146
Omega-3 index
    Gene Smart Diet increasing, 189
    for predicting heart attack risk, 153
Onions
    Roasted Vegetables, 263, 277
    Vegetable Scramble, 261
    Vegetable Scramble Wrap, 297
Optimal Maintenance Phase, **207**, 213, 216,
    234, 249
    breakfast recipes for, 306–8
    guidelines for, 304–5

Pork Sandwich, 262
    Spicy Maple Pork Medallions, 291
Portion sizes, 110, 250
Poultry. *See* Chicken
PPARs, as master health regulators, 55
Preconditioning menus, 248, 249, 252, 284–303
    Days 22 through 35, 284–303
Preconditioning Phase, **207**, 213, 216, 233, 238, 238
Processed foods, calories from, 110–11
Prostate cancer, 12, 13, 159, 177–78
Psoriasis, 7, 82, 159, 194
PUFAs. *See* Polyunsaturated fats
Pulmonary disease, omega-3 fatty acids and, 158

Q

Quadriceps, exercises for, 239–40

R

Raspberries
    Berries and Yogurt, 300
Reproduction, vs. cellular maintenance, 46
Resveratrol
    as bioactive, 70–72
    increasing exercise endurance, 70–71, 72, 170–71
    increasing life span, 70, 72, 170
    sources of, 170, 171, 185
    studies on benefits of, 170–71
    as supplement, 171
Rheumatoid arthritis. *See also* Arthritis; Osteoarthritis
    exercise for, 122
    Gene Smart Diet improving, 193–94
    inflammatory conditions occurring with, 82
    omega-3 fatty acids and, 158
    in young people, 29–30
Root vegetables
    Roasted Vegetables, 299
Rowing, 239

S

Salads
    Albacore Tuna Salad, 322
    Antipasto Salad, 294

Blue Cheese-Steak Salad, 286–87
Cabbage-Apple Salad, 274
Caesar Salad, 280
Chicken Salad, 271
Chicken Salad with Crackers, 263, 300
Citrus Salad, 300
Classic Caesar Salad, 276–77
Corn and Black Bean Salad, 278, 301
Curried Chicken Salad, 296
Curried Shrimp Salad, 316
Fried Oyster Salad, 325
Fruit Salad, 296
Greek Salmon Salad, 320–21
Grilled Tuna Salad, 320
Ham and Plum Salad, 297
Orange Salmon Salad, 265
Salmon Pasta Salad, 324
Salmon Pasta Salad with Crackers, 273, 290
Salmon Salad, 281
Seafood Pasta Salad, 314
Spinach Salad, 264, 299
Steak and Orange Salad, 272
Three-Bean Salad, 288, 296
Tomato-Bulgur Salad, 289
Tomato-Mozzarella Salad, 273
Tomato Salad, 279
Tossed Salad, 278, 298
Tuna, Apple, and Walnut Salad with Crackers, 270
Tuna Pasta Salad, 309
Tuna Salad, 288
Waldorf Tuna Salad, 318
Salmon
    Bagel and Lox, 262, 271, 278, 302
    Baked Salmon, 324
    Broiled Salmon, 319
    Greek Salmon Salad, 320–21
    Grilled Dijon Salmon, 289
    Grilled Salmon Dijon, 322
    Grilled Salmon Teriyaki, 309
    Orange Salmon, 264
    Orange Salmon Salad, 265
    Salmon Cakes, 310
    Salmon in Sun-Dried Tomato-Cream Sauce, 317
    Salmon Pasta Salad, 324
    Salmon Pasta Salad with Crackers, 273, 290
    Salmon Salad, 281
    Salmon Spread, 287, 296, 322–23
    Salmon with Lentils au Gratin, 280

Tomatoes
    Broiled Tomatoes Parmesan, 271
    Salmon in Sun-Dried Tomato-Cream
        Sauce, 317
    Shrimp and Vegetable Stir-Fry I,
        310
    Shrimp and Vegetable Stir-Fry II, 321
    Tomato-Bulgur Salad, 289
    Tomato-Mozzarella Salad, 273
Trans-resveratrol. *See* Resveratrol
Triceps exercise, 239
Triglycerides
    omega-3 fatty acids and, <u>210</u>
    reducing, 150, 173, 188, 189
Trout
    Lemon-Caper Trout, 282
    Lemon Fish en Papillote
        (Fish Cooked in Parchment), 262
Tumor necrosis factor-alpha (TNF), 21
Tuna
    Albacore Tuna Salad, 322
    Grilled Tuna Salad, 320
    Tuna, Apple, and Walnut Salad with
        Crackers, 270
    Tuna Melt, 298
    Tuna Melts, 315
    Tuna Pasta Salad, 309
    Tuna Salad, 288
    Tuna Spread, 293
    Waldorf Tuna Salad, 318

U

Ulcerative colitis, 8, 158
Unsaturated fats, 143

V

Vegetable oils, fats ratio and, 145
Vegetables. *See also specific vegetables*
    bioactives missing from, 168, 179–84
    in Gene Smart Diet, 227–30, 231, 232
    polyphenols in, 172, 185
    reducing costs of, <u>205</u>
    underconsumption of, 110
Vegetarian dishes, 304–5
Viagra, 80
Vioxx, 81
Vitamin E, increasing mortality, 69

W

Walnuts
    Tuna, Apple, and Walnut Salad with
        Crackers, 270
Weight gain
    age-associated, 29, 34
    development of diabetes from, 32
    from genetic drive to eat, 104–5
Weight loss
    energy equation for, 244
    exercise for, 118–19, 192
    fiber for, 135, 137–39, 191
    from Gene Smart Diet, 33, 62–63, 72, 100,
        112, 114–15, 116, 191–92, 244–50
    obstacles to, 195–96
    omega-3 fatty acids for, 159–60, 191, 192,
        245
    plateaus in, 304
    polyphenols promoting, 169, 178–79
    reducing inflammatory profile, 115–16
White blood cells, calorie restriction and, <u>40</u>
Whole foods, vs. supplements, 218–21
Wine, red. *See also* Alcohol consumption
    in Gene Smart Diet, <u>211</u>, 213, 223–25, 231,
        250
    health benefits of, <u>171</u>, 188, 189–90, <u>211</u>
    in Optimal Maintenance Phase, 305
    polyphenols in, 68–69, 72, 170, 231
    resveratrol in, 71, 185

Y

Yogurt
    Berries and Yogurt, 300
    Yogurt Sundae, 301

Z

Zucchini
    Vegetable Sauté, 283
    Veggie Frittata with Toast, 307
    Zucchini Broil, 261, 279

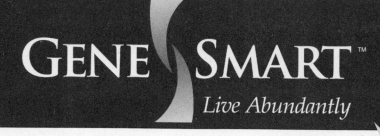
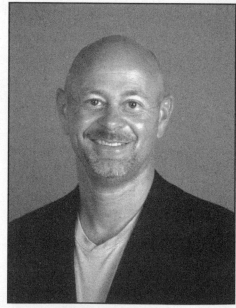